Healing Stories

Narrative in Psychiatry and Psychotherapy

Healing Stories

Narrative in Psychiatry and Psychotherapy

Edited by

Glenn Roberts and Jeremy Holmes

Department of Psychiatry, North Devon District Hospital, Barnstaple, UK

OXFORD UNIVERSITY PRESS
1999

Oxford University Press, Great Clarendon Street, Oxford OX2 6DP

Oxford New York

Athens Auckland Bangkok Bogota Buenos Aires Calcutta
Cape Town Chennai Dar es Salaam Delhi Florence Hong Kong Istanbul
Karachi Kuala Lumpur Madrid Melbourne Mexico City Mumbai
Nairobi Paris São Paulo Singapore Taipei Tokyo Toronto Warsaw

and associated companies in
Berlin Ibadan

Oxford is a trade mark of Oxford University Press

Published in the United States
by Oxford University Press Inc., New York

A catalogue record for this book is available from the British Library

Library of Congress Cataloging in Publication Data
Data available

ISBN 0 19 262827 5 (Hbk)

Typeset by Alliance Phototypesetters, Pondicherry

Printed in Great Britain by
Bookcraft Ltd., Midsomer Norton, Avon

This book is dedicated to
Ben, Laura, Martha, and Sam
in hope and love, for their still becoming lives

Foreword

Arthur Kleinman
Departments of Social Medicine, Psychiatry and Anthropology, Harvard University

Medicine is awash with stories, just like everyday life. We tend to treat stories as things individuals exchange with individuals. We emphasize the tale, the telling, the teller, the listener. Figuring particularly large is interpretation. Questions of interpretation preoccupy literary critics, philosophers, social scientists, psychoanalysts, and just about anyone who has taken narratives as their subject, including the authors of the chapters in this rewarding volume. Social theorists have even gone so far in their absorption with interpretation to liken life itself to a text with its requirements to be interpreted and for alternative interpretations to be somehow accommodated. But life isn't a text and interpretation needs to be understood as part of a larger process of engagement, negotiation, and action in everyday life. Medicine is made up of more than stories. So, how are we to understand the relationship of stories to suffering, healing, and everyday life?

People live in local worlds—families, neighbourhoods, networks, work settings, and institutions (including medical settings). These worlds are characterized by what is most at stake for their participants. What is at stake may be shared, such as status, resources, survival, or the desire for transcendence. But local worlds also greatly differ owing to the particularities of what is at stake, such as with respect to most meanings (mundane and ultimate). Local worlds, then, are moral worlds, because this is where people affirm, struggle for, and contest what really matters.

These moral worlds are the settings where suffering and healing, amongst many other human conditions, occur. Symptoms, and lay and professional responses to them, are part of the flow of interpersonal interactions in local moral worlds. That is to say, illness and healing are processes of interpersonal experience and they get taken up in what matters in local worlds. Suffering is one of the dangers of social life because it threatens what is at stake for stakeholders, who have crucial things to lose and preserve.

This is where stories come into the picture. Stories are, at the same time, a key component (but not the only one) of interpersonal experience and also a major way (but not the only way) that we learn about (or gain access to) worlds of experience. Stories do not exhaust experience, though they construct (and allow us to deconstruct) it. Stories are truly crucial for medicine, then, because this is an important way that we come to understand illness experience and experiences of care-giving and receiving. This side of stories is well illustrated in the chapters that follow. Several of the chapters also illumine professional practice via this same approach. But it is useful to remember that stories are told, retold, transformed, interpreted, misinterpreted, told by others second hand, and worked through in all sorts of ways in local worlds, where institutional, political economic, and moral processes shape their meaning and their uses. Stories divorced from this context, and addressed as isolated things in themselves, can distort clinical realities. Stories are powerful in medicine, as in life, because they bring us up against what matters in real situations for particular men and women. Thus, how we come to understand illness and healing narratives is as vital as the stories per se. This is why anthropology's methodology, ethnography, as well as the methods of biography and social history are of value to clinicians: they situate stories in the flow of interpersonal experience that is the very stuff of illness and healing. These ways of knowing give to stories their power to be clinically useful.

Preface

At the heart of any therapeutic encounter there is always a story. Patients seeking help bring with them stories, spoken or untold, fragmentary and whole, that collectively make up their own personal narrative. Whatever else their tasks, a central part of the doctor's or therapist's job is to facilitate the telling of these stories, to make meaning out of them, and to find patterns within them. The personal story draws us into a personal relationship, and the dialogue between illness and healing narratives provides the framework that guides both healing and suffering, and a means of integrating or detaching from that broad anthology which constitutes society's view of itself as a community of meaning.

The scientific culture of contemporary medicine has tended to displace the art of history taking, emphasizing objectivity and generalization at the expense of anecdote, metaphor, and the uniqueness of an individual life history. With a few notable exceptions, such as the work of Oliver Sacks and Lewis Thomas, the transposition of often inarticulate illness experiences into illuminating and iconic narratives has almost disappeared.

Even within psychiatry, perhaps the branch of medicine most naturally reliant on narrative, case histories are in danger of extinction and have recently been banished (albeit for good reasons of confidentiality) from the pages of the British Journal of Psychiatry. Only within psycho-therapy and psychoanalysis does narrative live on, each clinical case constituting a research enterprise of its own, yeilding a prototypical tale from which much is learned about similar cases with which the reader is struggling.

Ironically, while within medicine stories have retreated in the face of science's big guns, in other fields the 'narrative turn' has become a major academic paradigm. Anthropologists, ethicists, literary critics, oral historians, lawyers, economists, and sociologists all recognize the limitations of purely quantitative approaches and are interested in the work of Bertaux, Tonkin, Thompson, and other theorists of narrative.

Within the clinical environment there is an ever present tension concerning the status, utility, and application of narrative. This may be succinctly stated as the tension between fact and fiction—between evidence-based and narrative-based medicine. In seeking to tell a story about stories we are trying to negotiate and juggle this tension—what are the facts about stories? This is not a tension easily resolved. The story-teller's art constitutes a kind of honest seduction, the suspension of disbelief, an honourable smuggling, a bridging between inside and outside, indi-vidual and society, illness and health, as a means of reconnecting and reintegrating we contend that a narrative approach thus offers an antidote to the depersonalization of modern medicine. Stories can also be related to the new vernacular of 'evidence-based medicine', as we shall seri-ously consider the possibility that stories are a kind of evidence too, and contrast true stories with misleading facts.

As we open our story we are immediately faced with a parallel dilemma. What form or voice shall we adopt? Is it to be a scholarly review, or can we mirror the story-teller by drawing the reader into a journey, sufficiently signalled with scratch stones and way-marks to have some feel of familiarity and credibility.

If we *are* to find a voice, whose voice shall it be? As in any multi-author text, we have brought together a set of disparate themes, viewpoints, and authorial stances. If we aspire to science, the evidence might speak for itself, despite being delivered in many dialects. But in narrative, to a great extent, the medium is the message. Science is monistic, narrative inherently pluralistic— the varied voices of this text honour the multifarious nature of story, contained within a single volume.

Story telling is also by its nature selective. There is much we have left out, most notably in the psychotherapeutic field. We might, for example, have taken a look back to the common heritage of western medicine and narrative in Ionian Greece, and have stood with Ascelepius learning the divine art of healing from the Centaur Chiron, who's wound was his wisdom.

However, to have constructed a more elaborate structure built on more extensive foundations could have subverted our ambition to produce a relatively small book, which may stimulate our readers to dig their own foundations and re-survey the structures they already inhabit or aspire to. The present re-evaluation of narrative in psychiatry and psychotherapy is only beginning and *its* story cannot yet be told.

Authentic stories, are regarded by story-tellers as precious, and to be handled with great care. The Hippocratic impulse towards fidelity, integrity, and respect, and against self-motivated exploitation and personal profit, remind us that, within clinical practice, stories can be significantly misused. In telling the stories within this work each author has taken care to conceal identity or seek permission from those whom the stories belong to. They are retold rather than retailed.

In offering our book as a companion to the reader's thoughts and reflections, it is our guiding hope that it may provoke, or even inspire, debate, discussion, exploration, and the telling of other stories.

Barnstaple, U. K.
1998

G. R.
J. H.

Acknowledgements

We offer our thanks to the many friends and colleagues who have responded to our enthusiasm for stories and, through their engagement with our interest, contributed much to the thinking behind this book, particularly, Tony Clark, Monty Barker, Charles Montgomery, Arietta Slade, Sebastian Cramer, Paul Aylard, Tim and Ann Hockridge, Simon Nicholson, Phillip van Driel, Christa and Andrew Friend, Martin Mather, Charlotte and Richard McCaie, Michael Jackson, Brian Martingdale, John Strauss, Ann Colborn, Peter Whitfield, John Adey, and for early inspiration—James Phillips. It would not have begun without encouragement from Oxford University Press and has been sustained by the patient support and enquiry of successive editors. The project has been held together and brought to a successful conclusion by the efficient, cheerful, and ever willing help of Sue Bennett and the endless search for sources has been greatly assisted by our extremely able librarian, Alison Housley. Our thanks and gratitude also goes to the many people we have met as patients who, in the telling of their stories and their engagement in the shared struggle to make sense of experience, have given a great deal to what we have to offer here.

Contents

PART FOUR

Postscript

Contributors

Errollyn Bruce: Errollyn Bruce, Bradford Dementia Group, University of Bradford, West Yorkshire, BD7 1DP, UK

John Byng-Hall: Tavistock Clinic, 120 Belsize Lane, London, NW3 5BA, UK

Jeremy Holmes: Department of Psychiatry, North Devon District Hospital, Raleigh Park, Barnstaple, Devon, EX31 4JB, UK

Sushrut Jadhav: Centre for Medical Anthropology, Dept. of Psychiatry, University College, London Medical School, London, WIN 8AA, UK

Arthur Klienman: Department of Anthropology, Harvard University, William James Hall, Cambridge, Massachusetts, 021 38, USA

Roland Littlewood: Department of Anthropology, University College, London, WC1E 6BT, UK

James Phillips: 88 Noble Avenue, Miford, Connecticut, 064 60

R. Raguram: National Institute of Mental Health and Neurosciences, Bangalore, India

Glenn Roberts: Department of Psychiatry, North Devon District Hospital, Raleigh Park, Barnstaple, Devon, EX31 4JB, UK

Janet Sayers: Department of Social Work Studies, University of Kent at Canterbury, Canterbury, Kent, CT2 7NP, UK

Andrew Sims: Division of Psychiatry and Behavioural Sciences in Relation to Medicine, St James's University Hospital, Leeds, LS9 7TF, UK

Paul Thompson: Department of Sociology, University of Essex, Wivenhoopk, Colchester, C04 35Q, UK

Cover notes

Every picture tells a story
Every story paints a picture

Man the meaning-maker is forever trying to work out what is going on, and where in the world he is. For millennia he has assuaged his existential anxieties through the construction of stories and maps—which, from this point of view, are much the same thing. In this sense all stories can be configured as travellers tales, and all patterns of meaning, maps of the mind.

The Psalter map of 1250, used both on the cover and revealed in iterative succession through the book, is held in the British Library—a jewel like miniature within a book of holy songs, evocative and iconic, and typical of medieval maps of the world, the Mappa Mundae.

Its simplified form belies its contemporary status as an accurate map of the known world, which, in its confident delineation, is portrayed as the whole world. These Mappas were the products of a deeply xenophobic culture which felt a profound inhibition concerning exploration and experimentation—lest one heretically set sail to travel beyond the bounds of God's creation and encounter hideously deformed creatures at the edge of the world, before plunging into the surrounding and unfathomable Sea of Darkness. How much safer to confine seafaring to the familiar, womb shaped 'Mare Medi Terrain'—the sea in the middle of the land (Mediterranean).

The Enlightenment witnessed the recovery of Ptolomy's world map (AD 150), having been 'lost' for a thousand years which, with its awareness of incompleteness, was far more geographically accurate than its medieval successors, and once again men set out in boats to explore. The subsequent maps of discovery displaced these Mappa Mundae of conviction, which, despite their fascination and beauty, were revealed as dead icons, illustrating a stale story, ignorant of their own constructedness.

These artefacts of the medieval mind echo the mentation of both the fundamentalist and the psychotic, and thus serve as a window on the book. They illustrate our endemic need for meanings-to-live-by, the constructedness of those meanings, the inevitable tension involved in knowing and negotiating this, and the desire for truth. In the end, despite the warmth of their sanctuary, these images must be released in order to look further into the uncharted depths of reality. The songs continue, stories are revised, and new images are drawn.

Beginnings

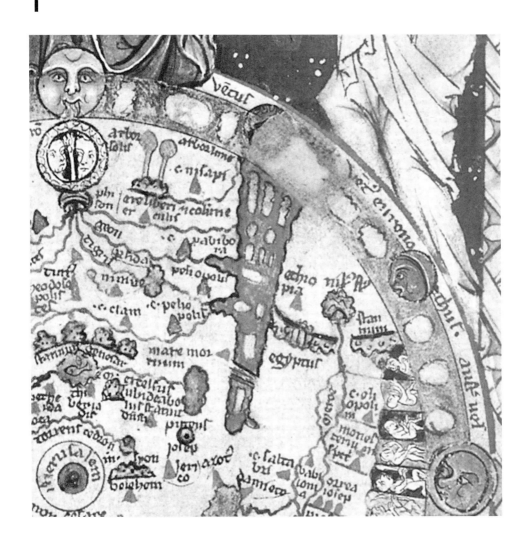

1 Introduction: a story of stories

Glenn Roberts

The significance of stories in psychiatry and psychotherapy is paradoxical and contradictory. They are at once ephemeral, 'only a story', flimsy remnants of an anecdote-based medicine, the stuff of propaganda and inculcation, arising from a flabby subjectivism, and seductive dis-simulations, and at the same time rich, iconic evocations of meaning, foundational and inescapable, accessing all that is unique and personal, containers of our origins, our tribal tales, and the myths we live by.

The wider story of medicine, containing those of psychiatry and psychotherapy (at least in their origins), finds itself increasingly preoccupied in the search for evidence and yet at the same time is being increasingly criticized for emptying itself of sustaining meanings. At this early stage the reader may find the assertion that, 'the Universe is made of stories, not atoms' (Muriel Rukeyser in Feldman and Kornfield, 1991), somewhat extravagant, as unacceptable as the notion that the moon is made of green cheese, and as redundant as belief in a flat earth. But if that is our most extreme boundary marker, you may be able to contemplate the more modest view's of Polkinghorne (1988) and Taylor (1996), that 'narrative is the primary form by which human experience is made meaningful', and 'our greatest desire, greater even than the desire for happiness, is that our lives mean something. This desire for meaning is the originating impulse of story.' And it is not only that we crave that our lives 'mean something' but that our suffering does also, for as Hauerwas (1993) has observed, 'the kinds of suffering that drive us mad are those that we say have no point.' Man cannot be healed by fact alone. Story is the warp to fact's weft, which together constitute a tapestry drawn from reality—but neither capture reality itself, the map is not the territory. Without facts there would be nothing to say, without story there would be no means of saying it: it may also be disconcerting, for some, to consider that facts may be stories and stories may be facts. In offering this suggestion we may, at first, appear out of step with the ascendant emphasis on 'evidence based' approaches driven by health economics and the need to prioritize 'scarce and costly resources'. We aim to take you, by cautious steps and reckless leaps, to consider the ubiquity, universality, and utility of story as a means, *the* means, by which we make meaning, and hence the unacceptable cost of loosing a narrative dimension to our practice and the potential of reinstating and enhancing it.

The loss of narrative

Scientific approaches to psychiatry and psychotherapy have progressively drawn away from the anecdotes and monographs of a former age, preferring the limited certainties of statistics and the double-blind trial (Murray, 1997). In throwing out the bard with the bath water, science risks loosing the meaning and significance of the very things it is so carefully measuring, and an awareness of the highly subjective means by which it chooses its object and method of enquiry. The scientific discourse factualizes information through the loss of a narrative context, and so creates an illusion of objectivity (Nash, 1994). We find ourselves situated between two unsatisfactory possibilities, between meaningless facts and meaningful fiction.

Case history and the loss of the person

The narrative theologian Hauerwas (1993), has spoken for many in complaining that 'there is no subject in the modern case history.' He comments on the risk of compounding our patients' sufferings by generating impersonal case histories that fail to illuminate the individual's experience as he struggles to survive his illness. He sees this dissociation from personal meaning as one of the major mediators in the experience of suffering, and the need not only restore 'the suffering, afflicted, frightened human subject at the centre', but also to search for a way of locating the individual's suffering within an 'ongoing story carried by a community that can make this suffering person's life its own.'

Oliver Sacks (1982) appropriated John Donne's words to underline this aspect of why the ill suffer through the attendant risks of isolation and alienation: 'As sickness is the greatest misery, so the greatest misery of sickness is *solitude* . . . Solitude is a torment which is not threatened in *Hell* itself.' Sickness creates a silence that is not easily shared, which is compounded by centring our accounts of sickness on disease and disorder rather than on the person. The clinical struggle is then with and against the illness rather than an engagement with the ongoing life of the individual (Davidson and Strauss, 1995).

Case histories are narrative constructions, the issue is how meaningful are they and to whom? In 'presenting a case history' there is a contrast as well as a tension between 'illness narratives', patients' own accounts of their experience, and the extracted, abstracted, clinical account that offers a formulation and points to a therapeutic approach (Frank, 1993). Both are necessary and there are risks in loosing the balance either way. If patients' accounts of their experiences are forever filtered through the idealized, approved, official textbook version of their illness, much that is of great personal significance will be ignored or lost, whereas it is difficult to integrate a meaning-laden, individualized description with accumulated knowledge, and the benefits of discerning common patterns. Whichever way we incline, balance is hard to achieve.

Contrast the following descriptions of Gilles de la Tourette syndrome. The first from an authoritative review (Singer and Walkup, 1991) in a respected international medical journal, the second from Oliver Sacks' (1985, p. 87) account of 'Witty Ticcy Ray'.

Singer and Walkup: 'Tics begin suddenly, in more than 50% of our patients as a simple eye blink, facial grimace, or head twitch. In the majority, motor tics progress in a rostral–caudal fashion, involving the face, head or shoulders before other parts of the body. Less commonly it presents with complex stereotyped movements or vocalisations. Some complex tics (e.g., touching or tapping) may be difficult to differentiate from compulsions.'

Sacks: 'He was (like many Touretters) remarkably musical, and could scarcely have survived— emotionally or economically—had he not been a weekend jazz drummer of real virtuosity, famous for his sudden and wild extemporisations, which would arise from a tic or a compulsive hitting of a drum and would instantly be made the nucleus of a wild and wonderful improvisation, so that the "sudden intruder" would be turned to brilliant advantage. His Tourette's was also of advantage in various games, especially Ping-Pong, at which he excelled, partly a consequence of his abnormal quickness of reflex and reaction, but especially, again because of his "improvisations", "very sudden, nervous, frivolous shots" (in his own words), which were so unexpected and startling as to be virtually unanswerable.'

How much sense does it make to discuss which is, more valid, i.e. truer? Both are needed, and each would be impoverished by the absence of the other. However, our starting position is in observing that accounts of illness experience are often detached from the context in which they are lived.

Meaningless medicine

There is growing concern that modern medicine evades the experience of illness that patients suffer from. Patients are offered a form of medicine that may be potent, but meaningless their lesions and disorders may respond, but the lived experience of illness is untouched and ununderstood. In acute illness this may be of little importance but the significance of this gap grows with the severity and chronicity of the illness, and how extensive the impact is upon the individual's life. Where modern medicine focuses on the disease at the expense of the person, it may, paradoxically, increase the suffering whilst seeking to relieve it.

Patients are increasingly complaining about this 'crisis of meaning' too. A recent review of the experiences of more than 500 service users in the UK (Rogers *et al.*, 1993) criticized the impersonality of psychiatric approaches which are referred to as 'mechanistic and dismissive of individuality.' Strauss (1994) offered an authoritative endorsement, that 'our field, reeling from the previous excesses of subjective reports and impressions, has now swung far to the other side, all but discounting the subjective in scientific and academic work.' This leads on, in his view, to 'the gross inadequacy in the mental health field, of our attention to the subjective side of the person's experience', and 'how little the psychiatric format—present illness, past history, family history, etc.—allows for noticing and recording the person's experience. From such a format, it is in fact almost impossible for the person to be discoverable.'

Meaningless training

Although medical education has broadly followed Sir William Osler's dictum 'that there should be no teaching without a patient as a text', there has been a progressive trend towards favouring short stories or even reviews and abstracts, rather than engaging in a long and complex biography. Klienman (1988, p. 258) has spoken of the incentives that may perpetuate it: 'Perhaps we should begin with the honest, if deeply upsetting recognition that at present many training programs tacitly inculcate values and behaviours that are antithetical to the humane care of patients.' He sees the dominant practices as driven by other motives, such as cheap manpower and financial considerations: 'if, by passing an endoscope, a clinician can earn in 15 minutes what he can make in half an hour of sensitive interviewing, then there is little chance that Psychosocial training will have any significant effect on healthcare behaviour.'

Some consequences: collusion with chronicity

If we are to consider seriously the rather unsettling question of how doctors and other therapists contribute to the chronicity of their patient's illness we need to reflect on the possibility that 'incurability' is an iatrogenic concept.

Klienmans's (1988, p. 180) particular insight into the anthropology of psychiatry, led him to observe that 'chronicity arises in part by telling dead or static stories, situating the individual in wasteland, a denervated place, robbed of its fertility and potential.' It is a sombre consideration that chronicity may be created out of the accumulated negative expectations that we imbue our clinical atmosphere with, and transact in our interactions with patients and staff. Possessing and perpetuating this narrative of 'incurability' may serve many protective and defensive purposes for the staff involved, and may even offer some comfort and orientation to the individual, but in doing so we may 'collude with building walls and tearing down bridges', exchanging the precarious and uncertain struggle for health with acceptance of meanings that forever constrain the individual's hope and potential.

Ron Coleman (Coleman and Smith, 1997), founder of the Hearing Voices Network, trainer of health care professionals, and voice hearer, tells the story of his renewal as pivoting around the day when he found a way of sloughing these constraints: 'I decided I didn't want to be a chronic schizophrenic any longer', and, in rejecting those meanings and attributions, became an 'empowered voice hearer', and the inimitable Ron Coleman, instead.

Oliver Sacks, doyen of medical story-tellers, began his enquiry into the neurology of the self at a hospital for chronic and incurable diseases. His patients' 'awakening' (Sacks, 1982) appeared to parallel his own. His subsequent studies and writings established him as a powerful advocate for recontexualizing illness experience in the lived story of a person:

> The 'unique case' maybe a nightmare for science, but is a necessity for medicine, where it is not just a question of quantities and systems, not just a question of applied physiology, but a question of individual economies and needs. I like to think that *Awakenings* has had some influence, not only in drawing attention to the complexities of treatment with L-DOPA, and all drugs; but to the current humane movement from an assembly-line to a personal medicine.
> (*Sacks, 1982, p. 35.*)

According to Wiggins (1975), the loss of story is itself 'a story to end all stories', and there is a broad contemporary countercurrent, a movement towards collapsing the 'fateful distinction' between fact and fiction, in view of the inability of *that* story to sustain life, and hence the resurgence of interest in story-telling.

Perhaps, 20 years on, I can make greater sense of my first psychiatric teacher's advice, to 'read novels'.

It would appear to be narrative's turn.

Reconciling fact and fiction: the perspectival world

Cox and Theilgaard (1987, p. 252) underline the way in which individuals each see the world from their own perspective and therefore each lives in a 'perspectival world'. Here, we are, for the most part, concerned about life stories or stories about lives, those basic configurations of meaning that we live in and through. However, few, perhaps none, present or experience their life story in a manner that could be considered objectively or historically accurate. What we possess is an interpretation of our life experience which we may tell quite differently at different stages of life, seeking to provoke or evoke different responses in our listeners according to our varying needs. There is inevitably a considerable difference between biography and autobiography.

Frank (1993) has asserted that, 'life stories are themselves highly selected and selective accounts: memory is strongly affected by the patient's motivations. A person's past history is essentially not so much remembered as constructed from the enormous number of experiences the person has undergone. It can therefore be viewed as an "apologia" to justify the person's present view of the world.' The Talmud puts it more succinctly (Rowe, 1983): 'We do not see things as they are. We see them as we are.' We also tend to see them as we want them to be, for, in commenting on the editorial processes at work in an individual giving an account of his life, Jean Peneff (1990, p. 38) has observed that most life stories contain few wrongful or immoral acts, unjust or violent practices, or deviant behaviour of any kind. They also tend to speak in an unconflicted way with a single voice and often whole periods of life are omitted, in particular painful episodes which could risk shame or disapproval for the speaker. He concluded that: '. . . the life history can be a way of excusing ourselves in public, an effective means of building an enhanced self-image.'

From what are our stories made: constructivism and classification

As soon as we catch sight of Adam (or Linnaeus) naming 'the beasts of the field and all the birds of the air', in the garden of Eden (*Genesis*, Ch. 2), we are ever after aware that we call creatures back to us by the names we have first sent them away with. Therefore, the meanings with which we format the world around us, enable us to be in relationship with it, but we easily loose awareness that these meanings are constructed and attributed, they are inventions not discoveries. They represent some interpolation of imagination, intelligence, memory, and choice, between raw sensory impressions, the experience of them, and the naming and recognition of them. A constructivist approach (Gergen and Gergen, 1988; Mair, 1988) leads towards the distinctly odd conclusion that meaning is always fictive, partial, and provisional.

Delightfully and inescapably we have story-telling brains, and in formatting and patterning the world around us we are little different from dream-time aboriginals (Chatwin, 1988), giving words and meanings to the landscape on which we shall then live. It is just so, and the best we can do. Our meanings are always provisional, and it corrupts the nature of those meanings if we demand from them some secure and final anchor-hold on reality; we necessarily live by faith. The post-Popperian scientist is denied any confidence in final truth (Wallace, 1988), and thus it may only be the deluded and the fundamentalist who *know* the truth, through their motivated conviction and effective exclusion of contradictory and dissonant information. However, the tension between fact and fiction will not be disposed of in favour of a ruthless subjectivism either. For there *is* 'furniture in the universe' (Whiteside, in Mahoney, 1991) and to have a low view of objective reality is constantly to risk falling over it. Hence, Jackson's (Jackson *et al.*, 1998) preference for a 'critical constructivism', as a practical and 'realistic' philosophy with which to underpin the treatment of highly disturbed adolescents in first-episode psychosis. For there are obvious dangers in abandoning all consideration of 'fact' and 'truth'; for example, Frank's (1993) view that 'the chief criterion of the truth of any psychotherapeutic formulation is its plausibility' may veer too far from the corrective notion of the elusive search for validation, and, at its extremes, risks the construction of a highly plausible but wholly false story which, in its fabrication, offers some new form of imprisonment.

From a narrative viewpoint it is easy to disparage classificatory systems, in their confidently asserted categories, as overdetermining boundaries and perpetuating the myth of knowledge. However, when the authors of contemporary classificatory systems are caught at work, in their grand attempt to map reality, and give names to what they find, they appear as latter-day Adams, which is not to devalue their heroic achievement, but to say it is just so. There may be no other way of sensibly talking about the meaning of things at all. Each word applied to an action or object is a symbol of some inarticulate and unfathomable mystery, and it is enlightening to realize that those who devised our present classificatory systems appear to be aware of this:

> A classification is a way of seeing the world . . . classifying means creating, defining and confirming the boundaries of concepts. These in turn define ourselves, our future and our past . . . no other intellectual act is of equal importance: if our classifications of things and people in the world around us were to collapse, the world would cease to be a coherent and organised environment and would become a nebulous agglomeration of rubbish-matter, people and things out of place.
> (*Sartorius, 1988.*)

If we allow it, we may now be able to see a narrative process at work in this most fundamental activity of naming. However, our comfortable consensus conceals our ignorance. Tightly held knowledge obscures. If asked to think, few would be satisfied with the conclusion that water comes from a tap, and if asked to think carefully, many could offer intricate and complex explanations of how water gets into a tap before getting out again. Our stories serve a purpose, many purposes, which is not to devalue them, as much as to enlarge our awareness of what it is that we transact meaning with, and through. However, such awareness risks robbing the story fabric, with which we clothe and protect ourselves, of its utility and strength, and us of our confidence in wearing it: insight is not without its cost.

In reality we may need to steer our rafts of understanding over unfathomable depths, our ignorance lending us some necessary courage and hope. For when our eyes are opened wider we may be burdened with the dizzying realization of our limited comprehension, and the depth of the waters beneath. The naturalist Annie Dillard (1976) writes engagingly of 'reeling with confusion' as she wrestles with the interaction between unconfigured sense impression (it out there) and the apprehension of meaningful patterns (what I make of it). She draws a provocative analogy by empathizing with amoebae which, lacking anything to think with, experience their environment directly and uncritically:

> I see the amoeba as drops of water congealed, bluish, translucent, like chips of sky in the bowl . . . Maybe I should get a tropical aquarium with motorised bubblers and lights, and keep this one for a pet. Yes, it would tell its fissioned descendants, the universe is two feet by five, and if you listen closely you can hear the buzzing music of the spheres.
> (*Dillard, 1976.*)

The realization that there is *only* story can be experienced as a confrontation with meaninglessness; what if we *were* to abandon all classificatory schemata out of dissatisfaction with their contrivance, and anthropomorphic imposition on the universe? Our storied lives constantly intersect with intimations and intuitions of profound and inarticulate truths, which our stories struggle to voice and draw into consciousness. Stories, in their telling, hold and preserve precious meanings; they are, chalices, cribs, and arks, ubiquitous and universal; as wayfarers they carry culture, seeding it in any fertile and receptive soil and leaving their traces as some kind of semantic detritus. True stories are anchored to the dark and mysterious depths of reality itself, and may survive decades or centuries of interpretation and reinterpretation. They stand as narrative icons, a revelation but seldom an explanation, offering instead an opportunity for connection, to touch and be touched, but by what and who?

In discussion with the author . . .

There is something disorienting and exciting when a post-modern author, within his story, exposes his reader to an awareness of himself writing it. In doing so he may also offer a particular insight into some of the processes and motivations at work in narrative construction, for his story is then as much about the making of story itself, as in his apparent subject. John Fowles (1969) provides a rich example when he looks out of Chapter 13 of his novel, *A french lieutenant's woman*, and, breaking the spell of narrative seduction, confesses to the reader that it is all imaginary. Having concluded the previous chapter with teasing questions concerning his main character: 'Who is Sarah? Out of what shadows does she come?', he then accurately anticipates the heightening of his reader's curiosity but says that he doesn't know. 'This story I am telling is all imagination. These characters I create never existed outside my own mind.'

What follows is a roller-coaster of revelation and relativism, as at different turns he engages the reader in a discussion on the modern novel and something of his own only partially understood motives in writing it. We are taken out of Victorian England and sit with the novelist, handling his manuscript. Although we appear to have been awoken from our naïvety, and robbed of the onward flow of plot and character, we are simultaneously engaged in another puzzle—that of the storyteller struggling with what he has written and why: 'for reviewers, for parents, for friends, for loved ones; for vanity, for pride, for curiosity, for amusement: as skilled furniture makers enjoy making furniture, as drunkards like drinking, as judges like judging, as Sicilians like emptying a shotgun into an enemy's back. I could fill a book with reasons and they would all be true, although not true of all. Only one same reason is shared by all of us: we wish to create worlds as real as, but other than, the world that is.'

Our engagement with *his* narrative process deepens when we realize that, by revealing himself at work as a writer, he has drawn us in, we have become characters in his story, and by demonstrating a constructivist perspective at work we are provoked into considering ourselves as story-tellers rather than readers. And he appears, for a moment, to worry about this, until we realize we are still on the hook: 'I have disgracefully broken the illusion? No. My characters still exist, and in a reality no less, or no more real than the one I have just broken. Fiction is woven into all . . . .' What may have begun for us as an entertainment or diversion, is rapidly deepening to an encounter with perspectival realism, leading him to confidently assert his fiction as factual within its own perspective, and for us to have difficulty in disagreeing.

In pursuing his exposé of 'the ghosts that are rattling their chains behind the scenes of this book', he challenges his readers to consider that they too are living within a story of their own construction. Eventually we are released from the glare and confusion of insight, as he leads us back into his character's lives and actions, and allows us to forget our own once more: 'I report then, only the outward facts: that Sarah cried in the darkness, but did not kill herself . . .', and although we have been caught up in a tale of mysterious romance, it is illustrative of the wider and deeper story concerning our main theme, which is the struggle with discerning reality and its narrative representation, and the difficulty of holding, in good faith, a commitment to the truth of the story, and an awareness, that in truth, what we have, all we have, is story.

Crites (1971) describes this well in asserting that, although it cannot be legitimately claimed that 'reality' is itself somehow possessed of a narrative form, nevertheless, 'our experience does have. Such that experience can be captured by narrative sequence and rekïndled, evoked, stimulated by narrative expression—when we speak about reality we do so in stories or fragments of stories.' It may be just this omnipresence of stories that serves to render them invisible, for, as Taylor (1996) has commented: 'we live in stories the way fish live in water, breathing them in and out, buoyed up by them, taking from them our sustenance, but rarely conscious of this element in which we all exist. We are born into stories; they nurture and guide us through life'—if we are fortunate.

Some purposes of story: what do stories do?

The storiographer Richard Bowman (1989) summarizes something of the potential of stories in giving cognitive and emotional significance to experience, as a means of constructing and negotiating a social identity and in orientating our travels over the experiential landscape, by attributing moral weight to actions and events. MacIntyre (in Taylor, 1996, p. 7) has emphasized that it may be through the hearing and telling of stories that children learn what a child and what a parent is, who the world around them is populated by, and what the ways of the world are. He warns that: 'Deprive children of stories and you leave them unscripted, anxious stutters in their actions as in their words. Hence there is no way to give us an understanding of any society, including our own, except through the stock of stories which constitute its initial dramatic resources.'

Bettleheim (1991) deepens this consideration when, as an educator and therapist of severely disturbed children, he considered his main task as the restoration of meaning to their lives. In pursuing this he places great emphasis on traditional stories as accessible resources of deep meaning, for he considered that these tales 'start where the child really is in his psychological and emotional being. They speak about his severe inner pressures in a way that the child unconsciously understands.'

Hearing stories, experiencing meanings

When we hear a story we experience it; 'In a very real way, we are imprinted with knowing just by listening to the tale (Estes, 1992, p. 387).' It is potentially liberating when these 'knowings' interlock with our unexpressed, unstoried experience. For some this is as effective as the accurate docking of a medication with its target receptor. I know of two people (both doctors) who were restrained from suicide through reading Tolstoy's (1906) *Twenty three tales*, and found sufficient warmth and hope to continue: one prescribed them to the other.

The recent popularity of traditional tales, such as *Iron John* (Bly, 1990) and those told by Clarissa Pinkola Estes (1992) in *Women who run with wolves*, attests to the acceptability of these stories to re-engage a contemporary readership. They may also bear witness to a growing preference for contextualizing our problems in living within an accessible narrative, rather than having them encrypted within the esoteric language of experts. Traditional stories are repositories of wisdom, offering an exposition of life problems and a method of approaching and resolving them, a source of identification, an opportunity for catharsis, a model of understanding and insight, and yielding a knowledge of motives, causes, and some kind of justification for otherwise unjustifiable and unmanageable turns of fate and fortune. Their capacity for containment and holding can either be seen as a means of dissembling, concealing the basic futility and purposelessness of human existence, in bad faith, or that they, 'bear witness to a strongly felt attunement to the actual hymn of the universe' (Gersie, 1992, p. 37).

Such folk-tales have been handed down from one story-teller to another for centuries they may provide prototypical maps and methods—none of which the hearer may be consciously aware of but may experience with an uncanny sense of salience and interest.

The ugly duckling

A young attractive and intelligent woman regards herself as utterly repugnant. She has learned to cope with her past experience by cutting herself in savage and provocative ways. In the context of a long-standing therapeutic relationship she accepted a copy of Estes (1992) retelling of 'The ugly duckling'. Without knowing quite why, she papered her kitchen with the photocopied sheets, sticking them to the wall alongside a copy of her father's death certificate, which she kept to try to remind herself that he was dead. Her experience was that he continued to wake her in the early hours of each morning, and all but suffocating her with his actions. She often cut in the early morning, making deep openings in her body until she felt cleansed by the flowing blood.

For many years after his death she remained hostage to her past, oscillating between feeling that she would do anything to be loved by him, which included killing herself so as to join him, and alternately that she had no family, and desperately needed to flee in the hope of finding a new life. She inspired affection in nearly all who met or worked with her, and yet remained convinced that she was repugnant, unacceptable, and unlovable—that she belonged and fitted in nowhere. Her imagery and predicament seemed to fit well with the story and she was unsure why she valued it, but read it daily.

The time came, as it did for the 'ugly duckling', when the risks she lived with seemed overwhelming, she frequently had a noose suspended from her ceiling, and at one point bought an electric hedge trimmer with which to amputate herself. A protracted struggle with Health and Social Services Authorities ensued (standing in here for the farmyard bullies, who variously neglected, harried, and persecuted the duckling, but eventually prompted its departure through despair), and it was possible to fund a residential placement in a creative, open, and therapeutic environment, where acceptance of her cutting, and interest in her as a person gradually created a thaw, the beginnings of trust, and self-acceptance. At the time of departure for this sanctuary she discussed what she had decided to take with her, which was very little but included her copy of the story. She felt she now understood more clearly what it had to say to her, which included the hazy and hazardous sense of the hope that lay ahead.

Held together by stories

Social groups, families, and couples are joined by their stories, and may be held together in proportion to the adequacy of their narrative to provide a shelter of shared meaning. These stories may be regarded as fulfilling a religious function, in that they bind together, and when they are absent or fail, or in some way unravel and no longer give a clear account of experience, the need arises for restoration, or for facing the probability of drifting or splitting apart. Laurens van de Post (cited in Cox and Theilgaard, 1987) has commented on the social and existential significance of stories: 'without a story one had no class or family; without a story of one's own, no individual life; without a story of stories, no life giving continuity with the beginning and therefore no future.' Our shared stories are the fabric of relationships and the basis for community.

Mair's (1988) views extend and widen this awareness when he speaks of stories as 'habitations' which we live in and through, and when stories fail, individuals and whole societies struggle to live by stories that cannot sustain them. The characteristic and disorienting revisionism of mid-life transitions (Stein, 1983) may result in couples, who formerly considered they had some form of shared life, 'loosing the plot'; re-evaluating and retelling the story they have lived; drawing out silent chapters; revealing concealed meanings, needs, and experiences; amplifying dissonance and re-editing earlier chapters out of a need, to clear their throat and speak with a clear voice, and to embark on the second journey in a different way and perhaps in different company. In its most hopeful form this process can apparently work as a means of revision and reconstruction—at least in fiction.

Michael Tournier (1992) gives an account of a couple living near Mont St Michael who have become weary and irritated with each other and are contemplating separation. Instead of grieving this they decide to celebrate it by offering a 'banquet of foreshore sea-food' to a gathering of all their closest friends on midsummer's day. The feast was intended to conclude at dawn the following day by their announcement of separation at sunrise. The friends gathered and as they ate and talked, began to tell stories, personal and traditional, short and long, and in the telling of these stories, which, as the night wore on, 'gained beauty and strength', they were provided with some form of supporting narrative by a compassionate community and, finding this 'house of words to live in together', they decide not to separate after all—this appears as a fable for - modern times but could also be seen as an analogue of couple and family therapy. Couples that do separate have the same need to formulate a story, or perhaps stories, to live by, that make sense of their experience, contain past pain and confusion, and enable release and opportunity for new experience.

Stories thus provide holding, containing structures of meaning. When an individual or shared story is coming apart and disintegrating it marks the entrance into some kind of rite of passage, a liminal and potentially transformative time of either drawing that particular chapter to a close, or else falling back on some broader deeper narrative able to hold the fractured parts together, a narrative scaffold, a sacred and sacramental tale. This process of renewal or emergence contains the attendant risk of unwittingly becoming hostage to the reconstructed story. Hillman (1983, p. 23) provides a cautionary note to how we select, hold, tell, and shape the stories we live by, for in his observation, 'the way we imagine our lives is the way we are going to go on living our lives. For the manner in which we tell ourselves about what is going on is the genre through which events become experiences.'

'Stories to live by', are ideally those that can support a continually changing life, those that are fecund and germinative, enabling and releasing. Mature stories are accepting of uncertainty, and integrate it *as* uncertainty suggesting a continuing journey rather than confinement and conformity to a new orthodoxy (Gersie, 1997).

Stories confer identity

Sacks (1985), writing on the predicament of amnesic patients who have 'lost their past', illustrates the need we all have for a story which confers upon us a secure sense of identity, 'we have each of us a life-story, an inner narrative—whose continuity, whose sense is our lives . . . to be ourselves we must have ourselves—posses, if need be repossess, our life-stories. We must "re-collect" ourselves, recollect the inner drama, the narrative of ourselves. A man needs a continuous inner narrative, to maintain his identity, his self.'

For some, the fulfilment of this need can be accessed by situating themselves within a secure and established narrative framework, they become 'people of the book'. For example, some of the most fractured and disorganized life patterns are associated with chemical dependency. Alcoholics Anonymous (AA), so named after the title of the first anthology of accounts from recovering alcoholics (Alcoholics Anonymous, 1993), has been built on a foundation of telling and hearing of stories. These stories of brokenness, spoken with vulnerability, are the established means of offering a bridge out of shameful denial and self-destructive alienation into a community of fellow suffers with a shared commitment to recovery. These holding and healing narratives serve first as a means of identification and then as prototypical stories offering hope and guidance. They are maps, which offer a means of locating oneself on some recognizable landscape—YOU ARE HERE—and then a structure with which to take up your own journey but in the company of a committed group of fellow travellers.

The AA story clearly draws directly from the Judeo-Christian narrative of brokenness leading to repentance and then salvation and restoration, putting AA's '*Big book*' within the covers of a bigger book. Many addicts have become dislocated from any deeper existential narrative. AA's story is of a crisis of meaning, offering a narrative means of escape from the repetitive drunkard's tale of denial and self-justification, to a story of restitution and spiritual growth.

Stories to live by: the containment of danger

Narrative responses to desperate circumstances offer a means of containing wild, threatening, and unpredictable experiences, and re-establishing some kind of order and relationship. As with Scheherazade, who told stories to save her life, the fictional will do every bit as well as the factual, if it is told with conviction and skill. Here we see story-making, as a life-supporting process, a psychic resource, a defence against futility, emptiness, and formless terror. And, if A. S. Byatt's (1995) views are correct, there is an intriguing and reciprocal relationship between the stories that we make and tell, and those that have been told to us, such that, 'we learn to interpret, and even to live our lives through the stories which have haunted the imaginations of our ancestors and of people from very different cultures and imaginative worlds.'

A particularly vivid and well-studied example of stories generated by threats to basic survival, is the evolution of a species of unfounded gossip, called 'Bobards', amongst concentration camp inmates (Bravo *et al.*, 1990). These were elaborate stories of military activity and political developments, the prospect of food arriving and conditions improving. Their baseless stories provided hope in a hopeless position and 'to back up the daily fight to hold on and to keep the hope of survival alive.' The authors conclude that, 'at the heart of these accounts we find a resource of the human mind which, impotent in the face of overwhelming force, instead drew on mythical hopes. These were hopes for actions and events which failed to happen or never could have happened.'

As examples of stories constructed out of desperate circumstances, a remarkable literary event was witnessed in 1993–1994, with the publication of successive memoirs from the Beirut hostages (Keenan, McCarthy, Waite). Each presented their experiences in very different literary styles. Terry Waite (*Independent*, Saturday, 1 October 1994) subsequently spoke about his writing, and described how he drew not on mythical hopes, but on story-making itself, as a means of surviving prolonged solitary confinement:

> I soon realised that if I was to survive, it was essential to maintain a strong inner life. I needed to tell myself stories. In telling myself the story of my life I was maintaining a lifeline with reality I had known and lived. Characters from the past emerged to comfort, amuse and haunt. Time took on another meaning. That which I called 'the past' was a part of me. My soul longed for harmony and rhythm . . . when I eventually emerged all I wanted was a pencil and notebook. The book was already written in my mind. One eminent reviewer described the book as being 'egocentric'. He quite failed to see that the writer was attempting to hang onto identity, because the threat of dissolving into madness was ever present.
> (*Waite, Independent, 1 October 1994*).

Illnesses, traumas, and life transitions may also conform to the pattern of 'desperate circumstances', carrying fundamental challenges to our hope and security, our sense of who we are, and what is going on.

Luria's (1973) account of *The man with a shattered world*, consists of a clinician's retelling of his patient's struggle to rediscover his identity by writing his life, an activity he had sustained for 25 years, resulting in a 3000 page document, which, because of his traumatic brain injury, he was unable to read. Luria believed that writing the story of his life gave his patient a reason to live, seeking to recover the man he had once been, and by telling others about his illness even to overcome it. At first the ambition, 'to overcome it', appears as a wish-fulfilling fantasy, and yet his heroic endeavour *did* enable some kind of immortality, first in inspiring Luria's account, and, in turn, providing a touchstone for Oliver Sacks, and other neurologists interested in re-centring case histories on people rather than lesions. Thus, in the preface of *The man who mistook his wife for a* hat, Sacks (1985) looks back to a Hippocratic tradition of medical story-telling, acknowledges its demise over the last century, and Luria's contribution in revitalising it:

> The tradition of richly human clinical tales reached a high point in the nineteenth century, and then declined, with the advent of an impersonal neurological science. Luria wrote: 'the power to describe, which was so common to the great nineteenth-century neurologists and psychiatrists, is almost gone now . . . it must be revived.' His own late works, such as The Mind of a Mnemonist and The Man with a Shattered World, are attempts to revive this lost tradition.
> (*Sacks, 1985*).

Narrative icons

Our stories do not only hold us together with their form but can guide and profoundly challenge us through their contents. The traditional invitations, 'Are you sitting comfortably . . .?', 'Once upon a time, . . .', or, 'In a land far away, . . .', are invitations to relax, de-defend, it is safe to settle down, and listen: you cannot be led into error because what is about to happen is defined as fiction, and you have confidence that you will be as free to walk away from it at the end as you were to sit down at the beginning. It has therefore been the vehicle through which many great teachers have sought to communicate difficult and provocative truths, a means of 'touching the depths without stirring the surface' (Bachelard, in Cox and Theilgaard, 1987). These sacred tales (see Sims, Chapter 6, this volume) or teaching stories offer a bridge between the lived story of the individual with the stories of others: 'A great story has the capacity to transcend the boundaries of our personal worlds, with their sorrows and joys, and introduce the universality of human experience' (Feldman and Kornfield, 1991, p. 7).

As well as encouraging and supporting, stories, as repositories of values and ethical imperatives, also challenge by introducing considerations of foreboding that carry a message or that bit of unbearable knowledge that has to be imparted. A story can thus contain within its framework the two seemingly contradictory elements of distancing and involvement.

The prophet Nathan (*Bible*, 2 Samuel, 12 vv. 1–7) provides a masterly example of story when he approaches King David to confront him with the complete unacceptability of his actions. His is the almost impossible task of confronting the all-powerful king of Israel who had taken the beautiful Bathsheba for himself and then contrived the murder of her husband on the battlefield after finding she was pregnant.

The prophet tells David a story: 'There were two men in a certain town, one rich and the other poor. The rich man had a very large number of sheep and cattle, but the poor man had nothing except one little ewe lamb that he had bought. He raised it, and it grew up with him and his children. It shared his food, drank from his cup and even slept in his arms. It was like a daughter to him. Now a traveller came to the rich man, but the rich man refrained from taking one of his own sheep or cattle to prepare a meal for the traveller who had come to him. Instead, he took the ewe lamb that belonged to the poor man and prepared it for the one who had come to him.' Having emotionally engaged David in the plot such that 'his anger burned against the man', he asks Nathan to name him, for surely David would act. 'You are that man,' says Nathan, and David is broken by the realization of his guilt and, in his repentance, becomes receptive to what Nathan has to say about his future.

The clinician and the story-teller

There are many patterns and dimensions of correspondence between the clinician and the storyteller. Clinicians have always had much in common with oral historians, who value the individuality of life stories, and, rather than seeing them as awkward impediments to generalization, view them as vital documents in the construction of understanding. Medicine's scientific bent meant that it took an eavesdropping professor of English to observe that, in reality, doctors devote their working days to a succession of narrative rituals, such that if they were required to cease story-telling they would be virtually struck dumb.

Kathryn Montgomery Hunter (1991) spent two years studying the narrative fabric of medical activity, and concluded that physicians habitually tell stories: case conferences, case reports, theorizing, and model making all have a narrative structure: 'They were stories, narrative accounts of the action and motivation of human beings, physicians and patients, who, variously were frustrated by circumstances, rewarded for effort, and plagued by fate stories . . . and how else', she asks, 'is the individual to be known but by a narrative account of his case?'

Telling a case: making a history

Case histories are not so much 'taken', or recorded by those whose job it is to 'clerk' a patient or assess a client, as elicited, moulded, shaped, constructed, and interpreted. Case history is a genre, a convincing and compelling manner of talking about the past (Charon, 1992, 1993; Susko, 1994), reinforced by the 'rhetoric of realism' (Tonkin, 1990, p. 29). For, as we have already argued, a truly objective account of another's life is an impossibility.

Hunter (1991) described this narrative transposition, between patient and clinician, from her systematic observations. It began with, 'the offering of a story of malady, to gain admission to the world of the ill', and she describes the activity of physicians who, 'take such a story, interrogate, and expand it and return it to the patient as a diagnosis, an interpretative retelling that points towards the stories ending'. As such she sees the centre of medical activity as transacted by narrative, 'a dialogue between illness and healing narratives', which provide a context for the interactions between clinician and patient, their roles, expectations, plot, and likely outcome. She also considers that these different stories lie in creative tension with one another and that patients come seeking precisely that difference, searching for a reinterpretation of their experience as a means of getting at the truth: 'the subjective, personal, patient story and the interpretative scientific medical story are not translations of each other but independently coexisting narratives.'

We are more accustomed to regarding these clinical accounts as records 'taken' from the patient rather than actively created illness meanings, arising from our dialogue; however, it is a common observation that different practitioners construct different stories even from the same patient, according to their particular interests, needs, and purposes, for how you listen influences and shapes both the telling and hearing (Klienman, 1988). Our conceptual models silently form and inform our observations and serve as guiding narratives which shape and influence our practice and research.

Psychopathology as 'dystoria'

Just as our diagnoses can be seen as highly condensed stories (Hillman, 1983, p. 15), so psychopathology can be seen as the consequence of living in the context of a story that is maladaptive and life-denying. Examples are given of stories that are experienced as poisonous and constraining, compulsive and dissembling, 'forgotten', and in their depths of unapproachable and inexpressible pain, have become an untellable, alienating silence. A common theme in many states of psychological distress is the interpenetration of current experience by past meanings.

Toxic stories

Some are simply cursed—they live with a toxic story, which configures meaning in a pattern that saps rather than enhances life, these are stories that disconfirm, reduce, shackle, and snare.

The Jungian storyteller Clarrisa Pinkola Estes (1992, p. 201) tells of the discoveries made by her friend, Opalanga, who was very tall and slender and, in addition to being mocked for being tall, as a child she was told that the split between her front teeth was the sign of being a liar. However, as an adult she had journeyed to the Gambia in West Africa and found some of her ancestral people, who had, among their tribe, many who were very tall and slender, and had splits between their front teeth. This split, they explained to her, was called Sakaya Yallah, meaning 'opening of God', and was understood as a sign of wisdom. Estes comments on the influence this process of detoxification and revision had upon her friend: '(her) stories which began as experiences both oppressive and depressive, end with joy and a strong sense of self. Opalanga understands that her height is her beauty, her smile one of wisdom, and that the voice of God is always close to her lips.' She offers an example of the process by which we so easily become 'caught in a story' (Byatt, 1992) and all the more so if told to us early and authoritatively.

People who (need to) tell stories

There are some people whose 'disorder' is that of telling stories (Nicholson and Roberts, 1994). They appear to be exploiting the lack of any objective means of verifying their account, by presenting with a persuasive narrative of simulated illness. They may be diagnosed as having a 'factitious disorder with psychological symptoms' (DSM–IIIR) and are characterized as purposefully pretending to have psychological symptoms, which are under voluntary control, but are compulsively driven by a psychological need to enter the sick role and achieve patient status.

The 'Falkland's veteran'

John presented through the accident and emergency department after a large overdose of paracetamol. He was an unemployed drifter, living alone in a damp bed-sit, and was greatly distressed. He reluctantly, and with much prompting, gave the junior doctor trying to assess him, a story of having served in the Falkland's war, and his deep remorse for having killed someone, whose death agony he continued to see in flash backs. A physical examination revealed numerous scars which he said were gained in active service and he described bearing an unmanageable guilt such that he wanted to take his own life.

His tragic story, apparent risk, and obvious distress produced an immediate admission which he gratefully accepted, and settled to the ward routine remarkably quickly. A psychologist with specific experience debriefing war veterans was asked for help. The implausible and contradictory account he then gave suggested that he had never been in the Falkland Islands. When confronted and simultaneously offered support and help, a different story emerged, of the breakdown of a very long-standing and somewhat demeaning relationship based on his dependency, a lengthy history of self-harm (the scars), and a past history of abuse. John was able to say that because he felt ashamed of his 'real story' and felt it would fail to elicit the care and support he so needed, he fabricated one which believed would suit his needs better.

The suspicion of simulation can create considerable confusion and division in the psychiatric team, provoking defensive or even hostile reactions and bring about the rejection of the patient, if he has not already packed his bags. And yet, the need to tell such stories appears to be a manifestation of highly disturbed individuals with great difficulty expressing their needs and problems. Patients who find some comfort and benefit in representing themselves as suffering from a major mental illness often feel threatened, abandoned, and overwhelmingly anxious. They often pursue a chequered career with multiple admissions, suicide attempts, forensic problems, and coincident or alternating presentation with episodes of diagnosable mental illness and undiagnosable physical symptoms, 'acting crazy may bode more ill than being crazy' (Pope *et al.*, 1982).

Angry rejection from staff may represent a repetition of the original developmental traumas. The classic, 'never darken our door again' response from many services to Munchausen patients is clearly inappropriate. At the same time, ineffective and sometimes massive consumption of resources must somehow be prevented.

A rational and compassionate approach hinges on mutual acknowledgement by patient and psychiatrist that the presenting symptoms are consciously produced and development of a broader narrative with an offer to negotiate care and treatment directed at their authentic problems. Therapy hinges on enabling the patient to acknowledge that he is caught in a story of his own authorship, and that the therapists central task is to help translate symptoms into problems that *can* be solved, or at least identified (Ritson and Forrest, 1970).

This realisation, that one *is* caught in a story, is disarming, disorienting, but ultimately hopeful, for it creates the necessary space to allow change and transition. If we are cloaked and protected by our narrative constructions it is understandably disarming and potentially humiliating to catch ourselves at it. However, the real hero in the story of '*The Emperor's new clothes*' (Anderson, 1992) was perhaps not the little child who declared the Emperor naked (although he did well), but would have been the unseen observer who at the close of the story stepped forward to share his cloak, covering His Excellency's embarrassment, offered time and care to help him come to terms with his predicament, and provided practical help in fostering his reintegration and rehabilitation.

People who loose their stories

When stories fail, the person's task is in coping with the process of becoming unstoried. The stories we live by may be cunningly tucked out of sight, mislaid by the right hand whilst the left hand is apparently unaware of what was going on; some fall into threads and fragments through the crude erosion and collapse of the architecture that supports them (See Bruce, Ch 9, this volume), others we are aware of, but in fear and shame, are unable to tell, and so are hostage to consequence.

The tale of Michael Barlow

Who was so called because, unable to remember anything about himself, including his name, he had been given the named Michael by the nurse who admitted him and subsequently took his surname from the psychiatric ward on which he found himself.

The police who found him were puzzled as to why this clean, tidy, well-groomed, middle-aged man was wandering around a small seaside town asking people who he was, and what he was doing there. The psychiatric nurses felt he was pretending, even their usually broad and tolerant minds were stretched to incredulity by his insistence that he knew nothing about himself or his past when there was clearly nothing wrong with his memory, for he instantly found his way around the ward, striking up affable relationships with staff and patients, and expressing benign confusion about his predicament.

During the three weeks of his stay he kept a journal, and noted carefully any reminiscent details, saying that he felt a real need to build up a life history for himself again. He returned in a naïve and strangely unconvincing state of delight one day, after confirming that the thickened skin on his finger tips may have been related to guitar playing, by visiting a music shop and trying one out. It all had the feeling of game and pretence. His journal took on a different character and he admitted that he was imaginatively filling in the gaps between bits of information, which he found gave a more satisfying story as he found the incomplete patchwork distressing.

It seemed equally incongruous that he started to express a willingness to establish a new life under his assumed name if he could not discover his own. However, the police eventually traced the keys, found in his pocket, to an abandoned car near to where he had been found. He did admit that it looked oddly familiar to him and on putting his key in the lock, not only did the car door open but also the shut door to his past memories and his identity.

Detail appeared to return gradually, like a landscape revealed by a rapidly lifting mist, hazy, fragments of recollection emerged, which he seemed curiously ambivalent about stringing together. Then came a realization that he had driven 100 miles from his home to the location of a fondly remembered holiday during better times, and that on the day of his travels he was due to face a disciplinary hearing at his place of work in relation to matters of a particularly embarrassing and humiliating nature. Instead, he had forgotten all of it, and appeared on our patch as the amnesic Michael Barlow.

The loss of his story fulfilled a transparent purpose, his three-week long dissociative fugue appeared to serve as a compassionate abdication of awareness, such that he could plan his return, and be received as a vulnerable person ready to face his responsibilities.

Unspeakable dread, nameless terror

For some, the issue is not that a story is fractured, mysterious or lost but that it cannot be spoken. The individual believes his experiences to be so unacceptable to others, or risk such negative reactions, that they are held with fear and shame, concealed, or hidden. Silencing seems part of all traumatizing or abusing experience. These silenced stories may be rehearsed inwardly, but the risks of saying them aloud seem too great, they are believed to be untellable for fear of the consequences, and there *are* many consequences. Silence is achieved at considerable cost, for if significant or even pivotal meanings in one's life are incommunicable then one is separated, even alienated, and little changes. The very meanings that would connect and create the possibility of attachment remain hidden, and people become invisible to each other (Harvey *et al.*, 1991).

Mollica (1988) has described his experience of responding to the needs of large numbers of Vietnamese refugees and the feeling of impotence and irrelevance of normal psychiatric practice:

> During the first year in our clinic, we were bewildered by 'what to do?', yet many patients continued to flow into the clinic quiet and depressed . . . little by little, like pebbles of sand poured into a pile on the beach, we began to listen to the stories of our patient's lives . . . finally we acknowledged that the majority of our patients had been tortured.
> (*Mollica, 1988.*)

These people had endured experiences and carried meanings that were untellable but also inescapable. They were trapped by what Mollica refers to as, 'the trauma story'. He commented that these stories had great power over the patients and could easily overwhelm the listener. Working empirically—trying to find an approach that worked—the therapeutic team progressively found their way to facilitating the telling of these trauma stories, whatever the orientation of the individual therapist, and discovered that this story-telling was at the heart of effective treatment. For, although it may have been hidden and desperately concealed from others, 'the trauma story is usually reviewed nightly in the patient's nightmares . . . a personal narrative in the mind that is retold daily as it is searched for new meanings and clues.'

Suffering creates a silence, and it is in naming that silence (Hauerwas, 1993) that the beginning, and only the beginning, of a healing journey becomes possible. The process whereby a person's unacknowledged experience becomes part of their acknowledged history has long been recognized as mutative (Campbell, 1998). Mollica (1988) found that certain patterns emerged in helpful or healing story-telling. The story needed to include both the events and how the refugees had been changed by them, and the reactions of those around them, which revealed the extent of the psychological impact of the traumatic events in their lives. This process nearly always resulted in an account that went beyond being overpowered and loosing control, to loosing their world: 'a subjective loss of one's own reality, a numbing and a paralysis of self reflection whereby the individual becomes trapped in the story or even becomes the story. These patients live in a world of traumatic images and memories in which nothing exists for them except the trauma story. Their psychological reality is both full and empty, full of the past and empty of new ideas and experiences. . . . the patient is silent. The trauma story becomes an inner personal obsession.'

In reviewing the theoretical foundations of traumatically induced dissociation, Mollon (1996, p. 36) has described narratization as a healthy defence, one that can be overwhelmed by unassimilable trauma. He looks back to Janet, who considered that traumatization resulted from the failure to take effective action against a potential threat, resulting in helplessness, which in turn led to 'vehement emotions' that interfered with memory storage. He suggested that memory itself is a kind of action—the action of telling a story. This action of creating narrative, by attaching words to the experience so that it can be made sense of, forms part of the wider action of responding appropriately to a situation. He argued that 'making intellectual sense of an unexpected challenge leads to proper adaptation, and a subjective sense of calm and control'. The 'vehement emotions' aroused by the frightening and overwhelming event prevent this process of adaptation; dissociation then occurs as a defensive means of uncoupling events and experiences from one another and inhibiting organized thinking. The traumatic experience is not lost from the mind, but persists as a 'subconcious fixed idea' that functions both to organize the memories of trauma, and to keep them out of awareness.

The limits of narrative: some cautionary tales

Tensions in narrative construction: the problem of 'truth'

There are considerable problems inherent in the otherwise simple notion of getting at the truth of any specific life experience; for memory is inherently revisionistic, shifting the balance and weight of significance attributed to past events, according to present needs and perceptions: 'Like myth, memory requires a radical simplification of its subject matter. All recollections are told from the standpoint of the present. The process of telling can serve many functions but preeminently in attempting to make sense of the past. That demands a selecting, ordering, and simplifying, a construction of coherent narrative whose logic works to draw the life story towards the fable' (Samuel and Thompson, 1990, p. 7).

We live in anthologies. Our stories nest in each other like Russian dolls, and we collect or recollect our life stories according to some organizing principle, a meta-narrative, which encourages the preservation of some information and the neglect of other.

Some ways of telling stories inhibit rather than enlighten. Alida Gersie (1997), as a mature story-teller, is aware that she *is* telling stories, and regarding the possibility of misapplication she warns of the endemic trend to attribute our sufferings to particular experiences, which may create 'shackling narratives which foreclose the future and condemn the past.' The clarity and simplicity of understanding we long for can be as much of an obstacle as confusion, if such clarity is forged at the expense of denying appropriate complexity, thus we are all prone to accept bogus interpretations as pertinent if they fit our expectations or preferences. Although in training we learn to structure our observations with familiar patterns and configurations of meaning, we run the risk of continuing to believe them, or at least to hold to them too rigidly. Some qualities of certitude are hallmarks of immaturity and insecurity rather than of wisdom.

Mary and the tapeworm

Although Mary had a long history of schizophrenia and many past admissions to hospital, she had for some years lived contentedly at home with her husband until he became ill. She coped fairly well whilst he was away, but created emotional scenes on the ward and also complained that she was affected by a tapeworm. Her distress was initially attributed to his illness and her consequent loss of support. It then emerged that she believed the tapeworm was travelling throughout her body and was in some way linked with her husband's illness. It was tempting to explain all of these difficulties as due to a relapse of her illness, especially as we knew she had neglected her medication whilst her husband was away, but there were some other puzzling features. Her erratic fluctuations of mood and behaviour continued, she appeared to the visiting nurse to have difficulty dressing herself, and was becoming progressively more forgetful. Her husband had been aware of this for a long time but had compensated for her. An electroencephalogram and various blood tests were normal, but despite the plausible story of a recurrence of psychosis, there remained a lingering uncertainty which prompted further investigation. A subsequent brain scan demonstrated a massive, benign, and slowly growing tumour (meningioma). It was successfully removed, but would not have been discovered if we had not doubted our narrative formulation, and preserved a vigilance for dissonant features.

This illustrates the need to be constantly alert for discrepancies, and rather than meet them with irritation, to value these intruders, which may disrupt and challenge our established patterns as offering guidance into a different, and perhaps 'truer' story. Indeed White's (1988) method of working with 'problem saturated lives', depends on searching for dissonant elements, which provide leverage to open up suffocating, constraining, and condemning stories.

Cultural relativism

The disposition to interpret the world around us through our dominant narrative can be tragic in its consequences. However, the cultural relativism of our guiding values, is often only revealed once that culture has itself moved on, leaving, sometimes literally, the broken ruins of its own confident creation. Robert Lacey's commentary (*Sunday Times*, 16 February 1997) on the inside story of the world famous auction house, Sotheby's, describes such a shift from the once eager and enthusiastic acquisition of ethnic and classical antiquities, supported by the narrative of Western superiority and imperialism, to the realization that such acquisitions represent the destruction of indigenous people's most sacred and precious artefacts. A pitiful and shameful scenario is offered of, 'a remote Indian village whose temple gods have been stolen and vandalised by antiquity traders. "How can you sell a god?" ask the villagers, as they sprinkle holy water and continue to worship in front of the rubble.'

Narrative seduction

Stories are also used to influence, and at worse to deceive and mislead. Narrating is never innocent (Brooks, 1993). It is less obvious that something is wrong when the story-teller is sincere and committed. The risks of naïve or motivated self-deception are all the more significant when they jeopardize others also. This occurs in its most concrete form when we are required to pre-pare stories for the courts. Kleinman (1988) warns that an 'ominous kind of retrospective nar-ratisation occurs in the tendentious reworking of an account of illness and treatment to fit the line of argument of a disability suit or malpractice litigation.' A similar risk may be at work in the current crisis over true and false memories in adult survivors of child sexual abuse.

Tony Madden's (1995) thoughtful review of *The falling shadow* exposes some of the problems in producing a too well-crafted narrative. The book followed the official enquiry into the mur-der of Georgina Robinson, an occupational therapist on the psychiatric unit where Andrew Robinson, her assailant, was being treated. It was written by the same highly respected investi-gators that conducted the inquiry. Madden sounds an alarm for those who would be swept along by the seduction of a well-crafted tale and lulled by its persuasiveness, which he fears may arise from the skilled injection of plot and purpose into the enquiry's material, its narratization, beyond what he believes can be reasonably drawn from the available data. He regards the gravest error is in the construction of a spurious sense of inevitability for, in his estimate, 'the most hor-rifying aspect of the killing was its unpredictability.'

He is able to stand aside from the content of the book and criticize the process of its con-struction, and in particular the risks of narrative devices giving a satisfying but spurious air of meaningfulness and causality, carrying its own grave and perhaps inappropriate attribution of responsibility and blame:

> The general problem is compounded in this book by the author's skill in fashioning a coherent narrative from the assembled facts. They create a sense of inexorable progress towards tragedy, exemplified by the metaphor of 'the falling shadow' which runs through the book. This is an effective literary device. It makes the book more attractive to the reader, but the sense of progres-sion is largely spurious. It could only have been imposed after the event, and it provides a mis-leading context in which to judge past action. It seems quite wrong that these journalistic devices should be used in reporting an inquiry that may blight careers, and whose priorities must be objectivity and fairness, with readability way down the list.
> (*Madden, 1995.*)

This cautionary note concerning the confidence we place in our stories also applies at the therapeutic interface. The novelist Fay Weldon (*Sunday Times Review* 29 February 1993), has presented an extreme viewpoint, based on her own experience, which caricatures the therapists behaviour, but in doing so she points to the risks patients run who experience poorly com-missioned the therapeutic narratives, through which the patient's needs are subjugated to those of the therapist. She complained that therapists try to 're-write the narratives of other peoples lives to their own satisfaction', and sees therapists as thwarted novelists using real people to con-struct their narrative:

> Eager for plot, hungry for emotion, randy for sexual detail, forever tying ends together to get their climax, the point, however spurious, of the work. And they should not do it. A writer of novels knows that real life is a hopeless basis for fiction. Real life is chaos, nothing fits. There is no point—that's why we need fiction . . . therapists think the plot they insert into other peoples heads will work out in happy endings, or what the therapist sees as a happy ending.
> (*Weldon, Sunday Times Review 29 February 1993.*)

Many would immediately complain that the target of her criticism should be identified as in-competent and misguided therapy, rather than therapy and hermeneutics *per se*. But, she makes a point none the less.

And in the end . . .

We have reached a beginning. The aim of this introductory chapter was just that, to lay a foundation, offer an oversight, mark some paths, point out some routes, and express some caution as well as curiosity, as, undeniably, inescapably, I have been telling you a story too.

Subsequent chapters will consider narrative both as a conceptual framework and as a therapeutic tool. There are important implications for training, for we would argue that induction into the story-tellers art, the acquisition of a continually expanding anthology of 'master tales' (Mckay and Ryan, 1995), and a deep awareness of the stories we are host and hostage to, are significant contributions in developing clinical maturity, and aid the delicate process of balancing the 'art' of psychiatry and psychotherapy with their complementary sciences.

This emphasis, on rekindling a narrative approach, is offered in part as a response to the critique of medicine and psychiatry with which we began, a means of recentring on the person, his experience, and the significance of his suffering. If this 'person-centred approach' is to be any more than flip jargon, or a nod to Rogerian allegiances, it will need to underpin the whole helping endeavour. A mature position may be to use both our stories and our narrative capacity as skilfully and compassionately as we possibly can in the service of our clients and patients, whilst at the same time inclining ourselves to suspect that we are wrong or at least only partly right, and thus allow for a healthy and potentially endless revisionism without being disempowered by our insight.

References

Alcoholics Anonymous (1993) G.B.: BPCC Hazell Books Ltd.

Anderson, H. C. (1992). The Emperor's new clothes. In *Fairy tales*, Everyman's Library. David Campbell Publisher's Ltd, London.

Bettleheim, B. (1991). *The uses of enchantment: the meaning and importance of fairy tales.* Penguin: London.

Bly, R. (1990). *Iron John: a book about men*. Element Books Ltd, Dorset.

Bowman, R. (1989). In *By word of mouth—the revival of story telling*, (ed. D. Jones and M. Medlicott). Channel 4 Television, London

Bravo, A., Davite, L. and Jalla, D. (1990). Myth, impotence, and survival in the concentration camps. In *Myths we live by* (ed. R. Samuel and P. Thompson), Routledge, London.

Brooks, P. (1993). The storyteller. In *Psychoanalysis and storytelling*. Blackwell, Oxford.

Byatt, A. S. (1992). The story of the eldest princess. In *Caught in a story—contemporary fairy tales and fables* (ed. C. Park and C. Heaton). Vintage, London.

Byatt, A. S. (1995). *Review of Hussein Haddawy's Arabian Nights*, Vol. 2, published by Norton, *Sunday Times*, 17 December.

Campbell, J. (1998). Remembrance of things past: reflections on the analytic process. *Group Analysis*, **31**, 21–34.

Charon, R. (1992). To build a case: medical histories as traditions in conflict. *Literature and Medicine*, **11**, 115–32.

Charon, R. (1993). Medical interpretation: implications of literary theory of narrative for clinical work. *Journal of Narrative and Life History*, **3**, 79–97.

Chatwin, B. (1988). *The songlines*. Picador, London.

Coleman, R. and Smith, M. (1997). *Working with voices: victim to victor*. Hansell, Cheshire.

Cox, M. and Theilgaard, A. (1987). *Mutative metaphors in psychotherapy: the aeolian mode*. Tavistock Publications Ltd, London.

Crites, S. (1971). The narrative quality of experience. *Journal of the American Academy of Religion*, **39**, 291–311.

Davidson, L. and Strauss, J. (1995). Beyond the biopsychosocial model: integrating disorder, health and recovery. *Psychiatry*, **58**, 44–55.

Dillard, A. (1976). *Pilgrim at Tinker Creek*. The Chaucer Press, Picador, Suffolk.

Estes, C. P. (1992). *Women who run with wolves*. Rider London.

Feldman, C. and Kornfield, J. (1991). *Stories of the spirit, stories of the heart*. Harper Collins, New York.

Fowles, J. (1969). *The French lieutenant's woman*. Johnathan Cape Ltd, London.

Frank, A. W. (1993). The rhetoric of self-change: illness experience as narrative. *The Sociological Quarterly*, **34**, 39–52.

Gergen, K. J. and Gergen, M. M. (1988). Narrative and the self as relationship. *Advances in Experimental Social Psychology*, **21**, 17–56.

Gersie, A. (1992). *Story making in bereavement*. Jessica Kingsley, London.

Gersie, A. (1997), *Reflections on therapeutic storymaking: the use of stories in groups*. Jessica Kingsley, London.

Harvey, J. H., Orbuch, T. L., Chwalisz, K. D., and Garwood, G. (1991). Coping with sexual assault: the roles of account-making and confiding. *Journal of Traumatic Stress*, **4**, 515–31.

Hauerwas, S. (1993). *Naming the silences: God, medicine and the problem of suffering*. T & T Clark, Edinburgh.

Hillman, J. (1983). *Healing fiction*. Stanton Hill, New York.

Holmes, J. and Lindley, R. (1997). *The values of psychotherapy*, (2nd edn). Karnac, London.

Hunter, K. M. (1991). *Doctors stories: the narrative structure of medical knowledge*. Princeton University Press, Princeton.

Jackson, H. J., Edwards, J., Hulbert, C., and McGorry, P. D. (1998). Recovery from psychosis: psychological interventions. In *The early recognition and management of early psychosis: a preventative approach* (ed. P. D. McGorey and H. J. Jackson). Cambridge University Press, Cambridge.

Klienman, A. (1988). *The illness narratives: suffering, healing and the human condition*. Basic Books, New York.

Luria, A. R. (1973). *The man with a shattered world*. Jonathan Cape, London.

Madden, T. (1995). The falling shadow. *British Journal of Psychiatry*, **167**, 827–8.

Mahoney, M. J. (1991). *Human change processes: the scientific foundations of psychotherapy*. Guilford Press, New York.

Mair M. (1988). Psychology as storytelling. *International Journal of Personal Construct Psychology*, **1**, 125–38.

McKay, A. E. and Ryan, S. (1995). Clinical reasoning through story telling: examining a student's case story on a fieldwork placement. *British Journal of Occupational Therapy*, **58**, 234–8.

Mollica, R. (1988). The trauma story: the psychiatric care of refugee survivors of violence and torture. In *Post traumatic therapy and victims of violence*, (ed. F. N. Ochberg). Brunner Mazel, New York.

Mollon, P. (1996). *Multiple selves, multiple voices*. Wiley, Chichester.

Murray, M. (1997). A narrative approach to health psychology: background and potential. *Journal of Health Psychology*, Vol. 2, **1**, 9–20.

Nash, C. (1994). *The use of storytelling in the sciences, philosophy and literature*. Routledge, London.

Nicholson, S. D. and Roberts, G. A. (1994). Patients who (need to) tell stories. *British Journal of Hospital Medicine*, **51**, 546–9.

Peneff, J. (1990). Myths in life stories. In *The myths we live by* (ed. R. Samuel and P. Thompson). Routledge, London.

Polkinghorne, D. E. (1988). *Narrative knowing and the human sciences*. State University of New York Press, Albany.

Pope, H. G., Jonas, J. M., and Jones, S. B. (1982). Factitious psychosis: phenomenology, family history and long term outcome of nine patients. *American Journal of Psychiatry*, **139**, 1480–3.

Ritson, B. and Forrest, A. (1970). The simulation of psychosis: a contemporary presentation. *British Journal of Medical Psychology*, **43**, 31–7.

Roberts, G. A. (1991). Delusional belief systems and meaning in life: a preferred reality? *British Journal of Psychiatry* **159** (Suppl. 14), 19–28.

Rogers, A., Pilgrim, D., and Lacey, R. (1993). *Experiencing psychiatry: users views of services*. MIND publications, London.

Rowe, D (1983). *Depression*, p-69. Routledge, London.

Sacks, O. (1982). *Awakenings*, (revised edn), Originally published 1973. Pan Books Ltd, London.

Sacks, O. (1985). *The man who mistook his wife for a hat*. Gerald Duckworth and Co. Ltd, London.

Samuel, R. and Thompson, P. (1990). *Myths we live by*. Routledge, London.

Sartorius, N. (1988). International perspectives of psychiatric classification. *British Journal of Psychiatry*, **152** (Suppl. 1), 9–14.

Singer, H. S. and Walkup, J. T. (1991). Tourette Syndrome and other tic disorders: diagnosis, pathophysiology, and treatment. *Medicine*, **70**, 15–32.

Stein, M. (1983). *In mid-life*. Spring Publications, Dallas.

Strauss, J. (1994). The person with schizophrenia as a person II: approaches to the subjective and complex. *British Journal of Psychiatry*, **164** (Suppl. 23), 103–7.

Susko, M. (1994). Caseness and narrative: contrasting approaches to people who are psychiatrically labelled. *The Journal of Mind and Behaviour*, **15**, 87–112.

Taylor, D. (1996). *The healing power of stories*. Gill and MacMillan, Dublin.

Tolstoy, L. (1906). *Twenty-three tales*, (trans. by L. and A. Maude). Oxford University Press, London.

Tonkin, E. (1990). History and the myth of realism. In *The myths we live by* (ed. R. Samuel and P. Thompson). Routledge, London.

Tournier, M. (1992). The mid-night love feast. In *Caught in a story—contemporary fairy tales and fables*, (ed. C. Park and C. Heaton). Vintage, London.

Wallace, E. R. (1988). What is truth? some philosophical contributions to psychiatric issues. *American Journal of Psychiatry*, **147**, 137–47.

White, M. (1988). The externalisation of the problem and the reauthoring of lives and relationships. *Dulwitch Centre Newsletter, Summer*. Dulwitch Publications, Dulwitch.

Wiggins, J. (ed.) (1975). Within and without stories. In *Religion as story*, ed. Harper Row, New York.

2 The psychodynamic narrative

James Phillips

Introduction

An account of the role of narrative in psychoanalysis and the psychodynamic therapies must begin with a recognition of the role of narrative and narrative identity in our lives in general. Considerations of narrative identity do not begin, after all, in the consulting room. They are with us, implicitly or explicitly, throughout our lives. We live in and through the stories we tell and imagine about ourselves. The narrative 'I' is that story-spinning self that tells stories about itself, exists in those stories, and conceives its identity in terms of those stories. To quote the literary critic Peter Brooks (1984) on this theme:

> Our lives are ceaselessly intertwined with narrative, with the stories that we tell and hear told, those we dream or imagine or would like to tell, all of which are reworked in that story or our own lives that we narrate to ourselves in an episodic, sometimes semi-conscious, but virtually uninterrupted monologue. We live immersed in narrative, recounting and reassessing the meaning of our past actions, anticipating the outcome of our future projects, situating ourselves at the intersection of several stories not yet completed.
> (*Brooks, 1984, p. 3.*)

In the most general terms the person requesting psychotherapy has a story to tell. It is generally a story that is not going well; otherwise the person would not be in the therapist's office. Again in general terms, the person about to become a patient brings in a wish that, at the end of the treatment, the story will have taken a turn for the better and will be now proceeding on a trajectory that promises success rather than failure. In the course of this treatment the narrative 'I' will have been transformed—if that is not too strong a word—from a narrative subject that can only imagine scenarios of defeat into one that can also imagine scenarios of triumph.

Whatever else it may be—and it is certainly much more—psychotherapy is a work with the patient's narratives and narrative identity. It does not, however, have a unique claim on narrative work. In a very general sense any form of psychiatric intervention will have its effect on the patient's narrative self. A depressed person who has been successfully treated with an antidepressant will not only have a different, more positive outlook at the completion of the treatment, but he or she will have a different story to tell: certainly about his or her future, but also perhaps about the past. The story of his or her past will have been recast from one that presaged only failure into one that, however, dismal, also allowed for a positive outcome. With respect to psychotherapy, let us keep in mind that we must correctly speak in the plural, for there are many forms of psychotherapy, and each will have its own distinctive approach to working with the patient's stories or narratives. In this chapter our focus will be on psychoanalysis and the psychodynamic therapies that originate in that tradition. Our subject will be the approach to narrative and narrative identity in this tradition.

Freudian beginnings

Our account of the role of narrative in the psychodynamic theories and therapies will appropriately begin with Freud. Although often only implicit, notions of narrative and narrative identity have been present in psychoanalysis from the beginning. Concerned as he was to establish psychoanalysis as a science, Freud placed a lot of emphasis on scientific-sounding concepts, such as mental structure, mechanisms of defense, and psychic causality. At the same time, however, he recognized (apparently to his surprise) that he was involved in telling stories. In *Studies on hysteria*, written at the beginning of his career, he wrote: 'I have not always been a psychotherapist. Like other neuropathologists, I was trained to employ local diagnoses and electro-prognosis, and it still strikes me myself as strange that the case histories I write should read like short stories and that, as one might say, they lack the serious stamp of science. I must console myself with the reflection that the nature of the subject is evidently responsible for this, rather than any preference of my own' (Bruner and Freud, 1895, p. 160). While Freud did not use the terminology of narrative, his entire enterprise was built upon the introduction of the unconscious to fill in the gaps of the patient's conscious narrative; i.e. the patient would attempt to tell a story, the story of his or her life. But the story would be filled with breaks, incoherencies, missing links, all of which Freud came to attribute to defensive processes that kept the missing portions out of consciousness. These breaks in the attempted story were usually marked by the eruption of symptomatic behaviour (e.g. the patient presents his story as a happily married man and then reports his incomprehensible and self-destructive visits to prostitutes). Freud treated the symptom as a break in coherence of the patient's consciously enacted life narrative and he argued that coherence could be restored through the insertion of unconscious content into the broken narrative. The patient came in with a story that did not make sense in significant ways, and the consequence of psychoanalytical treatment would be the restoration of sense. In this original formulation, therefore, the unconscious did not represent a limit to the life narrative; in fact, it represented the opposite, a fulfilment of narrative. The assumption of the unconscious was necessary, Freud said, 'because the data of consciousness have a very large number of gaps in them. . . . All these conscious acts remain disconnected and unintelligible if we insist upon claiming that every mental act that occurs in us must also necessarily be experienced by us through consciousness; on the other hand, they fall into demonstrable connection if we interpolate between them the unconscious acts which we have inferred' (Freud 1915, pp. 166–67). In its traditional, Freudian, formulation then, psychoanalysis treated the symptom as a break in coherence of the patient's conscious life narrative, and it argued that coherence could be restored through the insertion of unconscious content (a second or latent narrative) into the broken, conscious narrative.

Freud's account of the psychodynamic narrative can be illustrated through one of his case histories. For the purposes of this exposition we will do well to choose one of the shorter case histories from *Studies on hysteria*. Freud describes Miss Lucy R. as a 30-year-old governess who was referred to him in 1892 for symptoms of olfactory hallucinations, along with depression and fatigue. Once he decided that the woman's symptoms were hysterical in origin, he set about trying to figure them out. The story she presented was that of being the governess for the two children of a widowered businessman. The olfactory sensation was that of burnt pudding, for which she could offer no explanation. Operating on the assumption that the hysterically based olfactory hallucination was based on a forgotten trauma, Freud persisted in trying to get the patient to remember the traumatic scene that was associated with the smell of burnt pudding. As he wrote: 'Now I already knew from the analysis of similar cases that before hysteria can be acquired for the first time one essential condition must be fulfilled: an idea must be *intentionally repressed from consciousness* and excluded from associative modification' (Bruner and Freud, 1895, p. 116). As he worked his way back into the patient's history, Freud indeed uncovered three traumatic experiences. The first, associated with the burnt pudding, involved a scene in which the patient received a letter from her mother in England, during the reading of which the pudding she was making with the children burnt. The scene involved feelings of homesickness and leaving the children. When Freud surmised that these feelings were not enough to create the symptom and suggested that the patient was in love with her employer, she concurred, responding when asked why she hadn't told him that, 'I don't know—or rather I didn't want to know. I wanted to drive it out of my head and not think of it again; and I believe latterly I have succeeded' (Bruner and Freud, 1895, p. 117). With this revelation the smell of burnt pudding dissipated but was replaced by a smell of cigar smoke. Freud then pursued this symptom back to two other traumatic scenes, each of them involving the employer and the major one involving an experience in which her employer castigated her severely and in so doing dashed all her hopes that he might actually marry her and make her the stepmother of his children. Following these sessions she returned to Freud free of symptoms and in a much better mood. She declared that, while still in love with her employer, she had accepted the fact that she would not realize her fantasy but was not going to make herself miserable over it.

In this brief case history, then, we see Freud developing the presenting story into a much more complex narrative in which the perplexing symptoms are made to make sense through the interpolation of unconscious links that are initially out of the awareness of the patient. We should also note that in this brief case history Freud has not only offered a psychodynamic narrative of the patient's symptom formation, he has also offered a narrative of his treatment—in this case his abandonment of the hypnotic technique—and he has offered a further narrative regarding the development and pathogenesis of hysterical symptoms.

From a narrativist perspective three separate but related concepts emerge from Freud's work—all three, as just indicated, present in the case of Lucy R. The first is what we will call the psychodynamic narrative, i.e. a narrative that is marked by conflicts, elisions, emotional investments, unconscious defenses, etc. The second is the psychoanalytical developmental narrative, i.e. the story, told along Freudian lines, of human psychological development. The third is the treatment narrative. Let us discuss each of these in turn.

The first, the psychodynamic narrative, is the retelling of the patient's life narrative that emerges in the therapy process. This retelling includes not only the revised story-line but, in addition, the reasons for the omissions. It is thus a complex narrative of original version as corrected and retold, with the addition of conflict, defense, symptom formation, psychotherapeutic process, including transference repetitions of the conflict, and resolution of the underlying conflicts.

A further aspect of the psychodynamic narrative is that it is constantly changing in the course of the psychotherapy. Thus, the meaning of any event or memory in the patient's past is determined by the narrative context in which it is placed. As the narrative perspective is altered, so also is the meaning of the remembered event, and since the narrative is constantly being revised in the course of the therapy, so then is the meaning of the event. While Freud, as indicated above, did not speak in the terminology of narrative, his understanding of how memories are 'rearranged' or 'retranscribed' shows an awareness of these phenomena. As he wrote to Fliess in 1896: 'I am working on the assumption that our psychic mechanism has come into being by a process of stratification: the material present in the form of memory traces being subjected from time to time to a *rearrangement* in accordance with fresh circumstances—to a *retranscription*. Thus what is essentially new about my theory is the thesis that memory is present not once but several times over, that it is laid down in various kinds of indications' (Freud, 1985, p. 207). Freud is thus indicating that a memory or remembered event is not a photograph-like entity that is simply there for recall and always remains the same; rather, it is always recalled in some narrative context—the narrative of one's life as viewed from this present time—and it is altered or 'retranscribed' in this current context.

The second concept that emerges from Freud's work, related to the psychodynamic narrative but separate, is that of the psychoanalytical developmental narrative, i.e. the revised narrative that emerges from the treatment is not random or arbitrary. The analyst brings to the treatment situation a prefigured narrative schema. The patient's confused and confusing story is understood in terms of this prefigured narrative schema, and the revised narrative is told along the lines of the schema. For Freud, of course, the prefigured schema is pre-eminently the Oedipal narrative. The modal Freudian treatment is then one in which the patient's presenting story is retold according to the narrative lines of Oedipal conflict and resolution. According to Freud, this way of proceeding receives its ultimate justification in his conviction that the narrative schema brought to the treatment by the analyst *always* matches the ontogenetic development of the individual, even if the facts of the individual's upbringing do not fit the putative Oedipal developmental line. He makes this point in a strongly Kantian manner in describing the 'Wolf Man' case:

> I have now come to the end of what I had to say about this case. There remain two problems, of the many that it raises, which seem to me to deserve special emphasis. The first relates to the phylogenetically inherited schemata, which, like the categories of philosophy, are concerned with the business of 'placing' the impressions derived from actual experience. I am inclined to take the view that they are precipitates from the history of human civilization. The Oedipus complex, which comprises a child's relations to his parents, is one of them—is, in fact the best know member of the class. Whatever experiences fail to fit in with the hereditary schema, they become remodelled in the imagination—a process which might very profitably be followed out in detail. It is precisely such cases that are calculated to convince us of the independent existence of the schema. We are often able to see the schema triumphing over the experience of the individual. (*Freud, 1918, p. 119*).

It goes without saying that this approach to the treatment situation renders Freud vulnerable to the double criticism that the treatment result—the revised (Oedipal) narrative—is known from the outset, and that every patient's psychodynamic narrative will be the same. In this sense, then, the psychodynamic narrative and the psychoanalytical developmental narrative become conflated: there is only *one* psychodynamic narrative, namely the *Oedipal developmental* narrative.

Finally, the third narrativist concept that emerges from Freud's work is that of the treatment itself—the story of the treatment. In the typical Freudian case the treatment has its own narrative course and structure. In general terms the course is that of initial presentation and instructions for rules of treatment, with emphasis on: free association; emergence of symptomatic behavior, conflict, and transference; interpretation of conflict, defense, resistance, and transference by analyst; period of working through of interpretations and resistance; and, finally, resolution of conflict and termination of treatment. While the story of the treatment is, in obvious ways, different from the story of the patient, they are indeed related. The treatment story reflects the patient story—most concretely in the phenomenon of transference. If in the transference the patient enacts in the treatment setting essential features of his or her life and conflicts, the development of the treatment will, in important ways, parallel the course of that life and its conflicts. And since, as was indicated above, the patient's story, the psychodynamic narrative, itself reflects the psychoanalytical developmental narrative, we can now recognize an inherent integration of the three narratives—the psychodynamic narrative, the developmental narrative, and the treatment narrative. That said, it needs to be added that the critique articulated above regarding the predictable and stereotypic quality of the classical Freudian analysis can be directed also at the treatment narrative. Recognizing the unity of the treatment narrative with the other two—the way in which all analyses will uncover the Oedipal core at the centre of the patient's presenting conflict—must we not conclude that all good analyses will be much the same in their essentials and quite predictable in their results?

After Freud

While the Freudian paradigm held fast (with some important deviations such as Melanie Klein and Harry Stack Sullivan) for the first half of the century, resulting for some in a certain sterility of psychoanalytical thinking, the story of the latter decades is that of the break-up of the rigid Freudian paradigm. For a variety of reasons, including a reaction against drive theory and Freudian metapsychology, a questioning of the centrality of the Oedipus complex, and differing views of transference and countertransference, we have witnessed in psychoanalysis the emergence of what we can call theoretical and clinical pluralism. There is no longer one psychodynamic narrative, one developmental narrative, and one treatment narrative. There are now several of each. Figures such as Hans Kohut and Donald Winnicott are associated with approaches to theory and treatment that significantly alter the three narratives described above.

I would like to illustrate the situation of multiple narratives with two examples. The first is the reinterpreting of one of Freud's own case histories in the post-Freudian era. The second is a published exercise in the multiple viewing of a case presentation.

The Freudian (1905) case on which we will focus is that of Dora, published as *Fragment of an analysis of a case of hysteria*. Written in fact four years earlier, and thus shortly after the publication of *The interpretation of dreams*, and originally titled *Dreams and hysteria, a fragment of an analysis*, this short work clearly carries an agenda: to offer a concrete case demonstration of the theories presented in *The interpretation of dreams*, and to present case evidence for the sexual origin of hysteria. As Freud reports in a letter to Fliess: ' "Dreams and Hysteria" was completed yesterday. It is a fragment of an analysis of a case of hysteria, in which the explanations are grouped round two dreams. So that it is in fact a continuation of the dream book. It further contains solutions of hysterical symptoms and considerations on the sexual—organic basis of the whole condition' (quoted in Freud, 1905, pp. 3–4). For all the theoretical and clinical brilliance shown in this work, however, later readers have found Freud's treatment of Dora problematic, to say the least. They have offered other versions of the psychodynamic narrative, the treatment narrative, and the developmental narrative that help to understand this patient.

The treatment, which lasted only a few months, can be summarized very briefly. Dora was brought to Freud by her father with presenting symptoms of dyspnoea, migraine, a nervous cough, and aphonia. They first consulted Freud when Dora was sixteen, but the treatment only began after a second consultation, two years later. The circumstances of Dora's family arrangements quickly revealed themselves in the treatment. Dora's family were close friends with the K.'s. Frau K. had nursed Dora's father during a period of tuberculosis when Dora was six and had subsequently entered into a long-standing affair with the former. Dora had meanwhile grown close to Frau K. and shared her confidences with her. Herr K. had made a pass at Dora when she was fourteen and another on a lake walk when she was sixteen. Dora responded to the latter by slapping Herr K., who then denied that he had made the pass. Infuriated, Dora insisted to her father that he terminate his relationships with the K.'s. This demand, together with a suicide note found by her parents, are what impelled Dora's father to bring her in for treatment. He asked Freud to 'try to bring her to reason', to 'talk Dora out of her belief that there was . . . more than friendship between himself and Frau K.' (Freud 1905, p. 24). Freud's treatment, which was centred around the interpretation of two of Dora's dreams, focused on Dora's denial and repression of her sexual attraction to Herr K., and the resultant formation of hysterical symptoms. After about three months of treatment Dora announced abruptly that she had decided to terminate the analysis. In his study of the case, Freud attributes Dora's termination to a transference acting out of her revengeful feelings toward Herr K., and to his own lack of appreciation of the phenomenon of transference at the time of this analysis. Dora returned for a single session fifteen months later, informing Freud that she had confronted Frau K. with the fact that she and her father were having an affair and that she had got Herr K. to admit what had happened at the lake. At the end of the session Freud 'promised to forgive her for having deprived [him] of the satisfaction of affording her a far more radical cure for her troubles' (Freud, 1905, p. 122).

It would be fair to say that most contemporary readers of the Dora case would be struck by the insensitivity of Freud's treatment of his patient. It seems rather apparent from the information provided by Freud that her father has brought her in to silence her objections to the affair with Frau K., that he is willing to sacrifice her to Herr K. in order to preserve his liaison with the latter's wife, and that Freud, in pursuing *his* agenda in the analysis, colludes in this rather corrupt treatment contract. Likewise, the contemporary reader is hardly surprised that Dora breaks off the analysis prematurely. When Freud concludes with the statement that 'I do not know what kind of help she wanted from me' (Freud, 1905, p. 122), it seems clear that, for all the brilliance of his analysis of Dora's symptoms, he simply does not grasp that he has not responded to Dora's real needs and requests. Janet Malcolm captures the contemporary reader's reaction to reading the case.

> The Dora case—where Freud has not yet arrived at his final vision of the psychoanalytic case history and is still rendering the patient as a character in a nineteenth-century novel, and also as the

host of a kind of operable cancer—reads like an account of an operation being performed on a fully awake patient. Thus its agony and its horror. Every reader of "Fragment of an Analysis" comes away with the feeling that something awful has been done to the girl. The Dora case is known as the case that illustrates Freud's failure to interpret the transference in time; even more, it illustrates a failure of narration. Freud tells the novelistic story of Dora so well that the psycho-analytic story—the narrative of the analyst's probe into the patient's unconscious being—reads like an assault, almost like a rape; we cannot but feel outraged as Freud describes the girl's desperate attempts to elude him while he obscenely moves in on her.
(*Malcolm, 1990, pp. 318–19.*)

The revisions of the Dora narrative began with Erik Erikson, whose limited remarks on the case set the stage for most of the later commentary on the Dora treatment. Erikson focused on the fact that Dora was an *adolescent* and that adolescents have particular developmental issues that are involved in their pathologies and that need to be addressed in their treatment. With Dora, Erikson highlighted the issue of *fidelity* in Dora's adolescent life and development, for what was very striking about Dora's family setting was the way in which this virtue was being corrupted. In Erikson's words:

In fact, one might say, without seriously overdoing it, that three words characterize her social history: sexual *infidelity* on the part of some of the most important adults in her life; the *perfidy* of her father's denial of his friend's attempts to seduce her which had, in fact, been the precipitating cause of the girl's illness; and a strange tendency on the part of all the adults around the girl to make her a *confidante* in any number of matters, without having enough confidence in her to acknowledge the truths relevant to her illness.
(*Erikson, 1968, p. 250*)

According to Erikson, what Dora wanted and needed from Freud was an adult who would recognize her for the young girl she was, who would talk to her honestly about the deceit of the adults in her life, and who would, of course, not collude in her father's dubious treatment arrangement. In revisioning the case in this way Erikson is offering a different psychodynamic narrative of Dora's history, a different narrative of the treatment, and, finally, a significant addition, the adolescent phase, to the general developmental narrative propounded by Freud.

Following Erikson, papers by Glenn (1980) and Scharfman (1980) both developed aspects of Freud's therapeutic impasse as related to his treating his patient as an adult rather than as an adolescent. These papers, like that of Erikson, circumscribe their criticism of Freud in a context of deep respect. A more recent volume, *In dora's case: Freud—hysteria—feminism* (Bernheimer and Kahane, 1990), which gathers together a number of papers by scholars, primarily from literature departments, writing in a deconstructionist and feminist mode, takes a much less reverent attitude towards Freud in his treatment of Dora. Freud's sexism, aggressiveness, insensitivity, etc. are analysed at great length. Again, what emerges are different narratives of the patient and the treatment.

The second example of competing narratives can be found in a recent issue of *Psychoanalytic Inquiry* (Pulver, 1987) entitled 'How theory shapes technique: perspectives on a clinical study'. The journal issue consists of the presentation of clinical material from a single case by an analyst (Silverman, 1987), discussion of the material by a variety of other analysts of different theoretical persuasions, and an admirable effort by the issue editor (Sydney Pulver) and other discussants to make sense of the conflicting discussions. Silverman begins the journal issue by describing the patient as a twenty-five-year-old single woman who was referred for analysis by a psychiatrist with whom she had been in psychotherapy in college in another location. Her presenting problems were sexual and social inhibitions, masochistic tendencies, and chronic, neurotic depression. She described a rather unhappy childhood with an aloof, critical father, whom she loved and hated and to whom she assumed a rather masochistic posture. Her adolescent and early adult years were marked by shyness and heterosexual avoidance. Silverman reported that the analysis had progressed well for the first few years but that progress had suddenly stopped at a point at which the patient's father's health deteriorated and she had had to enter the family business. He described the current state of the analysis as one in which a strong transference neurosis had developed, with the patient treating the analyst as a parental figure to whom she could complain and whine and the analysis as a substitute and excuse for her not developing a real life outside the consulting room. Following his presentation of his notes of a recent week's sessions, the case was discussed by a variety of colleagues, a short sampling of which I will review. Given that Silverman is doing a fairly traditional analysis, Charles Brenner, not surprisingly, is in strong agreement with his approach. 'As you see, Silverman and I function as analysts in essentially the same way. We try to understand a patient's symptoms and characterological problems as compromise formations resulting from conflicts whose components are drive derivatives, anxiety and depressive affect, defense, and superego manifestations' (Brenner 1987, p. 169). Other commentators, however, are not so generous. Writing from a self-psychological perspective, Arnold Goldberg (1987) reinterprets the setback in the analysis as due, not to the external events impinging on the patient's life, but rather as a break in the analyst's empathic understanding of the patient. 'From this point, labeled a 'transference impasse', on we see the vivid reliving of a patient who feels misunderstood in interaction with an analyst who visits a personal set of theoretical ideas upon a bewildered soul. . . . we should conclude that there has been a break in the analyst's understanding of the patient. I believe that this is the case, and here is where a model involving selfobjects could be utilized' (Goldberg, 1987, p. 183). Finally, taking an interpersonal perspective, Edgar Levenson (1987) chastizes Silverman for not providing more detail about the patient and thereby making her more real. He then connects this failure to Silverman's reluctance to allow a full transference relationship to develop, and to his insistence on maintaining an authoritarian relationship with the patient: 'To put it succinctly, I would not see the patient as coming to therapy incapacitated by a fantasy ridden and inadequate perception of her world, but as a woman struggling with problems of identity and assertion, not so different from other women, in and out of therapy. The therapist is seen as a coparticipant, working to clarify his own preconceptions as they emerge from his life experience' (Levenson, 1987, p. 213).

What is most striking to the reader of these papers is the great diversity of opinion concerning both the dynamics and handling of Silverman's case. Each of the discussants has a different story to tell of the patient and of the treatment. As Estelle Shane (1987) summarizes: 'In summary, I would say that the diversity of opinions regarding the diagnosis and dynamics of Silverman's patient would suggest that one's theoretical stance takes precedence over other considerations' (Shane, 1987, p. 205). The influence of the theoretical stance is so strong that it affects the very perception of what is going on in the consulting room, leading Sydney Pulver to conclude: 'Facts, per se, do not exist. The very idea of what constitutes data and is thus worth recording is determined by the analyst's theoretical bent' (Pulver, 1987, p. 292). The summarizing commentators struggle admirably to find common ground among the discussants and to argue that the pluralism of perspectives and resulting narratives is not simply chaos. One commentator, Evelyne Schwaber (1987), sees the clinician as involved in a dialectical process, on the one hand informed with a particular narrative strategy, and on the other hand sensitive to the danger of simply imposing this particular narrative model on the patient regardless of what the latter presents: 'I argue, rather, for our recognition that no matter what theory we espouse, we run the risk of using it to foreclose rather than to continue inquiry, to provide an answer rather than to raise a new question. I speak for a search for ways to sharpen our attunement to hear new cues from the patient that may tell us that we have, even if unwittingly, superimposed our view and used our theory to justify it' (Schwaber, 1987, p. 274).

Narrative versus science

The emergence of multiple narratives in psychoanalysis and psychotherapeutic therapy has highlighted the conflict between narrativist and scientific aspects of the psychoanalytical therapies. Although we have found ample evidence in Freud of an appreciation of the narrative dimension of psychoanalytical treatment, he in fact favoured the scientific presentation of psychoanalysis. His 'discovery' of a unitary narrative of development and treatment allowed for an emphasis on the scientific grounding of the narrative. In the current atmosphere of a pluralism of narratives, however, the presentation of psychoanalysis as a positive science has become less convincing. Both psychoanalytical theoreticians and interested philosophers have begun to perceive psychoanalysis as having more in common with disciplines such as history than with the positive sciences. Since the former focus on the understanding and interpretation of meaning structures rather than the search for causes, psychoanalysis has for many come to be regarded as one of the hermeneutic disciplines (Phillips, 1991). It is in this context that the narrative dimension of psychoanalysis has come into prominence; hermeneutic and narrative readings of psychoanalysis clearly overlap. On the one hand, when we are trying to make sense of someone's life, we inevitably end up with a narrative account of that life. On the other hand, this is also inevitably an interpretive (and thus hermeneutic) proceeding, since we must always choose the rightness of one narrative account over another. We no longer enjoy the comfort Freud experienced in his one-size-fits-all approach to the unitary narrative. Since any person's life can be seen from many perspectives, and since the life story can be told in many ways, one must choose one's narrative approach and be prepared to defend it. This obviously involves many issues such as one's particular training, one's allegiance and sympathy to a particular school or approach, and one's personal reactions to the particular patient 't is clear, however, that no therapist approaches the patient in a completely neutral frame of mind. We all have our narrative strategies or schemata, our preconceived (and hopefully reasonable) ways of understanding human development, conflict, and treatment. It is hardly surprising, then, that a Kohutian analyst will have a different story to tell—a different psychodynamic, developmental, and treatment narrative—from a traditional Freudian, about the same patient.

The argument for psychoanalysis as a narrativist, hermeneutic discipline has predictably brought charges of relativism. Reading such documents as the issue of *Psychoanalytic Inquiry* discussed above (Pulver, 1987) and the voluminous literature on the Dora case makes such a reaction understandable. If more than one narrative account is acceptable—if, in fact, many are acceptable—what then is the limit? Do we not quickly reach a point where *any* narrative account is acceptable—mine, yours, or the postman's? The charge of relativism has been answered primarily by philosophers writing in the hermeneutic tradition. Richard Rorty (1979) has been a strong voice arguing for the inevitability of a fair amount of relativism in the human sciences—and for a resolution that relinquishes the wish for certainty and settles for a consensus of thinking individuals in open conversation. It is hardly surprising that other philosophers have found Rorty's 'anti-foundationalism' less than satisfying (Nagel, 1997). Another well-known philosopher, Richard Bernstein, has devoted a volume to this theme, entitled *Beyond objectivism and relativism: science, hermeneutics, and praxis* (Bernstein, 1983), in which he argues for a middle ground between the extremes of objective certainty and total relativism. Finally, I will mention the work of Paul Ricoeur, who, while thoroughly embedded in the hermeneutic tradition, rejects any rigid dichotomizing of hermeneutic and scientific approaches to disciplines such as psychoanalysis (Ricoeur, 1970).

If psychoanalytical and psychodynamic thinking are to claim a position 'beyond objectivism and relativism', this will mean agreeing at least on minimal standards for what might pass as an acceptable theory or narrative account. Such standards would include criteria such as internal coherence, therapeutic efficacy, verification through ongoing treatment, consensus among thoughtful observers, and conformity with established traditions. Each criterion could of course be attacked as not finally decisive in deciding between rival positions, and, indeed, it is of the nature of social sciences such as psychoanalysis and psychodynamic therapy that there will never be final agreement amongst all observers or participants about what is the correct account or psychodynamic narrative. The above discussion of the *Psychoanalytic Inquiry* and Dora cases bare ample witness to this fact. The issue of conformity with established traditions is an important one that in itself suggests all the ambiguity of the objectivism/relativism controversy. On the one hand, a tradition provides the security of working with principles that have been tried, tested, and found productive by a consensus of predecessors. The notion of tradition acknowledges the phenomenon of a community of investigators working out the established principles through ongoing dialogue and practice. On the other hand, the same tradition may also be a source of prejudice and unquestioned assumptions. We have in the unitary psychodynamic narrative of Freud an example of a tradition that became rigidified to the point of containing as much prejudice as truth. What we now have, as is especially apparent in the *Psychoanalytic Inquiry* discussion, is a plurality of traditions, each with its own claims to internal coherence and therapeutic efficacy, and each offering its own narrative account of the case in question. While there may be no standard for arbitrating which tradition is simply superior to the others, the criteria just mentioned may at least be used negatively to rule out clearly unacceptable theories. To say that we cannot declare one theory the best is *not* the same as saying that all possible theories are equal.

The crisis over narrative and reference

However successfully the conflict just described over the epistemological status of narrative has been resolved, a further, far more significant, conflict—related to the above conflict but more specific to narrative—has emerged over the *referential status* of narrative and narrative identity in psychoanalytical therapy. The issue here is the relationship of the narrative developed in the therapy to the actual life of the patient. This debate over narrative and reference within psychoanalysis is in fact reflective of a larger debate over the same issue in such disciplines as history, philosophy, and literary theory. It will thus be useful to begin this section with a brief review of the debate in the larger intellectual world before proceeding to a discussion of the debate within the narrower arena of psychoanalysis and psychoanalytical therapy.

The question posed in the debate over the nature of narrative can be stated simply: does narrative pertain only to fiction or also to life? Or, again, is the narrative account of a life merely a fictionalized construction or may it indeed represent the actual life in question? If the structures of narrative are only fictive and bear no reference to life, then a narrative identity can be nothing more than a fictive identity; it cannot be a way of analysing the real life of a real person.

Narrative in history has had its advocates and its adversaries. Pre-eminent among the latter has been the '*Annales*' group in France, who have been highly critical of narrative history, dismissing it as superficial in comparison with the study of long-term impersonal trends in demography, economics, etc. An ambiguous position is held by those historians who have defended the role of narrative in history but in turn argue for its fictive nature. Hayden White (1987), the most articulate of this group, writes as follows:

> What I have sought to suggest is that this value attached to narrativity in the representation of real events arises out of a desire to have real events display the coherence, integrity, fullness, and closure of an image of life that is and can only be imaginary. The notion that sequences of real events possess the formal attributes of the stories we tell about imaginary events could only have its origin in wishes, day-dreams, reveries. Does the world really present itself to perception in the form of well-made stories, with central subjects, proper beginnings, middles, and ends, and a coherence that permits us to see 'the end' in every beginning? Or does it present itself more in the forms that the annals and chronicle suggest, either as mere sequence without beginning or end or as sequences of beginnings that only terminate and never conclude? And does the world, even the social world, ever really come to us as already narrativized, already 'speaking itself' from beyond the horizon of our capacity to make scientific sense of it?
> (*White, 1987, pp. 24–5.*)

While the relationship of narrative to lived reality has been a matter of debate among historians, it is in the field of literary theory that the purely fictive nature of narrative has been most strongly promoted. In the Anglo-American world Frank Kermode (1966) has written forcefully of a longing for order that is found wanting in the world and is fulfilled only in fiction. It is in contemporary French literary criticism, however, that the breach between narrative and lived reality has been most stridently made. Roland Barthes (1977), who was highly influential in the matter, wrote typically with respect to narrative:

> Claims concerning the 'realism' of narrative are therefore to be discounted. . . . The function of narrative is not to 'represent,' it is to constitute a spectacle. . . .Narrative does not show, does not imitate. . . . 'What takes place' in a narrative is from the referential (reality) point of view literally *nothing*, 'what happens' is language alone, the adventure of language, the unceasing celebration of its coming.
> (*Barthes, 1977, p. 124.*)

Dismissing the referential or representational nature of fiction in another passage, he likened the work of fiction to an onion, 'a construction of layers (or levels, or systems) whose body contains, finally, no heart, no kernel, no secret, no irreducible principle, nothing except the infinity of its own envelopes—which envelop nothing other than the unity of its own surfaces' (Barthes, 1977, p. 125).

In the face of all this doubt concerning the reality claims of narrative, it is of interest that the strongest recent defences of narrative's connection to the real world have come from three philosophers, Paul Ricoeur (1984–1988), David Carr (1986), and Alasdair MacIntyre (1981), each of whom argues for the anchorage of narrative in practical life. In this synopsis I will focus on MacIntyre's analysis in his *After virtue*. In his analysis of narrative MacIntyre argues that human action is only comprehensible as intelligible action, and that this intelligibility means the embeddedness of action in a historical sequence: 'An action is a moment in a possible or actual history or in a number of such histories. The notion of a history is as fundamental a notion as the notion of an action' (p. 214). He describes this interconnection of action, intelligibility, and history further:

> It is now becoming clear that we render the actions of others intelligible in this way because action itself has a basically historical character. It is because we all live out narratives in our lives and because we understand our own lives in terms of the narratives that we live out that the form of narrative is appropriate for understanding the actions of others. Stories are lived before they are told—except in the case of fiction.
>
> (*MacIntyre, 1981, pp. 211–12.*)

Human activities are thus 'enacted narratives'. As such, they share some of the formal properties of narrative. They have beginnings, middles, and endings, as do literary works. They may be evaluated according to different genres—as, for instance, a particular sequence of events may be judged to be tragic or comic. And, as in literary productions, '[actual conversations] embody reversals and recognitions; they move towards and away from climaxes. There may within a longer conversation be digressions and subplots, indeed digressions within digressions and subplots within subplots' (MacIntyre, 1981, p. 211).

MacIntyre says further, of lived narratives, that they have both an unpredictable and a partially teleological character. The meaningfulness of a life is always in part a function of a projected future, but this future is marked by inevitable uncertainty. About the authorship of a lived narrative he says that one is never fully the author of the narrative that one lives out. 'We enter upon a stage which we did not design and we find ourselves part of an action that was not of our making. Each of us being a main character in his own drama plays subordinate parts in the dramas of others, and each drama constrains the others' (MacIntyre, 1981, p. 213).

Finally, MacIntyre associates the notion of *personal* identity with that of narrative identity, insisting that the concept of personal identity has no meaning if it does not include the idea of narrative intelligibility. The unity of an individual life is the unity of a narrative enacted through the course of that life. He concludes that '[t]he unity of a human life is the unity of a narrative quest' (MacIntyre, 1981, p. 219).

> When an occurrence is apparently the intended action of a human agent, but nonetheless we cannot so identify it, we are both intellectually and practically baffled. We do not know how to respond; we do not know how to explain; we do not even know how to characterize minimally as an intelligible action; our distinction between the humanly accountable and the merely natural seems to have broken down. And this kind of bafflement does indeed occur in a number of different kinds of situation; when we enter alien cultures or even alien social structures within our own culture, in our encounters with certain types of neurotic or psychotic patient (it is indeed the

unintelligibility of such patients' actions that leads to their being treated as patients; actions unintelligible to the agent as well as to everyone else are understood—rightly—as a kind of suffering), but also in every day situations. . . .In each case the act of utterance becomes intelligible by finding its place in a narrative.

(*MacIntyre, 1981, pp. 209–10*).

It is against this background of the general debate over narrative and reference that contemporary psychoanalytical accounts of narrative must be viewed. The relevance of the debate to psychoanalysis and the various psychoanalytical treatments is not difficult to grasp. The psychodynamic narrative is a narrative about the patient's past. If there is serious doubt about the reality basis of *any* narrative account of *any* life, that will certainly impugn the validity of the psychodynamic narrative. Indeed, most of the contemporary discussion of narrative among psychoanalytical theoreticians revolves around the questions just discussed concerning the nature of narrative. What is the referential status of the psychodynamic narrative? If the referencial link is not secure, is there still a place for narrative as predominantly fictive in the psychoanalytical treatment? And finally, may these questions be rendered unimportant by reducing the role of narrative in the treatment? In the remainder of this section I will describe the varied answers to these questions by a number of prominent psychoanalytical theoreticians. We will first look at the positions of the two theoreticians who have studied the question most intensively, Donald Spence and Roy Schafer, and examine the positions of two analysts, Jacques Lacan and Paul Grey, who, although deeply different in their views of psychoanalysis, come together in a kind of anti-narrativist stance.

Spence's ambivalent stance towards narrative is spread out over two books devoted to the subject, *Narrative truth and historical truth* (Spence, 1982) and *The Freudian metaphor* (Spence, 1987). His initial position is apparent in the title of the earlier book, *Narrative truth and historical truth*: namely, there is narrative truth and there is historical truth, and the two are not to be confused. Spence's point of view is here fairly close to that of Hayden White in his treatment of history. He shares White's scepticism about our ability to capture the actual past, but at the same time recognizes the importance of narrative structures and narrative identity in the psychotherapeutic process. The narrative account that is pieced together in the therapeutic process is thus important, but largely a fictive creation.

Spence recognizes Freud's effort to get at the historical truth of the patient's past and emphasizes Freud's fondness for archaeological metaphors as expressive of this historical quest. He then painstakingly shows how this historical endeavour is thwarted by actual psychoanalytical experience. The structure imposed on the data of free association does not emerge *from* those data, which are inherently chaotic, but rather from the theoretical, interpretive schemata that the analyst brings to the session.

Spence's analysis ultimately rests on a positivist view of the raw data of experience or memory. These are experiences 'too fleeting to be captured; they disappear from awareness before we can find the proper language. Others can perhaps be captured in words but not formed into sentences' (Spence, 1982, p. 41). Most problematic, memories are in their origin fragmented, visual phenomena. 'Patients' memories, if true, tend to resemble photographs—particularly if they are more or less faithful to the original experience' (Spence, 1982, p. 57). In this positivist vision, the discrete events that compose reality could only be reported accurately by someone directly witnessing them. The narrative coherence into which they are organized in an analysis is one imposed by the analyst. What all of this says, of course, is that the analyst's interpretations are actively constructed narrative structures that unify the patient's life but that reveal more loyalty to the aesthetic rules of narrative than to the reality of the patient's past.

A major consequence of Spence's position is that the Freudian unconscious has lost the role it had for Freud, and will have for Schafer, that of a second narrative. It is now reduced to the mute, inaccessible data of an inaccessible historical reality. In one of his scarce references to the unconscious Spence refers to the silent world of the senses. 'We not only try to arrive at an understanding of the world of the senses; we also try to put into words a completely separate domain which is, because it is unconscious, not accessible to awareness' (Spence, 1982, p. 162).

Spence's second book, *The Freudian metaphor*, is both a development and a more nuanced revision of the earlier book. Now fully adopting a hermeneutic reading of psychoanalysis, he recognizes that the rather absolute separation of historical and narrative truth espoused in the earlier book is not acceptable. If the narrative is a hermeneutically developed construction, it is neither simply fictive or realistic, but is in some way both:

> If our hermeneutic position is correct, then it must follow that the meaning of the material is highly dependent on who is listening to it, and that what was true for the treating analyst, at a particular time and place in the treatment, will never be true again.
>
> But what is bad news in some quarters is good news in others. The fact that the clinical data are theory-laden and context-dependent is no barrier to building them into a readable narrative; indeed, a narrative thrives on surplus meaning, and the richer the network of associations, the greater its aesthetic appeal. It could be argued that the very reasons that prevent us from uncovering reliable evidence and thus systematically validating the theory smooth the way toward constructing a plausible narrative.
>
> Narrative benefits by rhetorical elaboration; theory does not.
>
> (*Spence, 1987, p. 112.*)

It is in keeping with his new appreciation of the hermeneutic quality of psychoanalytical interpretation that Spence now disavows the implicit positivism of his earlier work. As he writes earlier in the passage just quoted:

> The belief in an archeology of the mind or of the session carries with it the idea that pieces of the past remain intact and can be recovered unchanged. The metaphor encourages us to look for tracings of the past, variously disguised but somehow recoverable, which could be used to validate the theory—both within the patient and within the session. But such a belief entails a kind of positivism which simply does not apply to the clinical material. The search for historical truth fails once we realize that the observer is always part of what is observed.
>
> (*Spence, 1987, p. 111.*)

What remains missing in Spence is a sense of human life described by MacIntyre (1981) as 'enacted narrative'. Because Spence places the origin of narrative in the activity of the analyst (or historian) rather than in the life of the patient, he clings to an understanding of narrative that remains highly aesthetic. The consequence is that, even in the later book, the therapeutic power of the psychodynamic narrative is its *aesthetic* appeal rather than its response to a deep need in the patient for a real revision of the distressful enacted narratives he or she has already been living with.

In Roy Schafer, the other psychoanalytical theoretician who has written extensively about narrative, we see another response to the critical debate over narrative and reference. While wholly rejecting Freud's positivist vision of psychoanalysis, Schafer remains loyal to the narrativist trend that is implicit in Freud. He considers the analyst's interpretations to be 'acts of retelling or narrative revision' (Schafer 1983, p. 187): this narrative revision representing a 'second reality' which is that of the unconscious. Like Spence in his later book, Schafer emphasizes the hermeneutic dimension of narrative structures. In fact, the words hermeneutic and narrative are almost indistinguishable in his discussion. There is thus no final, correct reading of a person's life, just as there is no neutral observation:

> Each account of the past is a reconstruction that is controlled by a narrative strategy. The narrative strategy dictates how one is to select, from a plenitude of possible details, those that may be reorganized into another narrative which is both followable and expresses the desired point of view on the past. Accordingly, this reconstruction, like its narrative predecessor, is always subject to change.
> (*Schafer, 1983, 193.*)

Although Schafer is in agreement with Freud that the unconscious is a second narrative that fills the gaps in the conscious narrative, he diverges from Freud in two significant ways. First, because his view of narrative is highly hermeneutic, he recognizes that the narrative strategy that will inform *his* interpretations—*his* version of a second reality—will be different from those of analysts of different persuasions. Thus there are many possible ways of retelling a life analytically. He acknowledges that his own approach favours the traditional Freudian story lines of sexuality, aggression, bodily zones, etc. Secondly, Schafer reverses the priority Freud gives to the past over the present. In Schafer's view, the history of the analysis itself assumes primary importance: 'Developing the psychoanalytic biography retains great importance, but what is more clearly recognized now is that the importance of this biography depends on the extent to which it enhances the understanding of the analysis itself' (Schafer, 1983, pp. 207–8). A consequence of this is a de-emphasis on linear, narrative time. For Schafer it is the *interpenetration* of the narratives of the past and the present that represents what is most unique about psychoanalytical narrative. The analysis of each informs and furthers the understanding of the other. And while the narratives of past and present each maintain a temporal dimension, Schafer points to the fact that psychoanalytical tacking between past and present 'is temporally circular rather than unidirectionally retrospective' (Schafer, 1983, p. 196). Psychoanalysis is thus distinct in being fully committed to narrative while at the same time uninterested in linear time. As Schafer says, '. . . in order to develop the transference neurosis as fully as possible, it becomes less rather than more important to think in terms of conventional linear time, less rather than more important to distinguish between past and present' (Schafer, 1983, p. 196).

Two further points may be made about Schafer's privileging the present over the past in his account of psychoanalytical narrative. The first is that he is able to escape much of the tension of the debate over narrative and reference. If the focus is primarily on the narrative of the treatment itself, this is a 'past' that is accessible to the two individuals who have lived through it. Recalling and narrativizing this 'past' does not carry the uncertainty that attends the same effort regarding events belonging to a past of 20 years ago. This is of course a matter of degree. As Schafer, with his strong hermeneutic stand, would agree, different analysts will narrativize their treatments (or the same treatment, as in the case of Dora) in different ways.

The second point is that in privileging the narrative of the present, Schafer is joining ranks with the majority of his colleagues who place greater emphasis on the transference/countertransference interactions of the treatment itself than on the exploration of the patient's past. In doing this he is effectively joining narrative theory with this current trend in psychoanalytical treatment. His approach does include the three dimensions of narrative described above in the section on Freud. The order, however, is now reversed. While the treatment narrative was the least important for Freud, for Schafer it is the most important. It incorporates both the psychodynamic retelling of the past as well as Schafer's own preferred developmental theory.

While Schafer adheres to a narrativist position in the psychoanalytical process, it is in fact a short step from the emphasis on the current analytical relationship to a disregard or outright dismissal of narrative as playing an important role in psychoanalytical treatment. I will conclude this section with one example of disregard and one example of dismissal. The first example is that of Paul Gray (1994), who centres the therapeutic analytical activity almost exclusively in the microanalysis of the patient's defenses *within* the session. For Gray it is this focus on the patient's *in vivo* experience of anxiety and defence that allows for real change. Understandably, with this emphasis on an analysis of the patient's mental activity *within* the analytical session, there is a corresponding de-emphasis on what is going on *outside* the session. Speaking of the 'outside' issues, Gray writes:

> I would hasten to agree that these aspects are all compatible with interpretations that could result in therapeutic gain, as is regularly true of much that is 'applied psychoanalysis,' psychoanalytically oriented psychotherapy, and so on. My thesis, however, is that what has just been described as 'outside' is peripheral to what is fundamentally psychoanalytic and consequently can unnecessarily dilute or distract from the analytic process and, in addition, strengthen the resistance against drive derivatives during the analytic hour and also against the degree of transference neurosis which might otherwise be achieved.
> (*Gray, 1994, p. 15.*)

With such an exclusive focus on analysing the ego and its defences, a formulation and analysis of the psychodynamic narrative will not have a very important place in this approach to psychoanalysis.

The example of an outright dismissal of narrative is that of Jacques Lacan (1977, 1978). For all his loathing of ego psychology and the work of analysts like Gray, the two in fact converge around the question of narrative—and its unimportance. Like Gray, Lacan did not focus on narrative as such. What he did, rather, was espouse a position that was at its core anti-narrativist, a position according to which any narrative ordering of the psychoanalytical data would represent all the superficiality of the secondary process, and according to which Freud's fundamental discovery, the unconscious, represents the limit and end of all possibility of a unified, narrative identity.

The point at which to approach Lacan on the issue of narrative is his point of view concerning the subject. For Lacan there is a major split within the human subject, between the conscious subject that goes about its daily life and that other, hidden, subject that is revealed through the chinks in the conscious narrative, through parapraxes, dreams, and symptoms. Describing this split in his favoured terms, the 'ex-centricity' or 'heteronomy' of the subject, Lacan writes:

> But if we ignore the self's radical ex-centricity to itself with which man is confronted, in other words, the truth discovered by Freud, we shall falsify both the order and methods of psychoanalytic mediation. . . .
> The radical heteronomy that Freud's discovery shows gaping within man can never again be covered over without whatever is used to hide it being profoundly dishonest.

> Who, then, is this other to whom I am more attached than to myself, since, at the heart of my assent to my own identity it is still he who agitates me?
> (*Lacan, 1977, pp. 171–2.*)

How may this unconscious, that is the subject's true centre, be further described? Lacan calls on the work of Saussure and Levi-Strauss to develop the notion of a 'symbolic order', transcendent to the individual, into which the individual is born, and which, through its play of signifiers, determines the individual rather than it being determined by him or her.

If the subject is thus 'decentred' towards the symbolic order of the unconscious, how may the conscious life of the self be described? For Lacan this is the false self of the ego or 'moi', a narcissistically structured persona that one presents to oneself and to others, and that is a product of the 'imaginary order'. Since the subject is alienated in this persona, the goal of psychoanalysis is not to strengthen the ego but rather to dissolve it.

The consequence of this division of the subject is that the notion of a unified or integrated subject—or, in our words, a narrative identity—is, for Lacan, an illusion. As he writes:

> Discontinuity, then is the essential form in which the unconscious first appears to us as a phenomenon. . . . Now, if this discontinuity has this absolute, inaugural character, in the development of Freud's discovery, must we place it—as was later the tendency with analysts—against the background of a totality?
>
> It is the *one* anterior to discontinuity? I do not think so, and everything that I have taught in recent years has tended to exclude this need for a closed *one*. . . . You will grant me that the *one* that is introduced by the experience of the unconscious is the *one* of the split, of the stroke, of rupture.
> (*Lacan, 1978, pp. 25–6.*)

If we replace Lacan's '*one*' with 'narrative identity' or 'narrative self', we can recognize in him a particular end-point in the psychoanalytical treatment of narrative—a point at which narrative and narrative identity are nothing more than comforting illusions that are not to be taken seriously psychoanalytically, except in their status as illusion and resistance.

Conclusions

In the concluding section of this chapter I would like both to summarize what has been said about the psychodynamic narrative and to offer a critique of its treatment by contemporary authors.

The notion of a psychodynamic narrative owes everything to Freud's notions that there is an unconscious dimension to human thought and behaviour and that the gaps in an individual's presenting story can be filled in through the interpolation of the unconscious links. Schafer's felicitous phrase 'second reality' nicely describes this notion of a retelling of the life narrative along psychoanalytical lines—a retelling that for both Freud and Schafer emphasizes (initially unconscious) themes of infantile sexuality, oedipal striving, etc.

Over the course of recent decades Freud's assertion of a single developmental narrative and a single psychodynamic narrative for each patient has given way to a recognition that the story of a life can be told in more than one way and that the kind of story that is told will depend a lot on the point of view of the person attempting to tell it. This does not mean that all narratives are equally valid and that therefore *none* is *really* valid. Rather, it is the task of the therapist/story-teller to justify his or her particular psychodynamic retelling of the patient's life history.

Such a justification will include elements of narrative fit, therapeutic efficacy, confirmation by the patient, confirmation through the transference, and allegiance to established psychoanalytical narrative traditions. That said, it is clear that different clinicians will offer differing psychodynamic narratives about the same patient and that these psychodynamic narratives will tend to follow the theoretical allegiances of the respective therapists. The work of Spence serves as a strong reminder of the degree to which a psychodynamic narrative may be imposed on the life of the patient rather than 'discovered' in that life.

Contemporary work in psychoanalysis and psychoanalytical therapy has shifted the focus of the work from an exploration of the past, as with Freud, to a focus on the ongoing interactions in the treatment itself. This has required a reformulation of the psychodynamic narrative, a task accomplished mainly by Roy Schafer. There is no longer a psychodynamic narrative of the patient's past and then a second narrative of the treatment itself. For Schafer the two are collapsed into one. The psychodynamic narrative is now a complex, interwoven tale, told along psychoanalytical lines, that intertwines themes from the patient's past with themes from the treatment itself, the emphasis falling on the latter rather than the former.

The preceding section concluded with examples of psychoanalytical treatment that prescind from an interest in the psychodynamic narrative—in the case of Gray because the essential work is focused on the patient's use of defence in the analytical session, and in the case of Lacan because the notion of a psychodynamic narrative implies a potential for self-integration that is simply illusory. For both these authors the notion of a narrative identity is not central to their work. In this they illustrate quite dramatically what in fact is true of even those psychoanalytical theoreticians sympathetic to a narrative dimension of psychoanalytical treatment—namely, that in a strong sense of narrative identity, narrative is not quite central to the psychoanalytical process.

To make this final point let me suggest a distinction between a strong sense of narrative and narrative identity and a weak sense of these phenomena. The strong sense would imply that narrative is at the core of human identity, that the terms narrative identity and personal identity become almost interchangeable. As suggested above, Alasdair MacIntyre is an example of someone who espouses such a strong sense of narrative identity. He writes of his '. . . concept of selfhood, a concept of a self whose unity resides in the unity of a narrative, which links birth to life to death as narrative beginning to middle to end' (MacIntyre, 1981, p. 205). And again:

> What the narrative concept of selfhood requires is thus twofold. On the one hand, I am what I may justifiably be taken by others to be in the course of living out a story that runs from my birth to my death; I am the *subject* of a history that is my own and no one else's, that has its own peculiar meaning. . . .. Thus personal identity is just that identity presupposed by the unity of the character which the unity of a narrative requires. Without such unity there would not be subjects of whom stories could be told.
> (*pp. 218–19.*)

As these quotes suggest, a strong sense of narrative selfhood places primary significance on human existence as temporal and historical, and on people as linguistically endowed story-tellers.

In contrast to the strong position, a weak sense of narrative and narrative identity would imply that narrative is a dimension of human identity, perhaps even an important dimension, but not the *defining* dimension of human identity. What I wish to suggest in these concluding remarks is that currently there are no psychoanalytically oriented theoreticians—Spence and

Schafer included—who have adopted more than a weak sense of narrative. The reasons for this are probably twofold. First would be the theoretical baggage that 'self' or 'identity' carry with them in the psychoanalytical tradition—baggage that includes such notions as psychic apparatus, internal structures, ego, id, superego, unconscious, representational world, internal objects, introjects, internalizations, incorporations, and self-objects, to mention only a sampling. With so many competing attributes for a definition of selfhood, it is hardly surprising that narrativity would not assume a position of primacy among them. Secondly, psychoanalytical notions of self and identity are generally not the products of philosophical reflection, as with MacIntyre, but rather are the products of clinical experience. The psychoanalytical notions will then reflect what has been found to be useful in the clinical situation. Thus the notions of self and self-object, as used in Kohutian self-psychology, are notions of personal identity that capture the clinical experience of practitioners working in that tradition. In her discussion of this issue Janet Malcolm argues that because of the complexity of both the patient's unconscious life and the treatment process itself, straightforward narrative is neither an adequate way to present a case nor is it the curative element in the treatment. Writing of Freud, who she claims shared this position, she says:

> He understood that he had to go beyond the novelistic plots and characters of the patient's present life and recent past, cross the River Lethe, and penetrate the obscure, inchoate, shade-populated region of infant sorrow where the patient was still haplessly living.
> In the Wolf Man and the Rat Man cases, Freud makes this crossing; in the writing of both case histories he eliminates almost everything pertaining to the patient's adult biography, and confines himself to the exotic inner world of the oedipal and preoedipal child. The only fully alive contemporary character in the Wolf Man and Rat Man cases is Freud, the narrator. The patient isn't there; he is like an anesthetized body on which an operation is being performed. . . .In his prefatory remarks to the Dora case, Freud explains that he has deliberately excluded from his account almost all mention of what he calls 'the technique of the analytic work'. We now know, as Freud was on the verge of knowing, how crucial this excluded portion is. It is in the particular, idiosyncratic, ineffable encounter between patient and analyst that the 'story' of an analysis is lodged. . . . A reading of these laconic, deceptively straightforward essays [the technical papers] quickly dispels the misconception that Marcus, among other literary Freudians, has given currency to— that psychoanalysis is a sort of cure by narrative. Peter Brooks, in his book *Reading for the Plot: Design and Intention in Narrative*, writes: 'There is in Freud's case histories an underlying assumption that psychic health corresponds to a coherent narrative account of one's life' (1984, 281–282) . . . But this 'underlying assumption' is nowhere to be found in Freud's writings. Quite on the contrary, Freud distinguishes between narrative closure and therapeutic benefit. Moreover— as both Brooks and Marcus refuse to notice—the protagonist of the Freudian case history is not an analytic patient trying to make a narrative of his life but a small child struggling (and tragically failing) to fathom the actions of his parents.
> (*Malcolm, 1990, pp. 318–23.*)

Where then might we turn for a strong sense of narrative in the psychoanalytical or clinical disciplines. First, ironically, we might, *pace* Malcolm, turn (back) to Freud. Although Freud does not frame his case histories in the language of narrative, he in fact comes closer than our psychoanalytical contemporaries to making narrative central to the psychoanalytical process. The reason for this has been suggested above: namely, his insistence on the importance of reconstructing the history of the patient as central to the treatment. Indeed, for Freud the formulation of the psychodynamic narrative—a narrative that is developed in the face of the patient's resistances and that includes those resistances within it—is the curative factor in the psychoanalytical treatment. In most contemporary versions of psychoanalytical treatment, with an increasing emphasis on the relational factors in the treatment process itself as the therapeutic ingredient, there has been a falling off of interest in the psychoanalytical narrative of the patient's past. Understandably, with this change of emphasis on what is important and therapeutic, the role of narrative in the strong sense has dimished in the psychodynamic and psychoanalytical therapies.

For a strong sense of narrative in contemporary clinical work and theorizing, we have to leave the narrow domain of psychoanalysis for other areas of psychology and clinical work. One such area is that called cultural psychology by Jerome Bruner. Bruner (1990) argues forcefully that the field of psychology should shift its focus away from the currently popular, computer-modelled, cognitive psychology and on to the study of the culturally mediated narrative-meaning structures that form our lives.

> Indeed, the very shape of our lives—the rough and perpetually changing draft of our autobio-graphy that we carry in our minds—is understandable to ourselves and to others only by virtue of those cultural systems of interpretation. But culture is also constitutive of mind. By virtue of this actualization in culture, meaning achieves a form that is public and communal rather than private and autistic. Only by replacing this transactional model of mind with an isolating indi-vidualistic one have Anglo-American philosophers been able to make Other Minds seem so opaque and impenetrable. . . .In this chapter, we shall be principally concerned with one crucial feature of cultural psychology. I have called it 'fold psychology,' or you may prefer 'folk social sci-ence' or even, simply, 'common sense.'. . . Since its organizing principle is narrative rather than conceptual, I shall have to consider the nature of narrative and how it is built around established or canonical expectations and the mental management of deviations from such expectations.
> (*Brunner, 1990, pp. 34–5.*)

For a more clinically oriented application of narrative in the strong sense, we can turn to the expanding treatment approach that goes by the name of 'narrative therapy'. Pre-eminent and typical is the work of David Epston and Michael White (White and Epston, 1990; Epston, and White, 1992). Narrative therapy, as understood by these and other practitioners of the field, can take place in a setting of individual, family, or group therapy. While this work certainly overlaps with some psychoanalytical and psychodynamic conceptualizations, it is not simply one more psychodynamic therapy. At its centre is a strong sense of narrative as the structuring core of a person's life and as the primary focus of the therapeutic work. With an emphasis on narrative identity and therapeutic change as a restructuring or rewriting of the life narrative, the clinical focus falls as much on the narrative future as on the narrative past. The therapeutic challenge, after all, is to loosen the sense of inevitability that is carried by the narrative of one's past so that the chapters that extend into the future are more under the authorial control of the patient.

With these new fields of cultural psychology and narrative therapy we leave the more narrow bounds of psychodynamic therapy and the psychodynamic narrative, so this is not the place to elaborate that field. I will conclude this chapter, however, by suggesting that a current challenge for psychoanalysis and the psychodynamic therapies would be to incorporate the productive contributions of these new disciplines. Doing so would clearly strengthen the narrative com-ponent of the former, and they would be the richer for it.

References

Barthes, R. (1977). *Image, Music, Text* (trans. S. Heath). Hill and Wang, New York.

Bernheimer, C. and Kahane, C. (1990). *In Dora's case: Freud—hysteria—feminism*, (2nd edn). Columbia University Press, New York.

Bernstein, R. (1983). *Beyond objectivism and relativism: science, hermeneutics, and praxis.* University of Pennsylvania Press, Philadelphia.

Brenner, C. (1987). A structural theory perspective. In *How theory shapes technique: perspectives on a clinical study*, (ed. S. Pulver), *Psychoanalytic Inquiry*, **7**, 167–72.

Breuer, J. and Freud, S. (1895). *Studies on hysteria*. In *The standard edition of the complete psychological works of Sigmund Freud*, Vol. 11, (trans. and ed. J. Strachey) pp. 1–241. The Hogarth Press (1955), London.

Brooks, P. (1984). *Reading for the plot: design and intention in narrative*. Random House, New York.

Bruner, J. (1990). *Acts of meaning*. Harvard University Press, Cambridge.

Carr, D. (1986). *Time, narrative, and history*. University of Indiana Press, Bloomington.

Epston, D. and White, M. (1992). *Experience, contradiction, narrative & imagination*. Dulwich Centre Publications, South Australia.

Erikson, E. (1968). *Identity, youth, and crisis*. W. W. Norton, New York.

Freud, S. (1905). Fragment of an analysis of a case of hysteria. In *The standard edition of the complete psychological works of Sigmund Freud*, Vol VII, (trans. and ed. J. Strachey), pp. 3–124. The Hogarth Press (1953), London.

Freud, S. (1915). The unconscious. In *The standard edition of the complete psychological works of Sigmund Freud*, Vol XIV, (trans. ed. J. Strachey.), pp. 159–216. The Hogarth Press (1957), London.

Freud, S. (1918). From the history of an infantile neurosis. In *The standard edition of the complete psychological works of Sigmund Freud*, Vol XVII, (trans. ed. J. Strachey), pp. 3–122. The Hogarth Press, (1955), London.

Freud, S. (1985). *The complete letters of Sigmund Freud to Wilhelm Fliess: 1887–1905* (trans. ed. J. Masson). Harvard University Press, Cambridge.

Glenn, J. (1980). Freud's adolescent patients: Katharina, Dora, and the "Homosexual Woman." In *Freud and his patients*, (ed. M. Kanzer and J. Glenn), pp. 23–47. Jason Aronson, New York.

Goldberg, A. (1987). A self psychology perspective. In *How theory shapes technique: perspectives on a clinical study* (ed. S. Pulver), *Psychoanalytic Inquiry*, **7**, 181–8.

Gray, P. (1994). *The ego and the analysis of defense*. Jason Aronson Inc., Northvale.

Kermode, F. (1966). *The sense of an ending*. Oxford University Press, London.

Lacan, J. (1977). *Écrits*, (trans. A. Sheridan). W. W. Norton, New York.

Lacan, J. (1978). *The four fundamental concepts of psycho-analysis*, (ed. J.-A. Miller, trans. Alan Sheridan). W. W. Norton, New York.

Levenson, E. (1987). An interpersonal perspective. In *How theory shapes technique: perspectives on a clinical study*, (ed. S. Pulver), *Psychoanalytic Inquiry*, **7**, 207–14.

MacIntyre, A. (1981). *After virtue*. University of Notre Dame Press, Notre Dame.

Malcolm, J. (1990). Reflections: J'appelle un chat un chat. In *In Dora's case: Freud—hysteria—*

feminism, (2nd edn), (ed. C. Bernheimer and C. Kahane), pp. 305–25. Columbia University Press, New York.

Nagel, T. (1997). *The last word.* Oxford University Press, New York.

Phillips, J. (1991). Hermeneutics in psychoanalysis: review and reconsideration. *Psychoanalysis and Contemporary Thought*, **14**, 371–424.

Pulver, S. (ed.) (1987) *How theory shapes technique: perspectives on a clinical study, Psychoanalytic Inquiry*, **7**, 141–298.

Ricoeur, P. (1970). *Freud and philosophy: an essay on interpretation*, (trans. D. Savage). Yale University Press, New Haven.

Ricoeur, P. (1984–1988). *Time and narrative*, (trans. K. McLaughlin and D. Pellauer), Vol. 1 (1984), Vol. 2 (1985), Vol. 3 (1988). University of Chicago Press, Chicago.

Ronty, R. (1979). *Philosophy and the mirror of nature.* Princeton University Press, Princeton, N.J.

Schafer, R. (1983). *The analytic attitude.* Basic Books, New York.

Scharfman, M. (1980). Further reflections on Dora. In *Freud and his patients*, (ed. M. Kanzer and J. Glenn), pp. 48–57. Jason Aronson, New York.

Schwaber, E. (1987). Models of the mind and data-gathering in clinical work. In *How theory shapes technique: perspectives on a clinical study*, (ed. S. Pulver), *Psychoanalytic Inquiry*, **7**, 261–75.

Shane, E. (1987). Varieties of psychoanalytic experience, 1. In *How theory shapes technique: perspectives on a clinical study*, (ed. S. Pulver), *Psychoanalytic Inquiry*, **7**, 199–206.

Silverman, M. (1987). Clinical material. In *How theory shapes technique: perspectives on a clinical study*, (ed. S. Pulver), *Psychoanalytic Inquiry*, **7**, 147–66.

Spence, D. (1982). *Narrative truth and historical truth: meaning and interpretation in psychoanalysis.* W. W. Norton, New York.

Spence, D. (1987). *The Freudian metaphor: toward paradigm change in psychoanalysis.* W. W. Norton, New York.

White, H. (1987). *The content of the form.* The John Hopkins Press, Baltimore.

White, M. and Epston, D. (1990). *Narrative means to therapeutic ends.* W. W. Norton, New York.

3 Defensive and creative uses of narrative in psychotherapy: an attachment perspective

Jeremy Holmes

Introduction

Joseph Conrad's *Heart of darkness* begins and ends on a packet ship moored on the River Thames, with the narrator Marlow sucking at his guttering pipe. In between the reader has been taken on a compelling and horrific journey into the interior. The book is a story within a story, framed by the river itself, whose reaches, unlike stories, are unpunctuated: stretching in a spacial continuum from London across the oceans to the heart of the Congo, and in time from the present day back to the Roman invasion of Britain.

This contrast between the structure and boundedness of the story, and the fluidity and formlessness of reality, forms the background to this chapter. There is also an opposition between artifice and nature, which can be expressed psychoanalytically as a contrast between the apparent actuality of the dream narrative and the patchwork of fragmented associations and 'day's residues' that a dream evokes. Bollas (1995) takes this as a general paradigm for the activity of the unconscious, which he sees as continuously fashioning lived life into stories, and then dismantling and dispersing those stories in the light of further experience. I shall follow this theme throughout this chapter which is both an exposition and a critique of the 'narrative turn' (Howard, 1991) in psychotherapy. I consider first some general aspects of narrative, and then its application to psychotherapy practice. My aim is to weave together contemporary psychoanalysis (Bateman and Holmes 1995), attachment research, and narrative theory into a common story.

My main argument is that narrative forms one half of a duality that lies at the heart of psychotherapy. This dichotomy can be expressed in a number of different ways: narrative and its deconstruction; prose and poetry; primary and secondary processes; story and image; 'when . . then' and 'present moment'; then and there and here and now. Things go wrong, I shall argue, when the balance of this duality is disrupted—too much prose and not enough poetry, or vice versa. Psychopathology, which I approach largely through attachment theory's distinction between the various types of insecure attachment, can be seen in terms of an excess of one or other element. Let us begin with two contrasting clinical stories.

Example 1: the constrictions of 'story'

Tom, an unemployed youth of 20 living with his parents and 15-years-old sister, was referred by his family doctor for help with his 'compulsive gambling' which was causing enormous concern within the family.

When Tom was interviewed on his own the story that emerged was as follows. He had been unemployed for most of the time since leaving college two years previously. Both his parents were working. During the day, while they were at work and his sister at school, he would take items from the house such as video machines or his father's tools, sell them to his friends and then proceed to spend the money on fruit machines. Things had come to a head when he had smashed the family car, which he had taken without asking and was driving without insurance, while on his way to a local gambling arcade.

Tom, a shy and young-looking 20-year old, described how difficult things had been since leaving college: how he had been unable to settle in a job, and how his father had had a period of unemployment which meant they had lost their home and had to move into a smaller house. He had missed his dad dreadfully when lack of local jobs meant that he had had to work away from home. When asked about his 'winning fantasies' in gambling, he spoke of how he dreamed of restoring both the family fortunes and his own reputation within the family.

When Tom was interviewed with his parents a rather different picture emerged. Tom's father, clearly a good man at the end of his tether, was constantly criticizing his son; Tom's mother was obviously depressed, sitting mostly silently with tears running down her face. They explained how they were convinced that Tom was 'on drugs': he was pale and tired all the time, irritable and monosyllabic, just like the descriptions in the leaflet a friend had given them. They were then asked to confront Tom with this possibility in the session. Tom denied using drugs (as he had in the individual session, apart from admitting to occasional cannabis), while the parents looked nonplussed. The therapist suggested that his exhaustion and irritability might reflect depression rather than drug dependence. As Tom's father continued to express his exasperation— saying how they had several times been on the point of throwing Tom out but could not bring themselves to do so—the boy became visibly upset. The therapist reminded him of what he had said about his feelings while his father had been away. 'I missed you dad . . .' he said tentatively. Father was stopped in his tracks and looked tearful. With prompting he began to say 'You're not a bad lad, son, it's just that you do bad things.' Tom went on to say how he felt an outsider in the family, while his parents and sister formed a cosy little threesome. Again mother and father looked upset, and mother began to say how she felt caught between her husband and son, and how, against her better judgement, she gave in to Tom's demands for money.

The session ended with the parents determined to be firmer with Tom, if necessary locking valuables away during the day, and with Tom and his father giving each other what seemed like a genuine hug of re-conciliation.

At the start of the session this family seemed trapped within a very restricted 'story' of their situation. Seeing Tom as a 'compulsive gambler' or a 'drug addict' made some sense of their distress, if only to medicalize it and so shape it in such a way that they could elicit help. The purpose of the psychotherapy was to introduce some perturbation into this rather rigid narrative, to disperse it for long enough for a new story to coalesce, one with more complexity, allowing for a greater range of emotional expression. The new story was one of a lost youth trying to rescue his family fortunes, of parents torn between lenience and violence, of the looming impact of unemployment. The crucial moment in the session came when Tom told his father he missed him, and his father responded by becoming tearful. At that moment he seemed to listen to his son again, and see him as a person, not as a clichéd 'story'. Momentarily, both escaped from their stereotyped version of events into a new envelope of shared feeling.

In this example there is a movement from a secure but narrow 'illness narrative', through the dangers but creative possibility of uncertainty and unstoried immediacy (which can be linked with Lacan's anti-narrative stance described in the previous chapter), to the possibility of a new and less constricted narrative. Here, then, there was an excess of 'story'. In the second example, by contrast, we see *un*storied disturbance and emotional danger in search of a therapeutic narrative that might provide a satisfactory fit with experience.

Example 2: searching for a story that fits

James, a successful teacher plagued by depression, arrived at his fifth session seven minutes late. Despite an apparently positive therapeutic alliance, the therapy had not been going well—therapist and patient struggled to find a real focus with which to work. James tended to tell lots of stories about his situation and his life, but no real pattern emerged, certainly nothing that could be useful to him. In this session, both James and his therapist knew he was angry with him—James had asked the therapist to run a seminar for a group of teachers at his school, but the therapist had declined, on the grounds that it would interfere with the therapeutic process.

James started the session by explaining that he was late because he had been helping a friend pull his car out of a ditch. The therapist mused to himself on the different possible stories of which this incident could form a part. He offered a fairly conventional transference comment: 'Perhaps you are hoping I will pull you out of the ditch of your depression—you are showing me the way'. No, this did not seem to fit. James spoke of his need always to be looking after others—family, fellow-teachers, pupils, and now the friend who was stuck in the ditch. This linked with James' childhood story: a feeling that his mother never really liked him, and was always fussing over his sister and brother. This led on to James' feeling of rejection over the therapist's refusal to speak at the seminar. Together, the therapist and James pieced together that by being late he was saying 'I am angry with you. You don't care about me. You are more interested in everyone else. Right, *I'll* show you how people should be helped. I'll get them out of their ditches even if you leave me in mine.' Next, James began telling the therapist how helpful something he had said in a previous session had been. The therapist commented: 'Do you notice how much your own aggression seems to threaten you? No sooner do you criticize me, than you have to tell me how wonderful I am, perhaps for fear I will retaliate or abandon you.' James laughs—a confirmatory response that the new story was on target.

Here, the affective response confirms that a story has been found that fits. This time, a narrative focus is helpful in filling in missing parts of a story, as described by Phillips as 'Freud's mission' in the previous chapter. The previous example seemed to illustrate the opposite: tears marked liberation from the constrictions of the old story. The work of psychotherapy is to find stories that fit with experience. This may mean disrupting clichéd stories, or reaching for a narrative that can better comprehend the confusions of everyday feelings. Affective responsiveness seems to be one way of gauging how successful this process has been. But how does one establish the truth or otherwise of a narrative? Can a story be emotionally true, while being factually incorrect, and vice versa?

Can there be a science of narrative?

Jerome Bruner (1986) argues that there are two kinds of approaches to truth:

> A good story and a well-formed argument are different natural kinds. Both can be used as a means for convincing another. Yet what they convince of is fundamentally different: arguments convince of their truth, stories of their lifelikeness. The one verifies by eventual appeal to procedures for establishing formal and empirical truth. The other establishes its truth by verisimilitude.
> (*Bruner, 1986.*)

As an advocate of narrative, Bruner's use of the word 'verisimilitude' is risky, given its definition *in the Oxford English Dictionary* of 'having the appearance of being real or true'. Critics of psychotherapy might argue that this is a concession that the stories elaborated in psychotherapy can lay no more claim to the truth than can myths or fairy stories. How can this charge be answered?

Bruner's response, I believe, would be that there *is* truth in myths and fairy stories—emotional truth rather than factual truth—which can be judged, not by scientific standards, but by such tests as whether the story rings true, feels 'right', is satisfying, coherent, or touches the listener emotionally. Ironically, a play has verisimilitude if it compels the audience to remain in a state of 'suspension of disbelief' for the duration of the performance. Similarly, psychotherapeutic case histories could be Brunerian 'good stories' which have a paradigmatic value in their own right, even though, by the standards of a 'well formed argument', by themselves they prove nothing.

The criteria of a 'good story' certainly apply to psychotherapy. Psychotherapists are constantly using their intuition to evaluate the patient's narrative, asking themselves if it makes sense or hangs together, questioning aspects that don't quite fit, probing clichés or phrases and well-worn narratives for what might lie beneath. The quest is always for a more elaborated, all-embracing, spontaneous, individualized, flexible story that encompasses a greater range of experience.

This evaluative activity, akin to aesthetics, is part of the 'art' of psychotherapy. But can there also be a science of narrative, including one that would encompass the narrative aspects of psychotherapy? One response that has gained in popularity recently is to concede that that the quest *is* fruitless and that there can be no science of psychotherapy. As discussed in the previous chapter the hermeneutic school of psychoanalysis, of whom Spence (1982) and Schafer (1992) are leading exponents, argue that what matters in psychotherapy is not objective or 'historical' truth, which is, in their view, in any case inherently unknowable, but 'narrative truth', i.e. something akin to Bruner's verisimilitude.

The main drawback of this position is the implication that a psychotherapeutic narrative is no more or less likely to be true than any other account of the patient's distress, whether religious, narrowly 'organic' in the psychiatric sense, or delusional. My objection to this position is not based on a fear of losing the respectability that the mantle of science confers. Nor would I want to deny that psychotherapy is, among other things, a moral rather than a narrowly scientific discourse, in which questions about what it is to lead a good life and to flourish as a human being are central (Holmes and Lindley, 1997). My main worry about the hermeneutic turn in psychotherapy is that it threatens to cut psychotherapy off from aspects of science—especially from evolutionary biology and developmental psychology—where dialogue is both necessary and possible.

The contribution of attachment research

While the immediate goal of psychotherapy may be to remove symptoms; behind that lies a set of more general and more ambitious objectives, namely, to help an individual to flourish, to foster well-being, and so on. These can be seen in terms of the development of a strengthened and more versatile set of selves: for example; a more secure self, a more creative self, a more coping self, a more resilient self, a more autonomous self, a self with a greater capacity for intimacy. As in the account of MacIntyre's theories in the previous chapter, and in contrast with the Cartesian *cogito*, narrative theory sees the 'I' not as a fixed and pre-existing entity, but as an autobiographical self, formed out of the interplay between agency and contingency, needing to be 'told' to another, or storied, before it can come into being (Brockmeier, 1997). The telling of a self implies a built-in dialogical structure. There is always an 'other' to whom the 'self' is telling his or her story, even if in adults this takes the form of an internal dialogue.

What are the origins of this 'self-story'? How do we begin to learn about ourselves and our feelings? For psychoanalysts, Winnicott's notion of maternal mirroring provides a model both of normal development, and of the possible role of therapy. When the mother looks at the baby, according to Winnicott (1967), 'what she looks like is related to what she sees there'. This clinical insight has recently been supported by Gergely and Watson (1996) who suggest that an attuned mother helps her infant identify feelings by mirroring behaviour that has two characteristics. First, the mother's facial expressions of emotion are '*marked*' by exaggeration, so that the child can see that they are 'pretend', not real. Secondly, they are *contingent* on the child's feelings, so that they arise only when he or she appears to be experiencing a particular emotion, a response which in itself has a soothing function. Here we see the beinnings of a possible representation of, or story about, the self and its feelings. 'Marking' is related to the highlighting, figure/groundedness of narrative; contingency is linked with the way in which, unlike real life, stories hang together in a coherent way.

Gergely and Watson's (1996) speculations are based on the three decades of research on infant–mother interaction arising from Bowlby's attachment theory (Holmes, 1993). Recent developments in attachment research have begun to link this understanding of early life with clinical narrative in adults. The *way* we tell stories reflects our fundamental stance towards the world. The development of the adult attachment interview (AAI) by Mary Main and her colleagues (Main, 1995) in the mid-1980s provided a scientific tool that was sophisticated enough to pick up some of the subtleties of the narratives that are the stuff of clinical reality.

The AAI was developed as an attempt to find an adult analogue of Mary Ainsworth's (1982) 'strange situation'. The 'when . . . then' of the 'strange situation' studies the response of one-year-old children to brief separation from their caregiver. Securely attached children protest on separation; on reunion, their protests are accepted, 'metabolized', and soothed by their caregiver (which includes the kinds of facial mirroring discussed above); they then return to exploratory play. Three patterns of insecure attachment are now recognized. *Insecure–avoidant* children protest little on separation, and on reunion with the caregiver hover nervously nearby; *insecure–ambivalent* children protest, but cannot be pacified when their caregiver returns, burying themselves in her lap or clinging furiously to her. The *insecure–disorganized* pattern was established after re-examination of videotapes of children who could not easily be classified as avoidant or ambivalent. These children show no coherent pattern of response, 'freezing' or collapsing to the ground, or leaning vacantly against a wall on reunion. In average populations about one-fifth of children are avoidant, one-sixth ambivalent, and one in 20 disorganized, although the proportion of the latter goes up dramatically in vulnerable groups, such as the socio-economically disadvantaged and where the mothers have been abused as children (Crittenden, 1988).

AAI is an audio-taped, semi-structured psychodynamic assessment session, whose aim is to 'surprise the unconscious' into revealing itself by asking detailed questions about relationships with parents and significant others, and about losses and separations and how the subject coped with them. Its system of categorization is similar to those developed for the 'strange situation'.

As a psychometric instrument, the AAI is original in that its scoring system is based not so much on content as on the form and structure of the subject's *narrative style*. Narratives are classified into one of four categories: 'secure–autonomous', 'insecure–dismissive', 'insecure–preoccupied', and 'disorganized' (or 'unresolved'). The key quality of *secure–autonomous* narratives is coherence: the subject is able to speak logically and concisely about their past and its vicissitudes, however problematic these may have been. *Insecure–dismissive* narratives (equivalent to avoidant attachment styles) are unelaborated and unrevealing: the subject may state that they have no memories of childhood before the age of 11, or that their parents were 'brilliant', without being able to amplify or produce relevant examples. By contrast, in *insecure–preoccupied* narratives (equivalent to ambivalent attachment styles) the subject appears bogged down in their history, telling rambling and inconclusive stories as though past pain was still alive today. The *unresolved* category is rated separately, co-existing with the others, and referring to points in a narrative where the logical flow is interrupted, broken, or disjointed. Main suggests that these narrative fractures may represent the emergence of previously repressed traumatic memories, and may be related clinically to dissociative states.

The AAI was developed within a theoretical framework that predicted that there would be connections between attachment experiences in childhood and narrative style in later life. This hypothesis has been supported by at least two sets of recent studies. First, Main and others have shown that, along with other measures looking at what I have called 'autobiographical competence' (Holmes, 1992), such as picture completion and 'tell-a-story' tasks, attachment patterns in infancy are remarkably predictive of adolescents' AAI status when measured some 15 years later (Benoit and Parker 1994). Fonagy *et al.* (1991) showed that the outcome of the AAI administered to prospective parents was a good predictor of attachment status of their subsequent one-year old children, 20 months later. Mothers with secure–autonomous narratives tended to have children who were secure in the 'strange situation', while dismissive parents tended to have insecure–avoidant infants.

Even more significantly, Fonagy *et al.* (1995) found that the capacity to think about oneself in relation to others—a capacity that he calls '*reflexive self-function*' (RSF)—is a key determinant of whether mothers whose own childhoods were traumatic will have infants who turn out to be insecure in the 'strange situation'. The capacity for RSF is a vital protection against psychological vulnerability in the face of environmental difficulty: an important finding for psychotherapists, since a large part of their work could be seen as enhancing RSF in their patients. Clearly, too, RSF is related to narrative competence: in order to tell a story about oneself in relation to others one has to be able to reflect on oneself—to see oneself, partially at least, from the outside—and this in turn depends on the experience of maternal mirroring.

Given their stability and predictive power it is reasonable to assume that attachment status and AAI classification are tapping into some meaningful psychological configuration. Attachment status seems to relate to patterns of parental handling in the first year of life, and is thus clearly an interpersonal phenomenon. Parental *responsiveness* to infant effect—of which the mirroring function is a central component—is a key determinant of secure attachment. In summary, environments may be *consistently responsive, consistently unresponsive*, or *inconsistently responsive*. Mothers of secure infants pick their babies up more quickly when they show signs of distress, play with them more, and generally seem more aware of them and their needs than the parents of insecure children. Parents of children who show the avoidant pattern are more brusque and functional in their handling, while parents of those who show the ambivalent reaction tend to be less attuned to their children's needs, often ignoring them when they are obviously distressed and intruding upon them when they are playing happily. The 'strange situation' measures the *enactment* of the child's relationship to her parents. The AAI by contrast defines individuals' *narrative account* of their experience—a movement from mechanism to meaning, from attachment behaviour to representation of attachments.

While attachment emerges from parental handling, narrative style has to do with individuals' relationship with themselves. Between the 'strange situation' and the AAI a process of internalization has taken place, which comprises an individual's awareness of themselves, their significant others, the relationships between them, and their awareness of, and ability to report on, these phenomena.

What then can we say about the origins of these kinds of awareness, and their relationship to security and insecurity? Here, Meares (1993) has developed an hypothesis based on what he calls 'self-narrative'. He starts from Winnicott's (1971) notion of the child's need to be able to play 'alone in the presence of the mother' if a stable 'true' (in attachment terms, secure) sense of self is to emerge. By providing a quiet background presence, the mother, in a typical Winnicottian paradox, enables the child to forget her, and to concentrate on the self-exploration that is the essence of solitary play. If, on the other hand, the mother is unavailable, or inconsistent, or unattuned, the child will be forced to think about his or her parent, and so be liable to develop a distorted representation of themselves.

Meares (1993) studied tape recordings of the type of speech used by 3–4-year-olds during this solitary play. Following Vygotsky (1962), he calls this 'inner speech', although at this particular stage in linguistic development it is audible, and therefore available for scientific study. Inner speech has specific features that differentiate it from social speech. Rather like Freud's (1911) contrast between primary and secondary processes, inner speech, unlike social speech, is disconnected and incomplete, words flowing into one another by association rather than following a logical progression. Audible 'inner speech' stops rather abruptly around 5–6-years-old. It is reasonable to speculate that self-awareness, which is so bound up with a sense of self, privacy, awareness of emotional truth and falsehood, and the ability to plan and to reflect on emotions, is a continuation of this play talk described by Meares.

What started as an interaction, shaped by the attachment dynamic, becomes internalized, so that the child now has within himself: (a) the vigilant yet non-intrusive maternal function; (b) the generative playful function; and (c) the capacity to put feelings into words. Acquiring inner speech means becoming intimate (to 'intimate' provides an etymological link between emotional proximity and communication) with oneself: knowledge of oneself goes hand in hand with knowledge of others. If required, the playing child can report on the goings on of the inner world: 'I was pretending the mummy had gone away and the baby was sad.' As an adult, perhaps during an AAI, they might be able to say: 'When my parents separated I used to pretend that my doll's mother had gone away and then returned.' Psychoanalytic psychotherapy recreates the childhood situation of being 'alone in the presence of another': 'free association' is, perhaps, none other than inner speech externalized once more.

The acquisition of inner speech is a developmental function. We can imagine how it could be disrupted in ways that might correspond with insecure patterns on the AAI. If the parent is unavailable, the child may be so concerned with maintaining proximity that he will be unable to play and so find his inner voice, leading to dismissive narratives and difficulty with intimacy. Preoccupied narratives may reflect unmetabolized pain that has not been transmuted into the metaphor of play: the sufferer is searching for a safe container and using whoever happens to be at hand for that purpose. If the parent has been intrusive the child's self-narrative may be contaminated with the parental narrative, always thinking and feeling what is expected rather than what might have emerged had more disinterested parenting been available. Finally, if the environment is traumatizing the whole 'containment/self-narrative' envelope may be obliterated, leaving lacunae and discontinuities in the texture of inner reality and its representation in inner speech.

These ideas can be linked with the notion of a child's 'theory of mind', as developed in the psychoanalytical literature by Fonagy *et al.* (1995), Leiman (1995), and Hobson (1993). Fonagy argues that traumatized children lack a 'theory of mind' in the sense that they have difficulty in seeing others as having feelings, intentions, and desires, any more than they can accurately define their own inner world.

Faced with aggressive or sexually intrusive parents, the normal process of 'secondary intersubjectivity' in which children share their experiences of the world with their caregivers via visual cueing, imitation, and so on, is inhibited. Leiman (1995) sees this in terms of inhibition of the normal mediating function of the parent, who, under favourable conditions, helps to create shared meanings in the transitional or interactive space between the child and their objects. To perpetrate cruelty, the abuser has to remove from their consciousness the knowledge that the child can experience fear, pain, disgust, and so on (the ultimate example of this is the abuser who then murders the victim in an attempt to obliterate mirroring altogether). The child grows up in a world in which their feelings, and meanings, are discounted or obliterated. At the same time the child is dependent on the abuser, and may indeed be strongly attached to them. There is often a vicious circle, based on the attachment dynamic, in which the more the child is traumatized, the more they cling to their attachment figure, who is thereby encouraged to perpetrate further abuse, and so on. The abused child is also likely to deny the existence of their abuser's mind, since not to do so would be to face the unacceptable fact that those one loves and on whom one depends have malevolent intentions towards one.

In summary, the findings of attachment research suggest that there may be objective criteria—coherence, succinctness, relevance, etc.—by which to evaluate the 'verisimilitude' of a clinical narrative. It also points to powerful links between the 'narrative truth' of the clinical situation and the 'historical truth' of the patient's actual biography.

The autobiographical self can be seen in terms of an inner object with which an individual has a relationship, comparable to 'external' relationships, which can be understood in terms of different attachment styles. At a clinical level, the psychological fluidity of the secure–autonomous individual can be contrasted with the relatively static (in psychoanalytical terms 'defended') positions of avoidant or ambivalent attachment.

Gergely and Watson's (1996) ideas suggest that there is a close relationship between the development of the self and secure attachment. 'Marking' enables one to distinguish one's own feelings from those of others, and is thus a bulwark against the excessive use of projective identification. Where 'marking' breaks down, which may be particularly the case in ambivalent attachment, the child may be unable to distinguish her feelings from those of the mother: 'Is it my feelings I am seeing myself in the mirror, or hers?'. Contingency is related to the 'truth' of one's feelings, helping one to ensure that there is a correspondence between an emotion and its representation. Here, avoidantly attached children may be especially vulnerable, since they have not had the wrappedness of attention that is needed for them to 'find' their feelings in the mother-mirror.

Those who are securely attached therefore can: (a) distinguish between their own experience and that of others; (b) represent and so tell the story of their feelings; and (c) have the capacity to break up their stories and reform them so they are more in keeping with the flux of experience. Ambivalent individuals are so close to their feelings that they cannot achieve the objectification—in White and Epston's (1990) terms, 'externalization', akin to Gergely and Watson's (1996) 'marking'—needed for a working story. Avoidant people, by contrast, cling to a stereotyped version of themselves and their past and feel threatened by the idea of the constantly updated narrative—again, in Gergely and Watson's terms, one that is checked for contingency—that is characteristic of creative living.

The linguistic triad and the triangles of psychotherapy

Patients seek help in a state of uncertainty and confusion. Something is 'wrong', but they do not know what this is, or what to do about it. Footsteps may have to be retraced: a story is needed which will both explain how they arrived where they are and point the way forward. Psycho-therapy, like art, 'holds a mirror up to nature'. The patient learns to put his or her feelings into words; these are then 'reflected back' by the therapist ('marking'); the patient then rechecks this reflection for its congruence/contingency/verisimilitude—whether it 'feels right'; finally a representation, or story is formed. In the remainder of this chapter I shall explore the formula: *raw experience plus meaning equals narrative*. The patient learns to build up a 'story-telling function' which takes experience from 'below', and in the light of overall meanings 'from above' (which can be seen themselves as stored or condensed stories) supplied by the therapist, fashions a new narrative about themself and their world.

This schema can be compared with the linguistic triad of signified, sign, and the lexicon from which the sign is drawn (Brockmeier, 1997). The sign is linked to the referent via the world of language. Similarly, a story is linked to what I am calling 'raw experience' via a world of meanings. It seems likely that the capacity to make this link is a developmental function, mediated by early attachment experience. The attuned mother responds to her infant's affective state, via identification, based on her *own* 'lexicon' of feelings (Fonagy's RSF). A 'story' is *offered* to the infant ('Oh you're feeling cold, bored, cross, wet, tired, hungry . . .' etc.) which in turn forms the germ of that *child's* RSF. If the caregiver is avoidant the range and complexity of the stories will be limited; if the caregiver is intrusive they will fail to match the child's experience. The caregiver does not just sooth the infant, they also *symbolize* the soothing process. In later life the child in whom this has failed may lack both the capacity for self-soothing, (so characteristic of border-line patients) and the ability to talk about, or symbolize their distress. Here we have a model for trangeneration transmission of psychopathology, and a picture of how psychotherapy might help break that cycle.

Narrative in clinical practice

How does the psychotherapist function as an 'assistant autobiographer'? In this concluding section I shall consider some ways in which the narrative principles so far elaborated impinge on the psychotherapeutic process.

Narrative as a therapeutic technique

The first task of the therapist is to assist the patient to tell their story. The starting point will be some form of distress: something is not right, things have gone wrong, the sufferer is not as they would like themselves to be. Desires have been thwarted, or hopes dashed. The attachment research outlined above suggests that secure attachment is marked by coherent stories that convince and hang together, where detail and overall plot are congruent, and where the teller is not so detached that affect is absent, is not dissociated from the content of the story, nor is so overwhelmed that feelings flow formlessly into every crevice of the dialogue. Insecure attachment, by contrast, is characterized either by stories that are overelaborated and enmeshed (un'- marked'), or by dismissive, poorly fleshed-out accounts, that lack contingency testing. In one it is barely possible to discern a coherent story at all; in the other the story is so schematic or vague that it lacks the detail upon which verisimilitude depends.

Starting with the assessment interview, the therapist will use their narrative competence to help the patient shape the story into a more coherent pattern. With an enmeshed patient the therapist will introduce frequent 'shaping' remarks or punctuations such as: 'We'll come back to what happened to you as a child in a minute; first let's hear more about what is troubling you right now. . .'. Note the 'We'll. . .', 'Let's. . .' construction in which therapist and patient are brought into an unitary position as joint students of the story. This is the beginnings of objectification, but also a model for an internal observing ego (or self-reflexive self) that can listen to and modulate feelings. Shaping a story is the narrative version of the modulation and responsiveness of the security-transmitting caregiver.

With a dismissive patient the therapist will elicit narrative in a different way, always searching for detailed images, memories and examples that bring perfunctory stories to life. 'What was your mother like. . .?'; 'Can you remember an incident that illustrates that. . .?'; 'When did you first start to feel so miserable. . .?'; 'When you say you feel depressed, what does that feel like. . .?'; 'Whereabouts in your body do you experience your unhappiness. . .?'.

In both cases, the therapist offers intermittent summarizing or 'marking' remarks, which serve to demarcate 'the story so far', and to confront the patient with a narrative construction against which to measure the raw material of their experience. Some of these comments may be purely, yet pointedly, descriptive: 'When you were talking about your relationship with your husband you appeared to be apathetic and defeated, yet when you started to tell me about your children you become quite animated!' Others will be more general and overarching: 'You seem to be confident about your relationships with women, including your mother and girlfriends, but to feel much more uncertain when you come to speak about men. . .'. These kinds of intervention would perhaps be classified as 'pre-interpretations', yet by translating a shared experience into verbal form they *are* interpretative in the sense of carrying over experience in one medium ('raw experience', affect) into another (words, narrative conventions). Here again we find a variant of the semiotic triad of signified, sign, and language.

As therapy proceeds the shaping process becomes less obvious, and is probably most evident in the therapist's rythms of activity and silence, the balance between verbal interventions and 'mmm. . .'s, grunts, and indrawn breaths. Like an attuned parent, the effective therapist will intutively sense when the patient needs stimulus and direction to keep the thread of narrative alive, and when they need to be left alone to explore their feelings without intrusion or control. Sometimes, especially when the therapy feels stuck, the therapist may simply describe, or tell the story of what has happened, either in a particular session or a sequence of sessions: 'You started off today seeming rather sad, and finding it hard to focus, then you began to talk about how difficult you always find Christmas, then you mentioned your friend's aunt who died suddenly. . . .' This story may well provoke a realization, or moment of insight such as: 'Oh . . . it was Christmas when my grandmother died, I always feel a bit down at this time of year. . .maybe that is why. . . .' This will mark the end of this narrative sequence; the narrative is dispersed [or 'cracked up', in Bollas' (1995) terms], mingled with new experience, until a new narrative sequence emerges.

In psychoanalytical psychotherapy the transference becomes a 'meta-story' which shapes the overall therapeutic interaction. Each session consists of a number of narrative episodes: what happened on the way to the session, an argument at work, something that happened with a partner, a memory from childhood, and so on. Luborsky (1984) has shown that most therapy sessions contain roughly three such episodes. Let us say the patient starts the session before a holiday break by talking about an incident at work in which his boss asked him to do a job, but without showing him clearly how it was to be carried out. The therapist might comment: 'There seems to be a story here about being left to fend for yourself without proper support. . . .' This might then prompt the patient to talk about how his parents left him in charge of his younger brother without explanation, and how frightened and angry he felt about this. This in turn may lead to a sudden realization about how upset he is about the coming break. A core story is emerging about abandonment and the response it evokes.

Implicit in my argument so far is the view that psychological health (closely linked to secure attachment) depends on a dialectic between story-making and story-breaking, between the capacity to form narrative, and to disperse it in the light of new experience. In Main's (1995) evocative phrase, the securely attached child shows a 'fluidity of attentional gaze', and in adult life narrative capacity similarly moves between fluidity and form, between structure and 'destructuring', construction and deconstruction. This capacity ultimately depends on being able to trust both intimacy and aggression (Holmes, 1996a), which form the basis of much psychotherapeutic work. Intimacy provides the closeness needed if meaning and experience are to be woven into narrative; trusting one's aggression enables these stories to be broken up and allowed to reform into new patterns. The attachment perspective I have adopted suggests three prototypical pathologies of narrative capacity: clinging to rigid stories; being overwhelmed by unstoried experience; or being unable to find a narrative strong enough to contain traumatic pain.

Nodal memories: deconstruction dismissive narratives

Just as language is infinite but based on a finite number of simple grammatical rules, so, despite the potentially limitless capacity of memory, most people have a small number of prototypical memories that epitomize their fundamental relationship to others and to the world. These often concern important transition points in their life history—the birth of a sibling, a first day at school, and so on. They might be called 'nodal memories' in the sense that they represent a concentration of the assumptions, fantasies, or working models about the self in relation to others. They may be actual or imagined. The subject usually 'reads' a particular meaning into them which acts as an organizing principle around which they organize their present-day experience.

One patient learned that she had been left in her cot for five hours after her birth: in her mind this represented (and explained) all her subsequent feelings of cut-offness and rage about being abandoned by lovers, friends, etc. Another dreamed that he was standing at the door of the flat in which he had grown up, with his mother holding his testicles: 'There you are', he would say 'they've got you by the balls.' A third focused all his feelings of being intruded upon by his mother, and lack of recognition for his achievements by his father, on his circumcision as a baby. Countless examples could be enumerated: the woman who had a terrible row with her mother the night before she died of a heart attack, and continued to blame and punish herself with depression thereafter; the young man thrown out of the house by his father whom he claimed dominated family life with his bad temperedness.

In the process of psychotherapy these nodal memories become reworked. First, they have to be unpacked—'cracked up' in Bollas' (1995) terms—and then reassembled, taking on a new perspective. The woman in the cot came to see that her mother was simply following the child-rearing fashions of the day, and that her furious attempts to be self-sufficient—to mother herself—had cut her off from the good things her mother did have to offer. The testicle dream became transformed into an image of a mother trying to protect her son from the harshness of the outside world. The same man had another dream which was simply an image of the post office tower: 'I suppose that's a phallic symbol', he said glibly. But what really seemed to fit was the tower as a symbol of communication, a way of linking with others which this lonely man so desperately craved.

The man who so resented his circumcision, now a successful test-pilot, came to see how his phallic prowess and fear of having his wings clipped flowed from his longing for a father to whom he could get access (the father had abandoned the family when the patient was 15) and who would see him as an equal. The depressed woman whose mother had died came to see her self-blame as a desperate wish that she could have at least some control over her fate, however painful. Finally, the man who rowed with his father saw how he might have provoked the argument in order to stimulate his normally conciliatory father to be more authoritative.

In each case the patient comes to see that there are many versions of the same story. Therapy provides an opportunity for the subject to begin to see himself from the outside; to forgive parents as well as to blame them; to see and own his contribution to circumstances, rather than viewing himself as a helpless victim; and to recognize that there are occasions in which fate deals us cards over which we have no control.

Example 3: changing the narrative context of memory

Dave was in his middle 50s when he suffered from a prolonged depression triggered by being made redundant from the firm in which he had worked his way up from the shop floor to be factory manager. His father had died in the war when he was two, and his widowed mother struggled to make ends meet for herself and her two children. He had always tried to be a 'good' boy, to help his mother, had worked hard, and was an indefatigable servant of his employers as well as father-figure to those who worked under him. In his depression he alternated between attacking himself for his failure to prevent the firm from going into receivership, and violently attacking his bosses for their financial mismanagement. In one typical state-dependent moment of recall he vividly and guiltily remembered an incident from childhood in which he had been at the cinema with some other boys. One of them proudly produced a half-crown which he stated that his Dad, whom he claimed was 'very rich', had given him—and then accidentally dropped it. Dave immediately offered to help him retrieve it, which he did, whereupon he walked out of the cinema with the money in his pocket. Fifty years later this scrupulously honest man was still berating himself for this callous act of theft. When the therapist gently suggested that perhaps he had felt that he, as a fatherless child, was entitled to purloin the money that this boastful son's father had given him, there was a sudden shift in the session as tears came to Dave's eyes. A new *context* for his depressive, guilt-laden, story had been created, one which encompassed his pain as well as his crime.

'Negative capability' and ambivalent narratives

This chapter began by contrasting the security of narrative prose with the poetic impulse to make contact with the 'thing itself', suggesting that psychological health might depend on a balance between these opposing psychic tendencies. The prosaic structure of narrative contains, reassures, sooths—but may also constrain, control, and distort. Lyric poetry can be a liberation from story, enabling us to see the world with fresh eyes, but its capacity to fragment meaning takes us dangerously close to the limits of understanding. In the previous section we saw how, starting from nodal memories, psychotherapy can help break up stories and so broaden the range of admissible experience. Equally, there is often a need to find ways of capturing the confusion and vagaries of overwhelming feelings.

Here Keats' 'negative capability'—the 'ability to remain in doubts, uncertainties and mysteries'—is vital. The therapist has both to be able to tolerate confusion, while trusting that a meaningful pattern will eventually emerge.

Example 4: finding a narrative thread

Naomi's sessions were confused and rambling, moving rapidly from topic to topic and from past to present and back again. She was tearful for much of the time, and seemed to 'flop' into her chair, gazing imploringly at her therapist, without ever clearly stating what was wrong or what she wanted. She 'didn't know why she had come . . . she had had a bad week . . . lots of worries about her 15-year old son who was getting nowhere at his school . . . it all started when she discovered that a friend had also been raped by the same man who had raped her when she was 17. . .her mother was dying then so she couldn't tell her or her father, they had too much to worry about . . . with two small kids and a new husband it's difficult to find time to talk . . . she met her first husband almost immediately after her mother's death . . . it was a relief to get away, the atmosphere was so sad . . . it was odd when her father remarried after her mother died, she couldn't get used to him holding hands with a new woman. . . .'

Gradually piecing together the story of the rape and her mother's illness seemed to help. She had left home at 16 after many rows with her mother and was working as a nanny. When her mother became ill she was expected to return home to look after the house. The rape happened on the way back from a party with a man she hardly knew. She described it in graphic detail. She arrived home. Her father called out: 'Alright?', as he always did. She could not bring herself to tell him, he was so worried about her mother. All this was 20 years ago, but it seemed like yesterday, she was not much older than her son is now. He is so difficult to talk to. Now things began to fall into place. The therapist commented: 'You did not talk to your mother, just rowed, and then she died; you could not burden your father; now you worry about your son, but can't talk to him; in coming for help you are looking for someone who will listen to the story you kept to yourself all those years ago.' 'I did tell my doctor—but he told me to forget about it, he wasn't much good, he committed suicide in the end.' Now at last a pattern was emerging—of painful feelings of loss and worry, of wanting help but never quite trusting it, of clinging on with words—the long rambling stories at least mean someone is there, even if they can't really hear what is said. The therapist mused: 'Perhaps you are wondering if I will be able to take it, or whether I will get angry, and let you down like the others, whether I am *really* prepared to listen to how distressed you are.'

Here there was a movement, from fragmentary and often poetic feelings, images, and themes, through a period of confusion, to a resolution in which a more solid interpretative story or pattern emerged. This is a familiar pattern with enmeshed narratives. The session starts with laying out the jigsaw pieces; an edge or container is formed; then images begin to come together—here a cloud formation, there a face; finally, there is a rapid period in which the pieces fall into place and the full picture appears at last.

Stories in search of a voice: working with trauma

The attachment framework I have adopted in this paper suggests four patterns of narrative styles in psychotherapy practice: secure, coherent; avoidant; ambivalent or enmeshed; and finally, trauma-organized narratives, often revealed by incoherence and fractures in an apparently smooth narrative envelope.

In the case above, Naomi had been traumatized by the rape, but she was able to talk about it to some extent, and with a little prompting could give a detailed and convincing account of what happened. For others, memories of traumatic events are associated with such unpleasant emotions that they are avoided in a phobic way. At the extreme of this is traumatic amnesia or repression. There is evidence that in these situations memory for trauma is organized differently from 'normal' memory. The subject will recall images, or physical sensations but not a coherent sequence of events. If they are asked to recall the trauma during neuroimaging there is activity in parietal regions of the non-dominant hemisphere (Van de Kolk and Fisler, 1996), while normal memories evoke dominant hemisphere activity. This suggests that traumatic memories have not been processed into a verbal, narrative, form, but remain in a 'raw' primary process state.

Trauma breaks through (or 'pierces', the etymological origin of the word) the self–other dialogue that underpins thought and language. The narrative self, is obliterated, and all that remains are dissociated images and sensations. When it is a caregiver who is responsible for the trauma, then this likelihood is increased since, as argued earlier, the perpetrator is the very individual whose responsibility is to help with the process of symbolization and soothing.

Feelings of shame, typical of trauma survival, are an elaborated version of this: the sufferer is an outcast, unworthy of attachment, rejected of men. Basic trust has broken down. Therapy can help, but often with extreme difficulty. The sufferer has to feel sufficiently held to risk the extreme emotional pain that may be associated with recall of the trauma. Some means of symbolizing or mirroring raw experience is required—often poetry, drawings or guided fantasy are first steps towards the elaboration of a coherent narrative of the trauma. The therapist becomes witness, but how can he or she, possibly grasp the unthinkable? The therapist stands for the part of the victims' self that could not bear to look at what was being done to them. By revealing the story to themselves the victims fear they will become enmeshed in the story, unable to escape.

Previous narrative defenses, such as psychic numbing, dissociation of feelings from story, selective forgetting, or even fragmentation of personality will be challenged as a more coherent and often unbearably painful account emerges, but one that seems to correspond more closely with experience.

Thus, trauma victims are often initially avoidant, and later become potentially trapped by their story. Turning trauma into narrative in therapy requires a sequential process, starting with the overcoming of avoidance by imagery, and later moving to a more objective, distanced position where the victim can identify with the therapist's benign concern. The fact that minor aspects of trauma can be played out symbolically in the transference helps with this process, since it becomes shared, and therefore potentially narratable (see the example below).

The role of the therapist

Working with traumatized patients tests not just the skills of therapists but also their personal strengths. Their moral maturity will be exposed, especially their ability both to use their own feelings in the service of the therapy, without allowing them to direct, dominate, or intrude upon the patient. Williams and Waddell (1991) traces the evolution of George Eliot's sensibility from the early novels, which, she argues 'suffer from an intrusive imposition of self, a persistence of personal elements that block her creative vitality', to her mature novels, which

> seem to produce a force and refinement of writing which is wholly distinct from that which seeks to express aspects of character which are superficially much nearer to her own experience in the sense of personal longings and aspirations. The danger *then* . . . is the imposition of feeling from the outside, resulting in sentimentality and pseudo-emotion. The emotional space necessary to, and produced by, that distinctness invites an identification on the part of the reader with . . . the inner qualities and characteristics of the object rather than the external and more available ones.

A similar maturity would be a goal for therapists who will inevitably draw on their own experience and preoccupations in their identification with patients, but at the same time have to find a distance—Waddell's 'distinctness'—that enables them to allow the patient's imagination to flourish, unimpeded by control or manipulation. Thus the therapist's attachment style, and *pari passu* their narrative style will be an all-important element in determining the outcome of therapy. Enmeshed therapists tend to impose their own narrative on patients, or get bogged down in interminable stories that have no end, while those with avoidant styles may fail to pick up on vital emotional cues, and jump to unwarranted conclusions. The therapist's task is to be attuned while retaining balance, a position I have called 'non-attachment' (Holmes, 1996a), as the following concluding anecdote tries to illustrate.

Example 5: non-attachment as trauma narrative emerges

After more than a year in weekly psychotherapy, Dave, already mentioned in example 3, revealed with intense shame that he had been at approved school in his late teens. He then said that he had been admitted to psychiatric hospital around that time, a fact he had only vaguely alluded to before. Then he spoke of the circumstances leading up to the admission. It seemed that he had doused some rags in petrol, wound them round his legs and set fire to them. As he spoke of this the therapist sat silently, rapt with attention, picturing vividly this now ponderous silver haired man in late middle age as a 17-year old. There was still a mystery to unfold. How did it all hang together? What 'made him do it'? Dave spoke of his naval school, to which, as a bright naval rating's orphan he had a scholarship, and the contrast between his schoolmates' parents who appeared on speech day in their officers's regalia, while his mother and step-father never came (they could not afford the train fares), and if they had would have shamed him with their shabbiness; of his envy and contempt for these well heeled lads who had no inkling what it was to suffer.

All this seemed relevant to his feelings about his 'posh-accented' therapist, to whom he was strongly attached, and yet could not fully trust. This too was sensed 'impersonally' by the therapist—he could *feel* the hostility, the longing, the envy, the dependency, but in an objective way that seemed to have little to do with him as a person. At this intense moment *he* did not exist; he was a projection of his patient's inner world, and yet at that moment felt intensely alive and very much himself. Then Dave made the missing connection: one of the staff at the approved school was sexually abusing the boys in return for cigarettes, and had made advances to Dave. He was deeply ashamed about this coersive propositioning which touched his longing for closeness (still speaking of his never-known dead father as if he were a close companion), his anger at the abuse of that craving, his embarrassment and confusion. This was what had led up to the episode of self-harm. As he listened, the therapist felt the story almost as if it were happening to him, yet impersonally—both fully involved and at the same time watching, observing, still able to protect the boundary of the session, both for himself and the patient.

This is an inadequate attempt to capture an intense moment in therapy—moments that occur regularly but infrequently. Perhaps, in the end, this is what therapy is *about*: the emergence of a story that is both intensely felt (captures 'raw experience') and has an objective validity (congruence, contingency, verisimilitude). The therapist's specific contribution to this process is as witness, holder of the narrative boundary, 'subjective-object' (in Winnicott's terms), facilitator, and one who is able both to loose himself and remain true to himself in the process. Winnicott writes of the importance of 'bringing the trauma into the area of omnipotence' (Winnicott, 1971; Bateman and Holmes 1995). In the transference the therapist becomes both the longed for and the abusive object—but because transferentially rather than actually so, one that is potentially transformational. Dave's therapist was responsible for creating a dependency, and with that the hope that, at last, Dave would have the enduring inner object, the missing father, he so longed for. At the same time that hope was constantly ('sadistically') dashed by the realization that his father *could* never come back to life again.

Conclusion

Such moments of insight, however significant, can never be points of arrival. Each story is there to be revised in the light of new experience, new facets of memory, new meanings. In this chapter I have tried to bring to life the cycle of narrative construction and deconstruction that I believe is central to the therapeutic process. I have argued that narrative has its psychobiological origins in the 'marking' and contingency of maternal mirroring. I have traced the links between infant attachment patterns and adult narrative styles. I have tried to show how, in psychotherapy, the therapist shapes the patient's story-telling and mirrors their affective experience in a way that leads to a more secure sense of self. My concluding hope is that some fragments of this story will coalesce in the mind of the reader to form the building blocks for more tales, as yet untold.

References

Ainsworth, M. (1982). Attachment: retrospect and prospect. In *The place of attachment in human behaviour*, (ed. C.M. Parkes and J. Sevenson-Hinde). Routledge, London.

Bateman, A. and Holmes (1995). London: Routledge.

Benoit, D. and Parker, K. (1994). Stability and transmission of attachment across three generations. *Child Development*, **65**, 1444–56.

Bollas, C. (1995). *Cracking up*. Routledge, London.

Brockmeier, J. (1997). Autobiography, narrative, and the Freudian conception of life history. *Philosophy, Psychiatry, Psychology*, *4(3)* 175–200.

Bruner, J. (1986). *Actual minds, possible worlds*. Harvard University Press, Cambridge.

Crittenden, P. (1988). Relationships at risk. In *Clinical Implications of Attachment* (eds. J. Belsky and T. Nezworsky.) Erlbaum, New York.

Fonagy, P., Steele, M., Steele, H., and Leigh, T. (1995). Attachment the reflective self, and borderline states: the predictive specificity of the adult attachment interview and pathological emotional development. In *Attachment theory: social, developmental and clinical significance*, (ed. S. Goldberg, R. Muir, and J. Kerr). Analytic Press, Hillsdale.

Fonagy, P., Steele, M., and Steele, H. (1991). The capacity for understanding mental states: the reflective self in parent and child and its significance for security of attachment. *Infant Mental Health Journal*, **12**, 201–18.

Freud, S. (1911). Formulations on the two principles of mental functioning. *Standard Edition*, **12**, 215–17.

Gergely, G. and Watson, J. (1996). The social biofeedback theory of parental affect-mirroring. *International Journal of Psycho Analysis*, **77**, 1181–212.

Holmes J. (1992). *Between Art and Science: essays in psychotherapy and psychiatry*, Routledge, London.

Hobson, P. (1993). *Autism and the development of mind*. Erlbaum, Hillsdale.

Holmes, J. (1993). *John Bowlby and attachment theory*. Routledge, London.

Holmes, J. (1996a). *Attachment, intimacy, autonomy: using attachment theory in adult psychotherapy*. Jason Aronson, New York.

Holmes, J. (1996b). Psychotherapy and memory: an attachment perspective. *British Journal of Psychotherapy*, **13**, 204–18.

Holmes, J. and Lindley R. (1997). *The values of psychotherapy*. Karnac, London.

Howard, G. (1991). Culture tales: a narrative approach to thinking, cross-cultural psychology and psychotherapy. *American Psychologist*, **46**, 187–97.

Leiman, M. (1995). Early developments. In *Cognitive analytic therapy: developments in theory and practice*, (ed. A. Ryle). Wiley, Chichester.

Luborsky, L. (1984). *Principles of psychoanalytic psychotherapy*. Basic Books, New York.

Main, M. (1995). Recent studies of attachment: overview with selected implications for clinical work. In *Attachment theory: social, developmental and clinical perspectives*, (ed. S. Goldberg, R. Muir, and J. Kerr). Analytic Press, Hillsdale.

Meares, R. (1993). *The metaphor of play*. Jason Aronson, New York.

Schafer, R. (1992). *Retelling a life: narration and dialogue in psychoanalysis.* Basic Books, New York.

Spence, D. (1982). *Narrative truth and historical truth: meaning and interpretation in psycho-analysis.* Norton, New York.

Van de Kolk, B. and Fisler, R. (1996). Dissociation and the fragmentary nature of traumatic memories: overview. *British Journal of Psychotherapy,* **12**, 352–61.

Vygotsky, L. (1962). *Thought and language.* MIT Press, Cambridge.

White, M. and Epston, D. (1990). *Narrative means to therapeutic ends.* Norton, New York.

Williams, M., and Wadell, M. (1991). *The chamber of maiden thought.* Routledge, London.

Winnicott, D. (1967). Mirror-role of mother and family in child development. In *The predicament of the family,* (ed. P. Lomas). Hogarth, London.

Winnicott, D. (1971). *Playing and reality,* Penguin, London.

II Middles

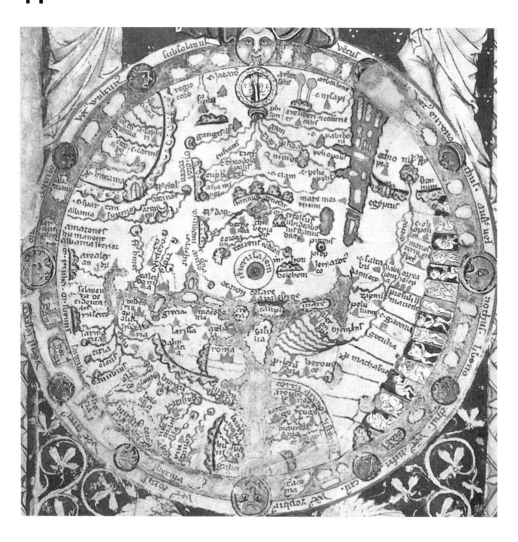

4 Gender Issues: Freudian and feminist stories

Janet Sayers

Freud notoriously narrated both sexes' psychology in terms of the male-centred myths of Oedipus and Narcissus. He rejected the suggestion that women's psychology might be better encompassed by the female-centred myth of Elektra. And he tended to focus on individual and intrapsychic issues to the relative neglect of interrelational and interpersonal issues now recognized by post-Freudian and feminist theorists to be crucial in shaping our adult lives and loves.

In this chapter, I seek to highlight the latter issues, and the rather different stories women and men often tell about themselves, with examples from culturally shared myths; published autobiography and fiction; dream stories anonymously written by pupils attending two parallel, single-sex, state secondary schools; and from the stories patients have told me in therapy.

I will argue that these narratives are means by which women and men defensively (in Freud's terms) or adaptively (in Jung's terms) seek to negotiate their closeness with others. I will also argue that, to the extent that these narratives fail in their defensive or adaptive function and contribute to the ills bringing women and men to therapy, therapy entails 'life-story elaboration, adjustment, or repair' (Howard, 1991, p. 194). It entails elaborating and undoing the patient's story, as Freud encouraged his patients to elaborate and undo their dreams (Holmes, this volume), so as to adjust and repair not so much divisions within the self, as Freud sought to do in helping his patients become conscious of the unconsious, as divisions in the patients' relationships with others as they surface in relation to their therapists in therapy.

Since Freud less often told women's stories, I will devote more space to them. I will begin, however, with men's stories.

Divided selves

Men often tell stories of being divided selves, which they link with memories of early separation from, and longing for, their absent mothers. A case in point is the narrator in Proust's autobiographical novel, *Remembrance of things past*, who again and again returns to just such memories in exploring the subsequent division in himself between his childhood and adolescent self.

Others dwell more on the 'Boys don't cry!' imperative stopping them expressing their upset at being separated from their mothers. They attribute to this factor their early suppression of, and division from knowing about, the tears and upset they might otherwise express, talk about, and share with others.

Freud described both sexes' psychology in these terms. He dwelt on the baby's early pleasure in breast-feeding. He claimed that the longing of both sexes to recapitulate this togetherness with the mother in her absence lies at the heart of the dream stories we tell ourselves each night. He wrote of the clash between the reality of the mother's separateness and the baby's wishful fantasy of being with her as primary cause of the repression of this fantasy into the unconscious. Herein, Freud (for example, Freud 1900) argued, lies the source of the division of the self into the reality-oriented conscious and wishful-thinking unconscious mind.

He added that children are yet further divided from consciousness of their longing for their mothers, at least in the case of boys, by fear lest realization of this longing be punished with loss of their penis (see, for example, Freud, 1923). He likened children in this respect to Oedipus, punished with loss of his sight for killing his father and having sex with his mother.

Feminists tell a somewhat different story. They prioritize our closeness with others, in the first place in mothering and being mothered. They draw attention to the pressure put on boys to separate themselves from early closeness with their mothers in the interests of forging a separate male identity (see Chodorow, 1978).

Certainly men often begin the tales of their lives with memories of just such separation, and of pressure to negate the feelings involved in the name of proving themselves to be manly, tough, and strong. In his autobiography, the psychoanalyst, Wilfred Bion, for instance, writes of being sent away from his mother and family in India to boarding school in England when he was eight. He reports the following conversation greeting him in his prep school dorm

> 'What's the matter?' asked one of the three boys . . . 'I don't know,' I wailed . . . 'Are you homesick?'
> 'Yes.' At once I realised what an awful thing I had done. 'No, B,' I hurriedly said
> (*Bion, 1986, p. 34*)

He adds, 'As my powers of deception grew I learned to weep silently.'

In her recent novel, *The Ghost Road*, Pat Barker, graphically illustrates the ill-effects on men of their 'silent' and suppressed weeping through the story she tells of the work of the psychiatrist W. H. R. Rivers in treating shell-shocked officers in the First World War. She reiterates Rivers' attribution of his patients' recurring nightmares to their having been trained at boarding school to suppress their feelings, and 'to meet without any manifestation of fear any occasion likely to call forth this emotion' (Rivers, 1920, p. 209).

She describes how, having thus learnt to repress and divide themselves from the fear and upset they experienced in the trenches, these feelings could only return when, falling asleep, their repression was temporarily relaxed. Hence the recurring nightmares constituting their 'war neurosis'. Hence too Rivers' tactic of seeking to free his patients from their night-time terrors by encouraging them consciously to share with him the otherwise repressed and unconscious feelings haunting their dreams. Barker writes:

> Every day of his [Rivers'] working life he looked at twitching mouths that had once been clenched. Go on, he said, though rarely in so many words, cry. It's all right to grieve.
> (*Barker, 1995, p. 96*)

Just as Barker, like Rivers, attributes the nightmares suffered by shell-shocked First World War officers to their early dividing themselves from expressing or even consciously knowing about their fears, Freud (1920) likened the recurrent nightmares of First World War soldiers to a game his 18-month-old grandson devised to master his anxiety at being separated from his mother.

Perhaps it is the continuing pressure on boys to master and repress their feelings about being separated from their mothers that accounts for young men today suffering recurring nightmares of maternal separation, akin to the nightmares suffered by soldiers in the First World War. Several boys in the above-mentioned secondary school study, but no girls, reported just such scenarios. A 17-year-old, for instance, wrote:

> I used to have a dream about being separated from my mother as she was taking me to school. There was always a very strong sense of loss in this dream—it was particularly vivid, and . . . frightening . . . [and] reoccurred very frequently for some time.

Unlike the girls, boys also reported repeated nightmares of explosions—of 'fire blazing across killing everyone', of bombs blowing up, of 'alien laser ships . . . vaporising people'. More often than the girls, they also recalled nightmares of being on their own—without their parents, friends, or anyone else they knew—and of being threatened and pursued in their isolation by uncontained, indefinite, impersonal, and unknown forces, animals, monsters, or by stereotyped cartoon, film, and video characters.

This difference in girls' and boys' nightmares can be understood in terms of post-Freudian theories regarding the importance to children of not being separated from their mothers. Perhaps mindful of the effect of being sent away from his mother to boarding school when he was seven, the Freudian analyst, John Bowlby (like other contributors to this volume; see, for example Holmes, Chapter 3), emphasized the importance to the child of experiencing 'a warm, intimate, and continuous relationship with his mother' (Bowlby, 1953, p. 13).

Similarly, Bion (1962), perhaps also mindful of the untoward effects of his early separation from his mother, stressed the importance of children's ongoing closeness with their mothers. He implied that this is necessary if the mother is to be affected by, take in, digest, and contain her child's projected feelings. Only then, he wrote, can the child repossess his feelings, not as monstrous and explosive (as in the above-quoted secondary school boys' dreams), but as containable and contained.

True, Bion was writing about babies and toddlers. But his emphasis on ongoing closeness with others surely also applies, even if only to a lesser degree, to older children? Yet boys, beyond earliest infancy, are often denied the continuing maternal closeness necessary, according to Bion, to their experiencing their feelings as containable and contained. The result, paradoxically, is that—having separated early from their mothers and from the feelings involved in the name of becoming manly and self-contained—many experience their feelings about the adolescent changes involved in becoming men as unmanly and uncontained. Hence, arguably, the frequency with which men, more often than women, tell 'out of body' stories (see Gergen and Gergen, 1993), of self-conscious division between their contained and uncontained bodies and minds. A 17-year-old in my secondary school study, for instance, wrote of this division:

> When I was five . . . I dreamt that I was asleep and standing by my self watching me sleep. Speech bubbles appeared. They said 'IS THIS ME?' At this stage the person who said the above woke up and was standing by another 'me' asleep. Again the 'This is me' reappeared . . . until I (real me) woke up! . . . *GROOVY!*

The Freudian analyst, Moses Laufer (for example, Laufer, 1989), attributes the adolescent's self-depiction as divided between his body and mind to an intrapsychic factor—to his being divided internally, like Oedipus, between wanting and not wanting incest. By contrast, the so-called 'anti-psychiatrist', Ronnie Laing (1959) attributed this mind–body split, at least as it occurs in schizophrenia, to an interpersonal factor.

Laing argued, in effect, that the schizophrenic tells himself a story of being divided between his mind and body to defend himself against the intrusion of his parents' annihilating indifference to, or hatred of, him. By telling himself he is divided from his body—from what his parents and others see and hear him say and do—the schizophrenic, wrote Laing, seeks to preserve his unembodied 'true self' from contaminating closeness with others. Often, Laing noted, it is the collapse of this precarious story—the dread of the inner self being invaded by their outer 'false self'—that causes divided self patients to seek help.

Faced with collapse of their divided self stories as defence against destructive closeness with others, Laing concluded, the answer lies in addressing such patients' dread of others' intrusion. It also means addressing their dread of being overwhelmed by envy of, and longing for, emotional closeness with others, as these anxieties arise in therapy.

Laing illustrated his claims with several examples. One involved an 18-year-old who recounted his divided self story in terms of being a man on the inside and a woman like his mother on the outside. Simon, a 19-year-old modern languages student, who I saw in NHS therapy, told a similar story.

Example 1: divided self

Simon was referred for therapy following his hospitalization after an attempt to kill himself. He began, like many of Laing's patients, by telling me about his mother's indifference to him, and frequent absence from his life. Her indifference included not believing him when he told her a man in the train had grabbed him, pulled his head back, and blown into his mouth, leaving his intrusive stink inside him.

Most of all, however, Simon complained of his father's hostile intrusiveness. He recalled his father calling him an 'alien', and 'the black sheep of the family'. He recalled him clubbing together with Simon's sister to castigate him as 'schizophrenic'.

It was to defend himself against his family's annihilating hostility and indifference that Simon depicted himself as a divided self. Or, as he later put it, 'I wanted to hide the real me behind something else'.

On the one hand he felt he was indeed the hated, alien figure his father took him to be. He remembered himself, aged 12 or 13, going home from school with his younger sister and encouraging her to go to a sweetshop with a stranger who had been courting them, only to feel he was the same as this stranger when, no sooner had he taken Simon's sister to the sweetshop, than he started abusing her. Simon felt he too was an abuser, paedophile, and rapist, not least because he had several times gone along with his brother's invitation to have sex with him.

On the other hand, he cultivated a contrary image of himself as a young woman—akin perhaps to the dead baby girl his mother had born his father and whom his father still grieved from early in their relationship together. Simon imagined himself being made love to as a beautiful young woman by another beautiful young woman. That was why he stole women's underclothes. Wearing them gave him sexual satisfaction. But he also hated himself on this account. Hence his suicide attempt.

He hated his sexual, bodily self. But he loved his intellectual, rational self. He regaled me with his near-perfect achievements at school. Now, however, he worried that he could not keep his body and mind divided. He worried that his bodily impulse to wear women's clothes had damaged his brain. He was convinced that a lump on his head was an effect of the bones of his skull being fed by excess sex hormones.

He had been to see his GP about it. But his doctor was no more understanding of him than his father. Simon could no more talk about his feelings with him than he could with his father or anyone else. His doctor would not tell him honestly what was wrong with him. He regarded him as a 'pest'. He was evidently discomfitted by being with Simon just as Simon's father was discomfitted by his attempts to share his feelings with him.

He complained he could not communicate with his fellow-students. Nor could he share his feelings with his lecturers. He had tried. But, like his mother, they did not believe what he said. They laughed at him behind his back. They treated him as beyond the pale.

If only he could establish the closeness he wanted with me, free of the division between being a hated man and loved girl—the division he portrayed as legacy of his parents' destructive indifference to, and hatred of him. He signalled his longing to be close, and for me to recognize his worth, by bringing a school photo of himself, aged 8, presenting his work—a beautifully detailed poem, quirkily about a poisonous snake—to a visiting dignitary, well known for her motherliness.

But he was also inhibited from talking about his feelings with me, just as he was inhibited about talking about them with others. Instead, he often wrote long letters to me about his feelings, especially about his hated, sexual self; his suicidal self-loathing at giving way to his urge to wear women's clothes; his rapacious, murderous thoughts about women and children; and about his attempt, aged 11 or 12, to kill and punish himself for stealing his father's typewriter and outdoing him as a poet in composing verses that had earlier won him the motherly dignitary's approval at school.

He felt diffident about confiding in me. He felt embarrassed being with me. He left sessions early. Later he wrote to me about his anger at my not taking in the fact of his initial 'crush' on me. Long separated from his mother, he wrote, 'I wanted to be close with you'. His longing had evidently been a major source of his nervous laughter when he was with me. I had not noticed. He told me he had concluded I did not take him seriously, that I had distanced myself from him out of fear lest he become too intimate and close. He was angry I did not understand.

But he was also more confident than with his parents that I might withstand 'the mess' of his trying to convey what he felt. He became hopeful that I might sustain his longing for, and hatred of me without rebuffing him. He wrote between sessions saying, 'I know that if I tell you what bothers me you will try to help'.

Perhaps it was his confidence of both of us being able to retain something of the closeness that—despite its conflicts—he had shared with me as his therapist that enabled him to leave therapy to pursue his studies first in another town in England and then in Germany. Before going abroad he wrote saying, 'You probably remember me . . . You are one of the few professional people who has known me.' He wanted me to endorse his passport photo.

When we met it transpired that he also wanted to renew his previous closeness with me—just as he renewed the closeness he experienced with the motherly figure at school by repeatedly returning to the photograph of them together. It was his answer to the disruption and separation from closeness with his parents, and his resulting 'keeping secrets and bottling things up', as he put it, that he had cultivated in the divided man–woman self story with which he began.

Boy crazy grandiosity

More often, young men describe themselves in terms of being gods and heroes. Freud argued that both sexes follow this path. He claimed that they quit early bits-and-pieces oral, anal, and genital autoeroticism for falling in love with themselves as a whole. He likened the process to the myth of Narcissus, son of the river god Cephissus, who became so enamoured with his reflection in a pool, and so much wanted to embrace his reflected self, that he fell in and drowned. Certainly many of the secondary school boys in my study told similar stories of themselves, as though they too were Narcissus.

My finding is consistent with the Freudian analyst, Peter Blos's (1967, 1984) account of male adolescence. He maintained that, in early childhood, both sexes separate and become independent of the mother by internalizing her control. He argued that, in adolescence, boys need to separate yet further from the mother by dislodging her as as an internal, controlling figure. But this unleashes divisions within the self that she previously contained—divisions that Blos claimed are unified through the adolescent boy identifying with his father as an ideal figure, and with others idealized in his stead. Blos implied that teenage boys, therefore, rightly narcissistic-ally fall in love with themselves as though they were their idealized fathers, or the idolized sports, film, and rock stars who take their fathers' place.

Similarly Jungians urge boys in adolescence to unify their otherwise divided selves, which Jung (1961) referred to in his own case as his No. 1 and No. 2 personalities, by modelling them-selves on mythical heroes. Or, as the Jungian psychiatrist, Anthony Stevens puts it, 'everyman', in youth,

> must undergo a second birth from his mother—a final breaking of the psychic umbilical cord. Victory over the dragon-mother often involves entry into her. Then, after a period in her belly, he succeeds in cutting his way out or causes her to vomit him up.
> (*Stevens, 1990, p. 125*)

Arguably, separating and freeing themselves from their mothers lies behind many teenage boys' stories of themselves as heroes and gods. Many teenagers from the boys' school in my study told stories of being super-successful sports or rock stars, and of thereby winning them-selves an ersatz princess, as in the following story recounted by a 14-year-old:

> I dreamt that I was playing cricket for England and got 600 runs and 19 wickets in the match and we won and I became world famous and married Michelle Pfeiffer.

Living out this story, however, which is very much sanctioned by the acclaim accorded men in male-dominated society, often causes women and men enormous problems. Imagining them-selves already to be the heroes of their dreams results in many young men not recognizing the shortfall between their actual and ideal selves necessary to begin to do the work necessary to close the gap. Doubtless this contributes to their scandalously poor performance, compared with girls, in recent secondary school league tables (see, Phillips 1993).

Proving themselves to be the heroes of their dreams as answer to unhappiness they might oth-erwise feel in their closeness to, and separation from, their mothers and others also undoubtedly contributes to the frequent macho delinquency of pre-teen and teenage boys, and to their sto-ries of themselves as delinquents, as in the following dream fragment from an 11-year-old:

> We started to annoy it [an 'unfriendly dog']. So it chased us. We all turned around and kicked it until it was unconscious and didn't move

Both sexes suffer from being victims, like the dog in this boy's story of men averting fear of others, by grandiosely arousing their fear and attacking it in them.

Other young men in my study told stories of failed grandiosity, of success turning to disaster. A 14-year-old wrote:

> I dreamt I had become a member of a really big rock/grunge band and that I was . . . in the mid-dle of singing . . . the '4th of July' . . . about the end of the world when everything in the song came true . . . and I was left alone on a completely deserted Earth.

Still others told nightmares of their triumphs not being noticed by others, or of others envi-ously attacking their success.

Grown men tell similar tales—of being damaged, or damaging others through their heroics at work, home, and in sex. They tell stories of suffering the ignominy of not being sufficiently glorious, of not being the gods, heroes, and saviours they and others, including their lovers, want them to be. Some, projecting their disappointment, blame others—rightly or wrongly—for stopping them achieving the glory they feel should be theirs. Or, like Willy Loman in Arthur Miller's play, *Death of a salesman*, they tell stories to themselves and others of being the greatest men ever, only to collapse into suicidal dejection at being nothing of the kind.

Others hate themselves in terms of prevailing stereotypes of masculinity for being homosexual, so much is homosexuality equated with being not a man but a wimp, woman, or queen. Lesbians too suffer from our society's ideals and stereotypes of men and masculinity. They suffer from the denigration of their desire as male not female. Lesbian and heterosexual women also suffer from trying to embody the ideals they learn as children, but above all as adolescents, that men look to them to realize. Women in turn make others suffer. They punish them for not being the ideal figures they imagine men to be in their dreams, daydreams, and stories of love and sex.

Hence the attraction for some feminists of psychoanalysis in so far as it seeks to undo the stories of men as gods and heroes contributing to many women's and men's ills. Some are attracted to the development of Freud's work by the French psychoanalyst, Jacques Lacan. Like Freud, Lacan compared women's and men's self-worshipping stories to the toddler, still the plaything of a welter of cross-cutting wishes and desires, falling in love, Narcissus-style, with his unified image in the looking glass, as though he and his imaginary mirror image were one and the same.

Lacan (1949) pointed out that this involves falsely unifying the division between oneself and one's reflection. It involves misrecognizing and alienating oneself through identifying with something other than oneself. It involves conflating one's actual and ideal self such that the gap between them—necessary to impel the struggle necessary to begin to close it, actually and in fact—is occluded. Lacan accordingly made it his business to disabuse his patients of being their ideal self, symbolized in patriarchy, he claimed (see Lacan 1958), by the idea of being or having the phallus.

Other Freudians focus less on divisions within the self (between the conscious and unconscious, actual and ideal self), and focus more on divisions in our relationships with others that are falsely unified or occluded in women's and men's self-aggrandizing image of themselves as heroes or gods. The analyst Henri Rey (1977) and his followers (e.g. Birksted-Breen, 1996) argue that this inflated image is often a defence against recognizing divided love and hate of those to whom we are closest and, in the first place, our separateness from our parents as a couple, through instead imagining ourselves to be unified, god-like, above it all.

Rey reports in these terms the following story told to him by a patient in recalling a dream of reaching to the heavens:

> he was balancing a long pole on his nose; it reached right to the sky and had a baby balanced on the end. As he awoke he said to himself, 'This fucking penis is good for nothing, it is so big that it is useless.'
> (*Rey, 1977, p. 33.*)

If the uselessness of such stories of phallic brag bringing patients to therapy lies in their falsely integrating or fleeing from, rather than confronting and working to integrate on a sounder basis their divided love and hate of others in being close to, or separate from them, then the answer lies in confronting these divisions. This includes confronting their manifestation in the relationship of patient and therapist in therapy. A case in point was Len, an architect in his mid-30s, whom I saw as a private patient.

Example 2: boy crazy grandiosity

An architect colleague had suggested Len might find that therapy might help shift him out of the rut he felt he was in both at work and at home. At least that was what Len said.

Like many men, as indicated earlier, Len went on to tell a story of himself that began with early separation from his mother. The separation had been total. His mother had died when he was 13. Her loss reminded him of other losses: the death of his older sister in childbirth when Len was 9; and the loss of his father to his stepmother on his marrying her a year after Len's mother died.

At some level Len worried that he might have contributed to the loss of his mother and sister. He worried that, like the damage he felt his architecture clients inflicted on him in intruding into his personal life, he might damage his wife in having sex with her when she was pregnant. He remembered dreading he might cause her, like his sister, to die in childbirth. He was horrified at the sight of his wife giving birth—her flesh putrid like that of his dying mother.

More often, however, his divided feelings of depression and guilt at the thought of damaging and contributing to the loss of those he both loved and derided were occluded by another story he told himself. He recounted how, following his mother's death, he became the supremo in his family. Just as he told me he converted vulnerability to attack by his peers by patronizing them as 'disadvantaged' and giving them cigarettes, he converted vulnerability to his mother's loss by patronizing his father as more bereaved than him.

Meanwhile at school he triumphed over any upset he might have felt at his mother's death by becoming a 'big deal' artist. He also became a Don Juan. Seducing women into crediting him with being the perfect lover kept at bay the discreditable hate as well as love of his mother and others he might otherwise have felt at losing them. Sex, he told me, is a 'fuck off' to death.

It was the same with his politics. He recalled a dream of his car being boxed in when he was visiting a friend, and of saving the day by giving the lads a loudspeaker. It was his solution to being 'boxed in' by closeness with, dependence on, and fear of others' loss. Rise above it all. Speechify. That was the motto impelling him to become a demagogue student activist. It had similarly impelled him to become a 'wild cannon' and 'maverick' at work. He kept the firm together, he told me. Without him it would collapse.

It was the same with his wife. Just as he had grandly taken his father under his wing when he was a teenager, he had grandly taken his wife under his wing in marrying her. Just as he derided his father's dependency on him, and his mother's nervous debility following the death of her daughter and father, and just as he derided his mother's fat and sweaty body before she died, he derided the dependency of his wife that led him to marry and save her from the abjection of growing up an unwanted foster child.

It was the same with me. He derided me. He had no respect for therapy. He bad-mouthed it as endless talk of 'murderousness and death'. He dismissed therapy with a two finger gesture of contempt. He called it 'furtive'. He likened me to the ignoramus who, going to the theatre, hangs up what little intellect he has along with his hat and coat outside. He short-changed me. He told me it was my fault, that I must have made a mistake in calculating his bill. He resented paying. After all he was 'a special case', too important to be bothered with financial triviality. He had no need of me. Rather I needed him. He spoke of my being lost without him when his work stopped him attending a session.

Slowly, however, his attitude changed. His grandiosity began to crumble. He began to face the separation and loss of his mother and others that he had long sought to escape by imagining himself, like Rey's patient, god-like superior to any such humdrum contingencies. Faced with the prospect of losing me over the Christmas break, he recalled a dream

> Mr B [a senior partner in his firm] and I were having Christmas lunch. But there was only very measly turkey legs . . . [and] I lost the turkey leg.

The loss of his 'measly turkey leg' was a striking contrast to his previous inflated image of himself as having the phallus, as Lacan might have put it. His dream reminded him of his broken-down car. He could not bear to lose it, he said. He assumed he could magically fix it, just as he imagined he could fix everything and everyone when his mother died. It reminded him of one of his clients who, when his job with him ended, could not bear to say 'Goodbye'. He talked of those who, rather than face threatened loss of those they love, escape into suicide.

Along with his dawning recognition of his own, as well as others' difficulties facing separation and loss came increasing recognition of the divided feelings involved. Now, as well as remembering his mother as someone he hated and despised, he also remembered loving her. He remembered her goodness. He wished she had lived to see his achievements so he could stop driving himself to ever more superlative feats.

He began to acknowledge his initial fear of depending on, and of losing his identity were he to become whole-heartedly involved in therapy with me. Having started idealizing himself, he now idealized me as 'an omniscient therapist' whom he also hated and wanted enviously to spoil and depose. Anxious about our work together, he recalled a recurring dream of being chased by a clown, of tearing off the clown's mask not so much to expose him as a fraud but out of 'livid' hatred of the clown, now equated with me, for making him feel so dependent on, and beholden to others working with him.

Following the next holiday break, he told me he had realized he valued and missed therapy when I was away. He confessed to having begun therapy in 'grandiose' fashion, and to now feeling quite the reverse— that he was not very 'adept' at it. He despaired of taking in anything good. All he seemed to imbibe was bad—cigarettes and beer. He was preoccupied with bad people, with two then-notorious child-killers. He became depressed lest, contrary to his former grand image of himself, as ensuring his teenage daughter's success where others failed, he could not get her through her exams.

He was laid low with flu. He worried lest his debility lose him his wife. He worried that she might heartlessly 'dethrone' and 'dispense' with him, as he had dispensed with his mother and others rather than countenance their loss. On the other hand, having previously dispensed with his wife as useless compared to him, he now acknowledged that she had also helped him. It was because she had suggested therapy, it now transpired, that he had first contacted me.

He now began to value not only her helpfulness, but also his father's ability to use help, unlike his own inability to use others' help when his mother died. He remembered his sadness at losing his father one morning when he was 8 when he had become separated from him in a crowded market. Facing his unhappiness at these and other losses, he acknowledged wanting therapy—its 'containment'.

He wanted me to keep an eye on him, as he kept an eye on his daughter, so as to work to resolve, rather than flee into self-glorification from his divided feelings about being with others and fearing their loss. He asked me to help him with his job. He also increasingly faced the fact of his poverty, which he had previously volunteered only to leave me to do the worrying on his behalf.

Beyond therapy, he set about remedying his indigence. He set about furthering the skills he needed to become the good son, husband, father, worker, and friend, he had previously imagined himself already perfectly to instantiate in the narcissistic story of 'boy crazy grandiosity' with which he had begun.

Divided loves

Freud (1914) claimed that women are even more prone to such stories of narcissistic self-love. He also claimed that, like the mythical Oedipus, women are divided within themselves between wanting and not wanting to kill one parent for love of the other. In fact, however, women more often begin the stories of their lives without stories of self-division giving way to narcissistic self-love. Nor do they often tell stories of early separation from their mothers. Rather, they often tell stories of divided love of their mothers because of their closeness to them.

Feminists draw attention to women's closeness with their mothers. They note that, unlike men, women less often remember being pressed into separating from their mothers in early childhood so as to forge a separate gender identity. Rather, some feminists argue (e.g. Chodorow, 1978), girls learn to become women through remaining close to, and imitating their mothers. This in turn results in women often telling a multiplicity of stories about their togetherness with others, whereas men more often retell themselves in terms of 'a single narrative line' or 'monomyth' (Gergen, 1992).

Women, it seems, from earliest childhood onwards, are both mindful of their closeness with others and of the divided feelings involved in making those with whom we are closest the repositories of our love and hate. Women's knowledge of, and frequent eloquence about their divided feelings about those with whom they are closest as girls, both at home and at school, has recently been highlighted by feminist psychologists on the basis of interviewing pre-teen and teenage students (see, for example, Brown and Gilligan, 1992) and their mothers (see Apter, 1990).

Women's ambivalence, as children and adolescents, about those with whom they are then closest is also graphically depicted in stories by feminist writers. In her recent novel, *An experiment in love*, for instance, the writer, Hilary Mantel, relates the excruciating embarassment of her novel's central, pre-teen protagonist, Carmel, already long-locked in divisive conflict with her mother, at feeling imprisoned with her mother in a department store changing room when she tries on the clothes she needs for secondary school. Carmel writes:

> I was shut up with my mother in my own cubicle, at dangerously close quarters. But she was all simpering smiles now: for the duration, I was her darling. She took off her coat and hung it on one of the hooks supplied, and at once her woman smell gushed out and filled the air: chemical tang of primitive deodorant, scent and grease of Tan Fantastic, flowery scent of face powder, emanation of armpit and cervix, milk duct and scalp.
> (*Mantel, 1995, p. 114.*)

Margaret Atwood similarly recounts in her novel, *Cat's eye*, the teenage fascination with, and horror of her novel's main character, Elaine, at her mother's and other women's bodies. Above all, she describes Elaine's divided feelings about the girls to whom she is closest and on whom she most depends, in both wanting them to be her best friends and recognizing they are her worst enemies in mercilessly inviting, attacking, and bullying her for her dependence on them.

Students in my secondary school study told similar tales. They reported nightmares of their friends turning their fellow pupils against them, of friends becoming enemies at sleepovers and on school trips. They recalled dreams of their best friends betraying, tricking, and laughing at them. They wrote nightmares of being ensnared by maternal and other female figures. A 12-year-old reported a recurring dream of being:

> on a giant web and there is a giant spider coming towards me . . . as she gets nearer she lets out a horrible scream . . . She gets really close to me and I am stuck on the web unable to move. She looks like she is going to kill me and then she scuttles back . . . puts on a smile, and it begins again.

They wrote nightmares of being engulfed or trapped with their friends' or their own mothers. A 14-year-old dreamt.

> My mum and I were in a house . . . Suddenly brown liquid started to roll down the hill towards the house . . . there was no way out

Women, as feminists have pointed out, often relate the teenage origins of the ills for which they seek psychotherapy in terms of feeling imprisoned with, or by, their mothers. The US feminist poet and therapist Kim Chernin (1986) writes of women's contradictory wish both to be and not to be with their mothers, contributing to their both reviving their childhood dependence on their mothers and punishing themselves for depleting them in this respect, and to their seeking to free themselves from their mothers through thin-making, self-punishing, and food-obsessed anorexia.

If eating-disordered patients' symptoms are due to not being able to deal with this contradiction—as feminist researchers find adolescent girls often deal with their contradictory love and hate of their mothers and friends by talking about, and sharing their divided feelings with each other—then the answer might lie in patients sharing such contradictions as they arise in therapy. An illustrative instance is Daisy, a lawyer I saw in NHS therapy when she was in her mid-30s.

Example 3: divided love

While Simon and Len related the 'divided self' and 'boy crazy grandiosity' stories with which they began therapy to early loss of, or lack of closeness with their mothers, Daisy related the 'divided loves' story with which she began therapy to unbearable closeness with her mother. Like many patients, as Freud (1896) initially found and then increasingly forgot, Daisy began her story not with early childhood but with her teens. She linked her presenting symptoms—her depression at so often falling short of her ideal of herself as perfect wife and mother in angrily shouting at her husband and children whenever they did not do her bidding—to her anorexic control over herself and others beginning when she was 16.

Writing about an 18-year-old patient, Dora, Freud (1905) attributed her anorexic symptoms to division between wanting and not wanting incest with her father through displacing her divided genital desire for him into oral preoccupation with sucking and feeding. Daisy, by contrast, said little about her father save to dismiss him for not protecting her from her mother, and to complain that he only related to her superficially.

Most of all she dwelt on her divided longing for, and loathing of her mother's involvement with her. She dwelt on this division driving them apart. She remembered her mother never cuddling her, being 'forbidding' and not 'warming to her'. She remembered her mother experiencing Daisy's yearning for love as 'insatiable', an 'encumbrance'. This was the reason, Daisy assumed, her mother quit home when Daisy was 16—to get away from Daisy.

Just as her mother seemingly could not abide the encumbering ambivalence of being with Daisy, Daisy could not abide being with her. She remembered her teenage dread of being overpowered by, or fragmenting in face of her mother's 'intensity'. It so contradicted her image of herself as 'happy-go-lucky'. She felt enmeshed with her mother. She likened being with her to a film of a Russian and American trapped in each other's country.

She talked of spurned love of her mother turning to virulent hatred of her. Like Gwendolen Harleth in George Eliot's novel, *Daniel Deronda*, confessing her conviction that she had willed her husband's death, Daisy confessed her conviction that she had willed her mother's death. Her mother dying when she was 20, Daisy told me, was her doing. How else but by making her die could she get away? Rather than staying together to sort out their divided love and hate of each other, she said, the only solution she felt as a teenager was to dispose of her.

Daisy not only remembered wanting her mother dead. She also remembered her mother wanting her dead. She compared her mother's eyes to 'laser beams' murderously penetrating into her. She remembered her mother's hateful 'physicality', her gestures, mannerisms, and 'thereness'. She remembered her mother imprisoning her in a suffocating cupboard, and 'in the bathroom, a small room, not being able to get away'. These images were so frighteningly vivid she had fled from them in her teens rather than talk about, and seek to resolve them with her mother.

Unlike the mothers and teenagers interviewed by feminist researchers as indicated above, Daisy felt unable to share with her mother the divisions between them. Years later, however, she shared these divisions with me. She told me of her teenage longing both to be and not to be the same as her mother. She told me how she had recently tried on an all-in-one slip of her mother's only to be bitterly disappointed that, despite now being a woman and mother herself, she still remained so different from her mother—a child, not 'rounded . . . womanly . . . grown up' like her.

She also told me of her teenage dread of being a woman like her mother; her horror of the uncontrollability of menstruation; her dread of suffering the same mental and physical ills and neediness that repeatedly led to her mother being hospitalized through Daisy's teens. She told me how she had accordingly reacted to her mother quitting home by anorexically controlling her own neediness. Otherwise, in her mother's absence, her needs would have become ungovernable. 'Anarchy'. So she controlled and drove herself to become 'the thinnest of the thin', 'self-sufficient', 'the cleverest of the clever'. Survival depended on excelling. It also depended on exciting herself, when she was 13, with stories of saving others in their neediness so as to be wanted by them, as their saviour, with every ounce of their desire.

Whereas she and her mother had evaded talking about their differences with each other when Daisy was a teenager, she shared these differences as they arose with me. On the one hand she told me she had no need of me. She arrived late for sessions: she only came, she said, because they were scheduled in her diary. She told me she distrusted me—my controlling, 'labelling', 'classifying', and hurting her with words as her mother had done.

She worried I would use words not to help understand what was going on between us but to distance myself from her as she used words to distance herself from me. On the other hand she wanted to be the same—a mirror of me. She wanted to be close. Often she ended her sessions in floods of tears—she was so loathe to leave.

I felt similarly divided. Her unhappiness made me want to hold her. But her cloying female sameness with me—her 'yucky', as she put it, detailing of her periods, for instance—together with her dismissiveness of therapy, intellectual superiority, and her making me feel redundant and useless also made me want to get away.

Perhaps it was my nevertheless being there for her week after week to share with her, rather than flee these divided feelings as she and her mother had fled them when she was a teenager, that led to a new story emerging. She had begun therapy with a tale of never being able to share and talk freely with her mother about their divided love of each other for fear of 'all hell breaking loose' and her mother being 'taken away'. She began with her mother's illness stopping her staying with, and trying to understand what was going on between them. She talked of how she had instead confided in her aunt until she too had given up on her. She talked of being an only child and therefore having no brother or sister with whom to confide. She talked of not being able to share divided feelings with other girls at school: she always felt so unwanted, rejected, excluded, and snubbed by them. She arrived at therapy complaining that, as a grownup, she could not talk with other women about their likes and dislikes of each other: being with them made her feel too 'uncomfortable'.

With therapy, however, as she increasingly shared her divided feelings about me and with me, her story began to change. She talked of not wanting to get away but of wanting to be together with me to sort out differences between us, and between herself and other women—in both not wanting and wanting to be with them, and in wanting them to want her to be with them. She talked of wanting to get back in touch with the good as well as bad, caring as well as uncaring figure she remembered her mother as being. She talked of making new friends. She talked of a new confidante she had made who, unlike the story of her mother and herself with which she had begun, happily stayed with rather than fled the divided loves and risk of being 'overwhelmed', as Daisy put it, in being together with her.

Boy crazy romance

Freud (1931) argued that women's divided love of their mothers is largely due to Oedipal rivalry with the mother for desire of the father. Women themselves, however, more often tell stories of divided love of their mothers not as an effect of Oedipal desire for their fathers, but as impelling them into desiring and wishing that their fathers and other men might save them.

Karen Horney, the first psychoanalyst to take issue with Freud's story of women's psychology as an Oedipal effect of penis envy, and one of the first to take issue with the heterosexism of post-Freudian psychoanalysis, argued that, to the extent that women become obsessed with seeking to escape divided love of their mothers through relentless pursuit first of their fathers and then of other men as their saviours, heterosexuality does them more harm than good (see Horney, 1934).

Horney traced this pursuit to adolescence exacerbating the girl's divided love of her mother in so far as she interprets her first periods as signifying that her mother has retaliated against her not only loving but also hating her by attacking and making her bleed. Horney (1935) traced what she termed the boy craziness of girls in adolescence to their looking to men to save them from their mothers' actual, imagined, or assumed vengeance and attack.

Subsequently, Lacan in effect recommended both sexes to look to men as saviours, specifically to the father and his successors to save them from damaging early closeness with their mothers. Lacan (1955–6) argued that the child is only saved from the grandiose ills risked by imagining himself to be everything his mother desires by her recognizing the law against their incestuous union represented by the father and symbolized by the phallus.

Kristeva

The literary critic and psychoanalyst, Julia Kristeva (1983), whose work has proved very appealing to some feminist theorists, similarly argues that the child is only saved from the horror of 'abjection'—of disappearing back into the mother's body—by the mother having an interest beyond herself and her child, again represented by the father. His intervention is crucial, Kristeva claims, if the child is to be saved from what the Freudian analyst Melanie Klein called the infant's 'paranoid-schizoid' fantasies about the mother, so as to recognize her separateness from them. Only through the separation introduced by the father, writes Kristeva, is the child impelled to use the 'semiotic' precursors of language to bridge the gap.

Boys, Kristeva writes, often grow up to find a lover to also bridge separation from the mother. Not so girls. They are less able, Kristeva claims, to recognize, countenance, or put something—represented by the father or later by a lover—as stand-in for separation between themselves and their mothers. Kristeva explains the greater frequency of depression in women in these terms, in terms of their being more wedded and addicted to 'the maternal Thing' (Kristeva, 1987, p. 71).

She illustrates this outcome in terms of Marguerite Duras's account in a film and novel, *The lover*, of her affair, (also retold in her later novel, *The North China Lover*) beginning in 1924 when she was 14, with a wealthy stranger from Manchuria whom she happened to meet on a ferry taking her from her mother's home in Sadec to her boarding school in neighbouring Saigon. Duras dwells on the background of the affair, particularly on her conflict between feeling hemmed in by her mother's depression—'the way she'd suddenly be unable to wash us, dress us, or sometimes even feed us' (Duras, 1984, p. 17)—and wanting to get away.

She attributes her mother's depression to Duras's father, 'the only man she had ever loved' (Duras, 1991, p. 23), dying 13 years before, and to her widowed mother then being oppressively taken advantage of by the Land Registry in Cambodia cheating her of the compensation due to her when the estates she bought in South Indo China were destroyed by floods. She also attributes her mother's dejection to her being yet further impoverished and drained by her older son, Duras's brother, Pierre's drug addiction and tyranny over her.

Duras recounts her hatred of him, her mother, and their common family fate of 'ruin and death which was ours whatever happened, in love or in hate' (Duras, 1984, p. 29). She writes of her teenage embarassment and shame at her mother's visibly oppressed dejection—the poverty of her clothes, her clumsy demeanor and bearing. She complains of her mother's 'incredible un-gainliness, with her cotton stockings darned . . . her dreadful shapeless dresses mended', her down-at-heel shoes, her awkward, painful walking (Duras, 1984, p. 106).

She portrays her teenage depression as her inability to restore her mother. She describes her-self as though she were someone else. She writes of:

> the loathing of life that sometimes seizes her, when she thinks of her mother and suddenly cries out and weeps with rage at the thought of not being able to change things, not being able to make her mother happy before she dies, not being able to kill those responsible.
> (*Duras, 1984, p. 106.*)

She likens her sense of being invaded by her mother's oppressed and oppressive depression to her terror of a mad woman, who lived near her family when Duras was a teenager, clutching at her in the street. She writes of her teenage, 'certainty that if the woman touches me, even lightly, with her hand, I too will enter into a state much worse than death, the state of madness' (Duras, 1984, p. 89).

Recalling her teenage dread of becoming the same as her mother, Duras also luxuriates in teenage memories of being with her. She remembers lying in bed with her mother—'she nestles up against her in tears' (Duras, 1991, p. 15)—crying that her mother loves her brother Pierre so much more than her. She remembers hugging her mother. She remembers her mother as dead to her: 'The mother doesn't cry—a corpse' (Duras, 1991, p. 16). She remembers her mother and her-self hugging each other, her 'mother still without a single tear. Killed by life' (Duras, 1991, p. 17).

She remembers lying in bed with her schoolfriend, Helene Lagonelle. She remembers ador-ing Helene's breasts and naked body. She describes their shared sexual confidences—including Helene telling her that some of their fellow boarders earn money as prostitutes. She recalls being wary of sharing with Helene, still a virgin at 17, the fact that she has begun having an affair.

Learning about prostitutes from Helene, she determines to become one herself, to get her lover to treat her as a whore. She wears a man's hat—a flat-brimmed, brownish-pink fedora—and flashy, garish, gold lamé shoes. She seduces him into having sex with her in his apartment in Cholon—then a Chinese enclave in Saigon.

Whoring herself to him, she identifies with her mother's shamefulness—her poverty, ruined lands, and loathesome son, Pierre. But through her affair she also distances herself from her mother, for her liaison involves courting a man who, unlike her mother, is not French but Chi-nese, not poor but rich. His father's wealth and influence also enables her literally to get away from her mother and her depression, equated with 'the horror of Sadec'. Her well-connected lover negotiates for her brother's debts to be paid, and for her mother to be refunded the money owing from her ruined lands so she can finance Duras's escape from Sadec to France.

Duras thus represents her North China lover as her saviour. But does his intervention do the trick? Not according to Kristeva. She argues that Duras's affair keeps her immersed with her mother. Just as her mother is dead to her, Duras is dead to her lover. Faced with his passion—with his telling her he loves her wildly—she remains silent: 'She could say she doesn't love him,' Duras writes. 'She says nothing' (Duras, 1984, p. 40). She tells him that her 'mother's misfortune took up the space of dreams' (Duras, 1984, p. 50). Necromantically falling in love with her mother's lifelessness and dejection, writes Kristeva, Duras is as lifeless to her lover as her mother is to her. She seeks to annihilate her deadly closeness with her mother by looking to him, only to be equally dead to him. Or, as Kristeva puts it,

> Destroy, the narrating daughter in *The Lover* seems to say, but in erasing the mother's image she simultaneously takes her place.
> (*Kristeva, 1987, p. 243*)

Kristeva quotes Duras's novel as evidence that looking to men to save her from abject oneness with her mother fails to individuate Duras from her mother. Ironically, however, Kristeva thereby contradicts her thesis, following Lacan, that men, in the first place the father symbolized by the phallus, save both sexes from grandiose or abject fusion with the mother. Whatever the function of the father in individuating the child from the mother, men do not necessarily serve to individuate and save girls in adolescence from fusion with their mothers, at least not in Duras's case according to Kristeva's analysis of the story she tells in *The lover*.

Others, accordingly, argue that the solution lies in returning to, and seeking to resolve through more certain means, the divided love of the mother, impelling women to live their lives in terms of stories of men saving them. Some feminists also argue that a major factor contributing to such stories of looking to men to save them from hated fusion and sameness with the mother is the negative image of women and mothers perpetrated by male-dominated society. One solution is therefore to affirm and attend to, rather than to negate and lose sight of, women's mothering.

Irigaray

This is the stance adopted by the feminist philosopher and psychoanalyst, Luce Irigaray. She counters Lacan's focus on the phallus by focusing on women's closeness with their mothers— including their simultaneous attraction and resistance to being close with them. She puts this division in first-person story form. Her story-teller urges her mother:

> Keep yourself/me outside, too. Don't engulf yourself or me in what flows from you into me. I would like both of us to be present. So that the one doesn't disappear in the other, or the other in the one.
> (*Irigaray, 1981, p. 61.*)

Her narrator threatens that, if she and her mother cannot become separate in being together, she will look to a man to save her. She tells her mother:

> if you lead me back again and again to this blind assimilation of you . . . I'll turn to my father. I'll leave you for someone who seems more alive than you.
> (*Irigaray, 1981, p. 62.*)

But Irigaray also entirely opposes this resolution of her narrator's and her mother's divided love of each other. She insists, contrary to Lacan, that mothers and daughters, and that women generally, can face and resolve their divided loves, and recognize that they are two not one, without looking to paternal or phallic intervention to save them. Addressing another woman, she writes:

> We are not voids, lacks which wait for sustenance, fulfilment, or plenitude from an other . . . No event that makes us women. Long before your birth, you touched yourself, innocently. Your/my body does not acquire a sex by some operation, by the act of some power, function or organ. You are already a woman; you don't need any special modification or intervention . . . No need to

fashion a mirror image to be 'a pair', or to repeat ourselves a second time. We are two, long before any representation of us exist.
(*Irigaray, 1980, p. 78.*)

Irigaray symbolizes women's already existing recognition of their separation from each other (prior to any phallic or paternal intervention), and of their divided loves in terms of the two lips of the labia. She counters Lacan's assimilation, akin to that of Freud, of women's to men's psychology by narrating it as a biologically gynocentric, not phallocentric, story.

Estes

Others answer men's male-centred stories less in terms of women's biology than in terms of culturally established, but now often forgotten, women-centred myths and legends. The feminist and Jungian therapist, Clarissa Pinkola Estes, opts for this solution in her recent American best-seller, *Women who run with the wolves*, (Estes, 1992) in answering, by implication, the male-centred stories recently popularized by the US poet, Robert Bly.

Like Estes, Bly draws on Jungian theory. Unlike Estes, he draws on this theory to oppose men's current emasculation, which Bly blames on our society dethroning men as fathers. Their demise, he says, has left us, like the fatherless Jack in the myth *Jack and the beanstalk*, 'stuck in the frightful scene in which the Giant [representing "adolescent envy and greed"] is eating and Jack is watching from his hiding place' (Bly, 1996, p. 43).

Bly (1990) argues that men should offset the strength acquired by women through feminism by strengthening themselves through following the myth of the prince in a Brothers Grimm folktale called *Iron John*. It is a tale similar to that of heroes freeing themselves from their mothers told by the Jungian psychiatrist, Anthony Stevens (1990). The Brothers Grimm story describes a prince taking a key from under his mother's pillow, and unlocking and freeing a Wild Man from a cage in which he is imprisoned, whereupon the Wild Man takes the prince into the forest and initiates him into the skills the prince needs to become a hero in battle, for which he wins a princess as his bride.

Bly argues that today's men, and that today's boys on the verge of manhood, like the prince in the Brothers Grimm tale, should similarly take the key, kept from them by the mother, and needed by them to liberate the Wild Man in themselves. He urges young men to leave their mothers and find older men to induct them into acquiring the strength they otherwise lack so as to become heroes.

Following Bly, Estes (1992) claims that, just as men need to reconnect with the Wild Man in themselves, women need to reconnect with their inner Wild Woman. She maintains, however, that women cannot look for guidance to the same legends that Bly recommends since these are steeped in the male-centred, anti-women terms of Christian theology. She recommends other, more woman-friendly myths, including a Russian version of the folk tale more more usually known in England as *Cinderella*.

The Russian tale is called *Vasalisa*. It begins with Vasalisa's mother dying and giving Vasalisa a doll, which she bids Vasalisa always to keep with her, to feed and nourish whenever the doll is hungry, and to consult whenever Vasalisa needs help. After her mother dies Vasalisa's father re-marries. Her stepmother and stepsisters cruelly mistreat her, and make her their household drudge.

Cinderella is saved, of course, by Prince Charming. Not so Vasalisa. According to Estes' account, Vasalisa is saved through countenancing rather than fleeing her love and hate of the mothers in her life. They are represented by the doll bequeathed her by her mother, and by a murdering witch, Baba Yaga, to whom her cruel stepmother and stepsisters send Vasalisa on the pretext that they need fire from Baba Yaga so Vasalisa can go on cooking their food, and heating their home.

Whereas Cinderella is saved by Prince Charming, Vasalisa is saved by the women in her life. She is saved by her stepmother stopping her remaining a victimized, innocent, downtrodden, too-good little girl. Through pushing her out of home and making her go out into the forest, her hated stepmother also makes Vasalisa confront another aspect of her mother in herself, represented by the murderous witch, Baba Yaga.

Through the help of the doll bequeathed Vasalisa by what Estes (following the psychoanalyst Donald Winnicott) calls her 'good-enough' mother, Vasalisa passes all the trials imposed on her by Baba Yaga. These include cleaning, cooking, and sorting poppy seed from dirt, which represents division and sorting of love and hate, good and bad, life and death. Having faced and worked with these divisions, Vasalisa is then urged and enabled by the doll to assume, rather than refuse, the strength symbolized by a fiery skull on a stick. It represents, says Estes, the 'ancestral knower' Vasalisa needs to confront and dispel the hate, as well as love, her stepmother and stepsisters signify.

Estes tells *Vasalisa*, and other similar female-centred stories, to draw attention to the strength and independence women can secure from each other, without recourse to idealizing myths about men as heroes and saviours. She shows that this entails confronting and doing the work needed to resolve the divisions of love and hate between women and their mothers in remaining close to, but also separate from, each other. In this, Estes's message is similar to that told by followers of Freud's disciple, Melanie Klein.

Klein

Melanie Klein argued, in effect, that men's phallic brag and women's idealization of men begins in childhood as escape from the depressive anxiety, guilt, and work involved in integrating love and hate of the women who first mother them. Kleinian feminists (e.g. Dinnerstein, 1976) and therapists (e.g. Temperley, 1993) seek to redress the harm done by this defence by enabling both sexes to recover and integrate on a sounder basis their divided feelings about those to whom they are closest. In therapy this involves enabling patients to take back, become conscious of, and rework feelings they otherwise split off from themselves, and project into the analyst (see Steiner, 1996). This is helped by the analyst sharing or 'containing' the patient's split off feelings. As Bion (see p. 71) claimed mothers contain their children's feelings, so they can be resumed and reintegrated as containable and contained (see Segal, 1997), rather than fled for boy crazy grandiosity or romance; as I will illustrate with one last example from my NHS work. It concerns a jazz musician in her late 40s whom I shall call Lisa.

Example 4: boy crazy romance

Like Daisy, Lisa, began the story of the symptoms bringing her to therapy—in her case, complete lack of confidence following the failure of her marriage—with memories of divided teenage love of her mother. But, whereas Daisy began therapy with a story of resolving this division through fleeing closeness with, and feelings of rejection by, her mother and others for anorexic self-sufficiency, Lisa began therapy with a story of decades of looking to men to save her.

She began with her teenage image of her mother, in contrast to her image of her mother's attentiveness to her as a younger child, as 'a blank', 'stupid', and 'dumb'. She remembered her father deriding her mother as useless and a nervous wreck. She remembered her mother's depression when she, Lisa, was 17. She remembered a nightmare of witches holding a market in the back garden, and recurring dreams of cooking and finding the shops closed so she could not buy the vital ingredient she needed.

By contrast with her nightmare images of her own and her mother's no-good cooking and mothering, she dwelt at length on her father, on how she had always sought to please him, and on her teenage excitement at his adventure stories of saving her from damning closeness with her mother, through himself and her running away to become free-as-air buskers.

Years later, in therapy with me, Lisa still wore the motley garb of the wandering minstrel. To this garb she had added the accretions of whatever else her father and her subsequent boyfriends, including the lover for whom she left her husband, seemingly most wanted her to be as the price of saving her from her mother.

She had taught herself chess, to be the sparring partner her father wanted, to prove himself 'champion of the world . . . of the universe even'. She had learnt Latin and Greek to become the classical scholar one of her boyfriends seemingly most wanted her to be. She became a financial genius to better another lover's previous girlfriend's City prowess. She pretended to passionate feelings her present lover apparently most wanted her to express.

She told her story in terms of a folk tale, recounted by Boccaccio and others, of a downtrodden peasant woman who is saved from abjection by passing each of a succession of tests a king sets her to ensure she meets the standard he requires to make her his queen. Her lack of confidence, she said, was chiefly constituted by her dread of failing the tests her boyfriend set her as the cost of saving her from fraught life with her husband, that had replaced the fraught life she had lived with her mother as a teenager.

Just as she was divided in her love and hate of her mother, she was divided in her feelings about me. On the one hand she treated me, like her mother, as a drudge with whom closeness was only bearable provided she enliven our togetherness with talk of her boy crazy affairs. Otherwise she hated being with me. She hated confiding her menopausal symptoms that made her so like her mother and so unlike the ideal she wanted her boyfriends to credit her with being. She hated confessing to a dream of her father returning from the dead to dismiss her, as he had dismissed her mother when Lisa was in her teens, saying, 'So that's what it's come to. You never did do anything. Just ordinary and middle-aged'. She hated sharing with me the fact that, far from being the wonderfully kind woman her men wanted to idealize her as being, she wanted cruelly to hurt and crush them in revenge for all the energy she expended in striving to be the princess of their dreams.

She also hated admitting the ordinariness of her problems, including her mundane preoccupation with being excluded by others. It had been horribly borne in on her, she said, when, aged 13, her father got together with her mother and, without any regard for her, uprooted and moved the family to the other end of the country to get himself out of a financial scrape. She hated confessing to me that, contrary to her earlier story of her father promising to save her from her mother, he and her mother were very much wedded to each other to the exclusion of her.

She hated her confiding closeness with me. But she also valued our togetherness. It would be paradise, she said, were I only to include her among my friends. She wanted to charm me just as she felt driven to charm her men. She read my books to make herself the patient I might most want her to be.

But then she hated me for seemingly having extracted this confession from her, for having 'the last laugh' as she felt her father had had over her. She sobbed that whatever she did would be done to please me, that nothing felt real, that she was just a hollow 'sham', an empty shell.

Just as she felt divided between love and hate of me, she made me feel divided between feeling full of her boy crazy stories, and as empty as she felt herself to be. Perhaps that was why alongside the warmth and brilliance of her talk I also felt inwardly shivery and cold as though it were I, not her, who, with her often diaphanous clothes and superficial play-acted roles, were inadequately attired.

Perhaps it was my containing these divided feelings—including feelings of coldness and warmth—that enabled her to repossess them as containable and contained. Perhaps it was her sharing her divided feelings as they arose in therapy with me that contributed to her retelling her story to incorporate her mother, not only as a hated incompetent from whom she had wanted to be saved first by her father and then by her succession of lovers, but as someone she also loved and remembered, unlike them, as always being reliably there for her.

She began to fashion a new story for herself of becoming closer to her mother and to other women rather than fleeing the divided loves involved for boy crazy romance. She represented it in terms of a jazz improvisation on which she now worked—on the theme of 'London Bridge is falling down'. It was a fitting epitaph to the monument she had previously made of herself as a phallic ideal—as Lacan might have put it—of men's desire that had caused her the loss of confidence with which she had begun.

Conclusion

If therapy helped Lisa and the others described in this chapter to recognize the collapse of the stories contributing to their ills, and to rework the interpersonal divisions involved, this was largely due to their security in sharing these divisions as they arose in therapy with me. Arguably their security in this respect was largely a result of their knowing that, whatever divided feelings they aired about me and others, I would be reliably there, session after session, to go on sharing and working with them, to resolve the contradictions in their lives on a firmer basis than that afforded by the stories of divided selves and loves, and of boy crazy grandiosity and romance that brought them to therapy.

One-to-one therapy is similar in this respect to the 'secure base' families and family therapy described by John Byng-Hall (Chapter 7, this volume). He points out that they provide the assurance their members need to contain and confront differences with, and about, each other in the knowledge that they can be explored without driving them apart.

In summary, in retelling the stories of my patients—together with the stories told by secondary school students, autobiographers, novelists, and post-Freudian and feminist theorists—I have sought to highlight the means by which therapy often entails undoing our 'story lines', as the psychoanalyst Roy Schaffer (1992) puts it, so as to tell and retell in terms of the developing relationship of patient and therapist, our ambivalence about each other, dating from our ambivalence about our closeness with, and separation from continuing containing closeness with, the women who first mothered us. It means ending, if all goes well, with a more forward-looking interpersonal prospect than afforded by the backward-looking individualistic prospect of the heroic 'monomyths' (Gergen, 1992) of Oedipus and Narcissus with which I began.

References

Apter, S. (1990). *Altered loves*. Harvester Wheatsheaf, Brighton.

Barker, P. (1995). *The ghost road*. Viking, London.

Bion, W. R. (1962). A theory of thinking. In *Second thoughts* Karnac, London, 110–19.

Bion, W. R. (1986). *The long week-end 1897–1919*. Free Association Books, London.

Birksted-Breen, D. (1996). Phallus, penis and mental space. *International Journal of Psycho-Analysis*, **77**, 649–57.

Blos, P. (1967). The second individuation process of adolescence. *Psychoanalytic Study of the Child*, **22**, 162–86.

Blos, P. (1984). Son and father. *Journal of the American Psychoanalytic Association*, **24**, 301–24.

Bly, R. (1990). *Iron John*. Random House, New York.

Bly, R. (1996). *The sibling society*. Hamish Hamilton, London.

Bowlby, J. (1953). *Child care and the growth of love*. Penguin Books, London.

Brown, L. and Gilligan, C. (1992). *Meeting at the crossroads*. Harvard University Press, Cambridge.

Chernin, K. (1986). *The hungry self*. Virago, London.

Chodorow, N. (1978). *The reproduction of mothering*. University of California Press, Berkeley.

Dinnerstein, D. (1976). *The mermaid and the minotaur*. Harper & Row, New York.

Duras, M. (1984). *The lover*. Flamingo, London.

Duras, M. (1991). *The north China lover*. Flamingo, London.

Estes, C. P. (1992). *Women who run with the wolves*. Rider, London.

Freud, S. (1896). The aetiology of hysteria. *Standard Edition*, **3**, 191–221.

Freud, S. (1990). The interpretation of dreams. *Standard Edition*, **5**, 4–5.

Freud, S. (1905). Fragment of an analysis of a case of hysteria. *Standard Edition*, **7**, 7–122.

Freud, S. (1914). On narcissism. *Standard Edition*, **14**, 73–102.

Freud, S. (1920). Beyond the pleasure principle. *Standard Edition*, **18**, 7–64.

Freud, S. (1923). The Ego and the Id. *Standard Edition*, **19**, 12–66.

Freud, S. (1931). Female sexuality. *Standard Edition*, **21**, 225–243.

Gergen, M. (1992). Life stories. In (ed. G. C. Rosenwald and R. L. Ochberg). *Storied lives*, Yale University Press, New Haven.

Gergen, M. and Gergen, K. (1993). Narratives of the gendered body in popular autobiography. In (ed. R. Josselson and A. Lieblich) *The narrative study of lives*, Sage, London.

Horney, K. (1934). The overvaluation of love. In *Feminine psychology*. Norton, New York.

Horney, K. (1935). Personality changes in female adolescents. In *Feminine psychology*. Norton, New York.

Howard, G. S. (1991). Culture tales. *American Psychologist*, **46**, 187–97.

Irigaray, L. (1980). When our lips speak together. *Signs*, **6**, 69–79.

Irigaray, L. (1981). And the one doesn't stir without the other. *Signs*, **7**, 60–7.

Jung, C. (1961). *Memories, dreams, reflections*. Fontana, London.

Kristeva, J. (1983). *Tales of love*. Columbia University Press, New York.

Kristeva, J. (1987). *Black sun*. Columbia University Press, New York.

Lacan, J. (1949). The mirror stage as formative of the function of the I. In *Ecrits*. Tavistock Publications, London.

Lacan, J. (1955–6). On a question preliminary to any possible treatment of psychosis. In *Ecrits*. Tavistock Publications, London.

Lacan, J. (1958). The signification of the phallus. In *Ecrits*. Tavistock Publications, London.

Laing, R. D. (1959). *The divided self*. Penguin Books, London.

Laufer, M. (1989). Adolescent sexuality: a body/mind continuum. *Psychoanalytic Study of the Child*, **44**, 281–94.

Mantel, H. (1995). *An experiment in love*. Viking, London.

Phillips, A. (1993). *The trouble with boys*. Pandora, London.

Proust, M. (1913–1927) *Remembrance of Things Past*, Chatto & Windus, London

Rey, H. (1977). The schizoid mode of being and the space-time continuum (beyond metaphor). *Journal of the Melanie Klein Society*, **4**, 12–52.

Rivers, W. H. R. (1920). *Conflict and dreams*. Kegan Paul, London.

Schaffer, R. (1992). *Retelling a life*. Basic Books, New York.

Segal, H. (1997). *Psychoanalysis, literature and war*. Routledge, London.

Steiner, J. (1996). The aim of psychoanalysis in theory and in practice, *International Journal of Psycho-Analysis*, **77**, 1073–83.

Stevens, A. (1990). *On Jung*. Penguin Books, London.

Temperley, J. (1993). Is the Oedipus complex bad news for women? *Free Associations*, **4**, 265–75.

5 Circles of desire: a therapeutic narrative from South Asia—translation to creolization

Sushrut Jadhav, Roland Littlewood, and R. Raguram

The same breast which was originally sucked: by pressing well what is akin to it one derives pleasure later. Out of which genitals one was born: in the genitals of the same kind the same one revels. Who was mother becomes wife in her turn and who was wife becomes mother verily. Who is father becomes the son again and who is son becomes the father again. In this manner, revolving in the cycle of birth and deaths, even [just] as the pot in the pulley of the well, people attain series of births from several genitals and deaths. While matters stand thus, having heard from the scriptural texts and from the mouth of the preceptor that there is nothing other than the Brahman, the Yogin attains the superior worlds.

Yogattatva Upanishad (Ayyangar, 1952)

A medical narrative

In summer 1985, as a junior doctor in psychiatry at the Indian National Institute of Mental Health in Bangalore, one of us (SJ) was running his out-patient clinic, clerking his patients, and discussing them with senior psychiatrists. We usually saw about 20 to 35 people over a period of four hours in a clinic shared by four residents and two consultants. People came from long distances, often with packed food as gifts for the doctors and porters, and with a determined hope for relief from their sufferings.

In what we might perhaps now regard as an arrogant style, our diagnostic interviews demonstrated adherence to the western canon: for India's mass suffering could be helped only by the application of scientific medicine and therapeutics. As doctors we were the authors of our patients' trajectories of sickness (*cf.* Kleinman, 1988); our mission, to relieve their pain through the individual psychological models of Freud, Meyer, Maslow, Erikson, and Piaget, and through a phenomenological understanding of psychopathology derived from Kant and Jaspers. No room here for any local models of liberation from the human condition, for we prided ourselves on our knowledge of the cutting edge of western medicine; alienated from our own local understandings we did not think they should find any place in our therapeutics.

On one morning, Andhaka* was brought to us by his family. A grim-faced mother and several cousins stood in the doorway whilst his anxious father remained outside in the corridor.

---

* The name 'Andhaka' is a pseudonym for our patient. When referring to Andhaka, the son of divine Shiva, the term 'mythical Andhaka' will generally denote his identity.

Andhaka's mother related the calamity in her family but it took a while to piece together the puzzle: Andhaka had taken a serious overdose of medical drugs the day before and had been rushed to a general hospital. The doctors there had treated him and then asked the family to consult us. The mother had no idea about any possible problems and appeared quite helpless. She brought with her a few papers detailing the medications and procedures at the hospital, along with a referral letter from the physician asking us to provide further care: no account of any reasons for the overdose except for a list of depressive symptoms which highlighted the seriousness of his condition.

Andhaka was interviewed. He had been plagued with distressing thoughts that led to the decision to end his life. His problems had begun about a year and eight months before, when he argued with his adoptive mother over what he termed an innocuous issue, during which she had accused him of staring at her as if she were a 'street woman' (prostitute). Accused of harbouring a sexual intent towards her, Andhaka was to be plagued by repeated distressing thoughts, arising against his volition, compelling him to stare at the 'private parts' (breasts and genitals) of women between the ages of approximately 35 and 45 years. This led to severe disruption in his life. He had held a job selling newspapers in a relative's shop but could not continue because many of the customers were middle-aged women. He could not stay at home because there again there were too many women of this age group, nor could he talk about his situation to anyone. He lost sleep and then his appetite, and was continually tormented by these thoughts. Trapped within this preoccupation and now seriously disabled, he had taken a large number of paracetamol tablets to escape his predicament, yet seemed almost glad to have survived. In our psychiatric terminology, his mental status examination revealed severe obsessional ruminations that compelled him to stare at the genital region and the breasts of middle-aged women, leading to secondary avoidance of any social contact with them. Guilt, a sense of profound shame, and other depressive symptoms, together with suicidal thoughts, completed the clinical picture.

Our interventions followed rapidly: a severe obsessive–compulsive disorder with secondary depressive features and a high suicidal risk argued for hospital admission. The family gladly accepted this decision and appeared relieved. Senior colleagues approved. The dramatic nature of such a presentation was matched by our inability to think of any very obvious psychodynamic interpretation. Our western textbooks of psychiatry simply prescribed admission, antidepressants, and supportive therapy; the (cultural) content of his symptoms did not matter as long as the form (the biology) was targeted by our scientific rationale (Littlewood, 1996a). Our treatments were explained to the patients in Indian English mixed with Kannada phraseology when appropriate. Discussion with colleagues and in supervision always took place in English, and, like this paper, was written and validated within the space of Western academic assumptions: a process not dissimilar to, and one that reflects, the wider academic research currently conducted by our Indian and British colleagues and, indeed, in the international collaborative studies of the past few decades. (We shall return to this matter at the conclusion of this paper in attempting to relate these issues to the translation of local narratives).

Later that evening, Andhaka was offered antidepressant medication and reassurance on the ward. This was now an illness that we could take care of. No need to worry; a week of antidepressants and his symptoms would improve. A few days later, however, Andhaka continued to say he felt tormented by his thoughts.

His family history had now been explored: Andhaka was born in a lower middle-class *marathi-kannada* joint family living locally in Bangalore. He was the eldest of four siblings and grew up with 18 other relatives—his father, mother and siblings, his father's sister and her husband, and several other paternal aunts, their husbands and children. The grandparents were dead. Their extended household was patrilocal, with cooking carried out within the domestic space of each subunit (a married couple with their children). As space was limited, all the parents and children slept on the floor of two large rooms without segregation of gender or age. Apart from the customary tensions between various in-laws that are characteristic of the Indian joint household, there was an important and continuing conflict that was of particular importance for Andhaka. His father's sister had no children and this posed a threat to her whole marriage, and thus to all in the household, because of the possibility of her husband seeking a divorce, thus bringing shame upon everybody. The family (chiefly Andhaka's father and the father's sister's husband) resolved this through giving away Andhaka in adoption to his paternal aunt in return for Andhaka's adoptive father arranging a lucrative government clerical job for his birth father. Andhaka was already 18 when this took place. At the time of the adoption, the family told him that he had no cause to worry, for his own parents would continue to look after him and this decision would save the family from breaking up if his now adoptive father should annul the marriage with Andhaka's aunt. In later sessions, he revealed a strained relationship with his own mother: he had stopped talking privately with her since he was 12, following a minor quarrel which he revealed later in therapy. Andhaka's personal history was characterized by other, traumatic, sexual events which we reconstructed in our further sessions.

Plagued by severe obsessive doubts and ruminations occurring since puberty, together with Andhaka's avoidance of his own mother since he was 12, led to an initial psychodynamic hypothesis: an unresolved early sexual inclination towards his mother had become generalized to other women of the same age group. In sessions, Andhaka resisted any attempts to explore his relationship with his mother, questions about which led to missed sessions or else extended digressions (in the form of queries about his therapist's own background and status in the hospital).

Andhaka's resistance to verbal exploration was dramatized a few days later when, one evening, at around 11 p.m., SJ was given an urgent message to come down to the wards, as Andhaka had gone missing. He had left a note behind pleading 'to be forgiven' and requesting the staff not to bother searching for him. Realizing the seriousness of the situation, SJ rode off on his moped towards the highway to Vellore and found Andhaka lying in the middle of the road. On this dark highway, he anxiously approached the prostate body. Spotting Andhaka's silhouette by the beam of his moped, he pulled up and parked by the side of the highway. Andhaka continued to lie on the road but moved to the side on SJ's request. A short intervention by the side of the highway followed. Reluctant at first, but then wavering in his intent to return (against the background of highway traffic roar and beams that intermittently lit the scene), Andhaka eventually acceded to SJ's request and returned to the hospital:

SJ: I have come to help.

ANDHAKA (sobbing): No. No one can help me. I deserve to die.

SJ: Can you at least help me understand?

ANDHAKA: It does not matter any more.

sᴊ: How can I then understand?

ᴀɴᴅʜᴀᴋᴀ (still sobbing): I have committed a great sin and deserve to die.

sᴊ (perplexed, trying to recollect events over the past few days on the ward): What is it? What did you do?

ᴀɴᴅʜᴀᴋᴀ (nodding his head sideways in a pathetic manner): I can't tell. Please forgive me (sobbing again).

sᴊ: Look. I have come here all the way in search of you. I am relieved to see you alive. We were all very worried at the hospital. (In the authorative voice of a doctor): Get up and sit on the moped and we will go back.

Andhaka, in a robotic manner, got up and sat on the pillion clutching SJ tight as they retraced their path. SJ felt Andhaka periodically embrace him with now less frequent but deep sobs: a mixture of relief and gratitude. As they enter the driveway of the ward, a crowd of nurses in starched white sarees and ward boys (porters) greet them with loud cries of relief. SJ feels he has returned from a hard fought battle with a trophy snatched from demonic enemies. It is now well past midnight. As they entered his room Andhaka threw over a comic magazine, *The demon son of Shiva* (Pai, 1985), crying 'You want to know why I wish to die? Here! This is the reason!' Exhausted and tired from the events that night, SJ took the magazine and returned to his hostel after ensuring Andhaka went to bed.

A mythic narrative

Next to his English texts on psychiatry and the social sciences, within the secular space of the hostel room, SJ stood and looked at the magazine. It was a well-known children's comic book serial, popular in the country for its ability to retell Hindu mythology at a modest price, with brightly coloured illustrations recalling those of Euro-American 'sword and sorcery' comic books. Indeed, homes in South India with children would invariably have single issues either bought or borrowed from friends and neighbours. Its appeal lay in a clear and lively depiction of the classic Indian myths in English; and was (and still is) considered by parents—and the publishers—to be of immense educational and moral value. The story of the mythic Andhaka is briefly summarized at the beginning.

> Andhaka is the offspring of Shiva and born ugly. When given away in adoption, he lives surrounded by the crudeness and arrogance of the Asuras. But his origins being divine, there is a different destiny in store for him. Through a boon, he gains physical beauty, but his heart continues to harbour evil. His parents themselves are instrumental in bringing about his ultimate spiritual transformation. Andhaka's story aptly traces the journey through fire that a soul must make before attaining liberation.
>
> Hearing of the beauty of Mount Mandara, Lord Shiva came there with his wife, Parvati, and his ganas [attendants]. One day when Parvati was in a playful mood, she brought forward her hands and covered all three of Shiva's eyes. At once the world was plunged into darkness. Held over the fiery third eye of Shiva, Parvati's hands began to perspire. The perspiration flowed out and fell upon the ground and suddenly there arose from it a weird being. As Parvati stared at it, the omniscient Shiva smiled and said, 'My dear, it is you who closed my eyes, so this is your work.' At this Parvati smiled and uncovered Shiva's eyes. In the returning light, the creature looked more horrible than before and Parvati is horrified, but Shiva persuades her to accept him with compassion as a son, explaining that he was born of the sweat of her hand and the heat of his eye in

the darkness, hence the child is called Andhaka—'the blind one'. Parvati accepts Andhaka as their son but soon the couple give him away to the childless King Hiranyaksha of the Asura Kingdom as a reward for his austerities and prayers to Shiva.

Hiranyaksha is joyous but now grows arrogant and launches a campaign to conquer the three worlds. This terrifies other kings who plead with [the god] Lord Vishnu for help. Lord Vishnu manages to destroy Hiranyaksha and makes Andhaka the king in his stead. However, his adoptive cousins tease him for being blind and mock him for his ugly looks. Unable to stand their onslaught, Andhaka retreats into penance in the deep forest, standing on one leg with arms raised until he is reduced to a near skeleton. In response to his suffering, Lord Brahma [the supreme divinity] grants him any boon of his choice. Andhaka chooses two: undisputed control of the three worlds and immortality. Brahma grants the former but requests Andhaka to reconsider the latter for 'whoever is born must die' and therefore asks him to select the manner of his death. Andhaka chooses in what appears to be an impossible manner: 'Let the most excellent of women in the world, whatever her age, be like a mother to me and should I look upon her as anything but mother, let destruction befall me instantly'. Surprised at this strange request, Brahma grants him this wish but advises him to 'always fight with heroic persons' and touches Andhaka's body to make him strong and handsome—and then gives him sight when Andhaka cleverly argues that without this he would be unable to fight with any 'heroic person'.

Andhaka returns to his kingdom where he is now accepted, yet like his adoptive father he craves for power and conquers Heaven, Earth and Hell until he is Master of All. Still not content, he then indulges in pleasure, bad company and sinks into decadence to be hated by everyone. His pride 'blinds him to the destiny he had chosen for himself'. One day, his soldiers spot a beautiful woman tending to a meditating hermit in the forests. When Andhaka hears of this, he orders his men to bring her to his palace with the excuse that a hermit with his eyes closed in meditation does not do her justice if he has not looked at her. When Andhaka's men try to take her away, the hermit protests that she is his wife and asks them to tell Andhaka that he ought to come personally to take her. Blazing with anger like [sacrificial] 'fire fed with ghee', Andhaka attacks the hermit who takes leave of his beautiful wife to 'perform the most severe austerities to free her from Andhaka's threat'. He leaves behind his guard, Viraka, who fights a lengthy and courageous battle that leaves everyone dead, except for Viraka who is buried under the huge pile of weapons. Realizing her imminent danger, the beautiful maiden is joined by the three divine beings Vishnu, Indra, and Brahma, disguised in female forms, who fight off Andhaka's army with 'streams of energy' until the hermit [now disclosed as Shiva himself] appears and praises the courage of his wife [Parvati]. Andhaka renews his challenge to Shiva. A final battle ensues and 'in one movement, Shiva pierces his trident into Andhaka to scorch him under the sun until his body withers once again to skin and bone', magically transforming Andhaka's character from 'arrogance and hatred' to 'humility and devotion'. Andhaka asks for forgiveness and Shiva, acknowledging his courage, not only forgives him but asks Andhaka to choose a boon. Unaware of his origins and his destiny, Andhaka asks for Shiva to accept his eternal devotion and for 'the Mother of the Universe [Parvati] not to be angry with me, but to look on me with compassion. Let me see her always as mother'. Shiva grants him this wish and then 'merely turns his benevolent glance upon Andhaka, and Andhaka remembers the full story of his birth'.

Andhaka tells Shiva that he would have been dead by now according to the destiny he had chosen for himself if it were not for Shiva's grace. He bows before his father and mother and 'knows happiness at last'.

Over the next few weeks, Andhaka argued the parallels between this story and his own. With intense anger towards his biological mother, he recalled how she had teased him as a child for being ugly and dark complexioned, and on one occasion humiliated him in front of other family members for his expressing a wish to suckle her breasts soon after the birth of his younger brother. There were other occasions when she had caught him attempting to masturbate on the

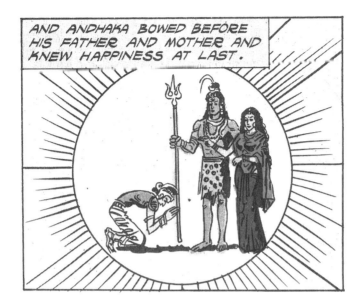

floors of the family house whilst sleeping in close proximity with his cousins and aunts (and stimulated by observing their sexual acts). During our conversations, he would express intense guilt and remorse for what he had done, and said suicide was the only way out of his predicament. It was only then that it became apparent that although he knew the general outline of the myth, Andhaka had read only the first few pages of the comic version and had stopped before the point when Brahma grants the mythic Andhaka the boons that he chooses. Guilt precluded further reading, as, unlike the mythic Andhaka at that point, our patient had become aware of 'the destiny he had chosen for himself' (he used the same words as the book). He had then decided to write his final note and fled the hospital to end his life.

Further therapy sessions involved a fuller examination of the mythical story of transformation (Barthes, 1974) that ended with the sense of relief for the mythic Andhaka as he knelt for the final act of forgiveness and blessing by Shiva and Parvati. This was coupled with the suggestion that sexual strivings towards older women were part of normal psychosexual development and that this was natural and expected. By this time, Andhaka's symptoms had slowly started remitting although his relationship towards SJ was characterized by periods of anger at what he thought was our harsh response when he broke accepted social boundaries in the hospital and 'manipulated' the hospital staff. In this transference, in which he experienced his young doctor as a parental figure who, like his parents, judged his behaviour as 'bad and unforgivable', SJ wished he could forgive him as Shiva does the mythical Andhaka at the very end of the story. Andhaka had begun delving into other spiritual and mystical books, often bringing into therapy material that resonated with his own sense of despair. Thus, he spoke of going into *vanvas* (exile in the forest) to do penance and seek forgiveness from the gods for harbouring evil thoughts, which fate had unleashed on him. In his quest for penance, he inserted himself into the queue for the ECT clinic: when dissuaded, he constructed his own machine complete with batteries and electrodes to 'burn out' his thoughts, recalling the mythic Andhaka scorched (and redeemed) under the rays of the sun (Jadhav, 1994).

He described how he had categorized his two mothers as good and bad: the former being his adoptive mother, the latter his biological mother. His adoptive mother, always his favourite aunt, he viewed as warm, nurturant, and caring, whilst his biological mother had failed for it was she who had first roused his sexual feelings and then had rejected him in preference to his siblings, and it was she who had given him away for adoption. In the hospital, at visiting time, Andhaka took great pleasure in playing what he called 'the power game between my two mothers to seek me'. Often this took place through deliberate avoidance of his biological mother's affectionate gestures towards him. He spoke to us of dreams in which he had intercourse with both of them, and related childhood memories of erotic stimulation when they bathed and dressed him. His hostile and erotic drives towards maternal objects were defended against through psychological splitting. Terrified of his sexual feelings for his own mother and their more accessible transference to his adoptive mother, he had developed a phobic attitude towards all sexually active women of their age. Unable to possess her, he had created a fantasy through which he could control her sexuality. Caught in their struggle for their claim to the eldest son, he seemed to manipulate this conflict through his symptoms, to gain some power over them as retribution for what they had done to him.

It is noteworthy that Andhaka never expressed overt anger nor hostility towards his father, although his expression of such feelings about his doctor suggested an active displacement of such potentially dangerous aims from their principal object. Andhaka's father was a distant and rather authoritarian figure who briefly dropped in during visiting hours to express formally his sincere hopes of his son's recovery in our able hands. Indeed, SJ's idealized position with his family was confirmed when during one such family visit to him in the midst of a busy out-patient clinic, both parents proposed marriage between him and their niece (who was conveniently sitting just outside the clinic). By this time, Andhaka had begun addressing SJ as 'Dada' (a term customarily reserved for respected elders in India) and despite rather naïve attempts to reflect back this popular paradigm of autocratic father and apparently submissive son, he continued to use this term throughout the therapy.

In the meantime, reports from both mothers suggested some improvement in his behaviour towards them. He no longer avoided eye contact on their regular visits to the hospital, had apologized for his bad behaviour in the past, and had begun expressing a wish to return home. As concerns over his suicidal intent diminished, together with the improvement in his mental state, we were able to negotiate his discharge from hospital. Three months after his admission, he was discharged with an arrangement to continue with regular out-patient appointments. Soon SJ was to leave the country for Britain and planned termination of the sessions. Andhaka wept as he expressed his gratitude for what he identified as divine help in bringing about his transformation, and he enthusiastically posed for a photograph of the hospital ward taken by SJ for a conference in the United States.

We are not claiming that Andhaka was fully 'cured' in a therapy he had initiated himself: recent reports from colleagues in Bangalore suggest he does periodically return to the out-patient clinic for support. We do propose, however, that a culturally sensitive way of deploying popular mythical material appeared to be 'therapeutic', even if it was Andhaka who first proposed it, albeit rather laterally. It was Andhaka himself who introduced the mythical story in therapy when he felt overwhelmed by verbal explorations into his own inner conflicted life. This could also be construed as Andhaka's effort to retain some control over the therapeutic encounter. An 'encounter' with the therapist's westernized self, both engages the therapist and encourages him to become more reflective about local meanings and their shaping of indigenous psychologies. If the myth had not been brought up in therapy, further sessions would have continued along classical psychodynamic lines in addressing the internal resistance of the patient.

Secondly, the myth of Andhaka was useful in dealing with the resistance that came up in therapy at the very outset and facilitated the open recognition of difficulties that would otherwise have been unmanageable, given the social prohibitions against speaking of sexual desire for maternal figures.

A third point: Andhaka's emotional distress was objectified and rendered culturally meaningful through the mythic drama that was strikingly paralleled in his own life. The story of transformation and reconciliation provided a healing narrative in which Andhaka's own closed personal script was recontextualised and structured through an alternative resolution that provided hope of a recovery, as in the mythical narrative. Resolution of what we might term a developmental conflict was through a mechanism described in Hindu culture as 'identification through submission' (Obeyesekere, 1990, p. 84), which, like its European counterpart in psychoanalytical thought, allows introjection of parental and societal values.

Myth, narrative, and healing: the global and the local

Popular tales and mythology have often been a focus of interest both for local healers and, more recently, health professionals (Sarbin, 1986; White and Epston, 1990; Freedman and Combs, 1996; Gersie, 1996): in particular for psychotherapists working with patients from a 'traditional' cultural background who themselves often bring such material into the clinic (Verma, 1988; Bilu and Witztum, 1995; Mishara, 1995; Kakar, 1997). The classic instance of healing through myth is Lévi-Strauss' (1968) rather literary and much criticized structural analysis of the shamanic healing of a woman in obstructed labour in rural Central America. Resolution of the problem involves the shaman in the recitation of a mythic narrative about a quest to find the abode of the female divinity who was responsible for the formation of the fetus, and who, now jealous, is unwilling to release it out into the world. The shaman's recitation is lengthy and involves his manufacture and dramatic deployment of small figurines, which represent the mythic protagonists whose symbolic attributes are expressed in appropriate shape, colour, texture, and material. Together, patient and healer participate in a narrative quest in a shared cultural idiom, 'recreating a real experience' (Lévi-Strauss, 1968, p. 194), linking current physiology (obstructed birth) with its cognitive representatïon. The healer 'rapidly oscillates between mythical and physiological themes, as if to abolish in the mind of the sick woman the distinction which separates them' (Lévi-Strauss, 1968, p. 193).

How may myth—a sacred or moral schema in a narrative mode [as a sequence of events that organize and convey meaning (White, 1987)]—facilitate healing? Tantalizingly vague as to the actual mind/body interactions presumed in his account, Lévi-Strauss proposes that in small-scale 'tribal' and non-literate societies, healing stands for the concordance between individual experience and the cognitive norms represented in a society's standardized myths. By contrast, he argues conventionally that in psychodynamic therapy in Euro-American societies, the patient is encouraged to elaborate a personal myth, verbalizing and objectifying the unspoken and thus gaining some control over it (Lévi-Strauss, 1968, p. 198). In both instances we might note that the narrative presents a story in linear time, with a situation, a crisis, and its resolution. Freud's own interest in recapitulationist theories condenses in a single tale of human history and individual development, with cultural variation and individual psychopathology as dramas along this route. Dow (1986) has proposed the term *symbolic healing* (including shamanism and western psychotherapy) for a general model that similarly places together individual experience and autobiographical memory along with shared and standardized concerns. His four, rather general, stages of symbolic healing comprise:

1. The experiences of healer and healed are already to be found in a generalized form in a set of 'deeper', shared, culturally meaningful narrative schemata, which Dow terms myths: in which key symbols couple together personal experience with the shared social order. Life is experienced through such stories, which contain certain locally accepted (and hence possible) actions exemplifying individual identity, moral action, suffering, and restitution. In other words, they offer a local psychology.

2. A suffering individual comes to the healer who defines the presenting problem for the patient in terms of the myth, not just explicitly through verbal narration but through actions that recall and make real the myth for the patient. Whether physical or non-physical, these procedures employ the existing assumptions about the nature of mythical interactions and precipitating experiences, including notions of causality, time, space, agency, and of crisis and redemption.

3. The healer transfers the patient's personal emotions, which are still bound up with the presenting problem, on to transactional symbols which are particularized as the case demands, from the general myth. This might involve direct instruction, clarification, confrontation, example, paradox, down-playing other procedures, or through the patient forming an attachment to some figure (real or fantasized) that encapsulates the myth.

4. The healer manipulates these transactional symbols to assist the patient to transact his or her emotions.

In an overview of the paradigms of Hindu identity, written for their psychiatric relevance, Guzder and Krishna (1991), like Kakar (1981), Erndi (1993), Kurtz (1992), and Bracero (1996), emphasize that local models for experience and self-identity, particularly those for Indian women, evoke and reframe powerful mythological images which are already well known in the community. The classic instance is Sita as the ideal of female self-renunciation in the Ramayana epic. Standardized mythical narratives, proposes Dow, help patients articulate and objectivize inchoate personal experiences, serving as templates for providing explanatory schemata for personal distress in a setting where western psychological idioms are alien. Given the highly westernized psychiatry that has been grafted on to India (for a variety of political and economic reasons that are beyond the scope of this chapter), the place of cultural understandings is generally marginalized locally by doctors who consider them irrelevant to the understanding and treatment of psychiatric disorder. In this context, even in psychotherapy, normative psychological schemata for western experience are encouraged in local settings, despite their inappropriateness. Andhaka's problems, if they are to be interpreted in a western psychodynamic idiom, may be easily conceptualized as standard Oedipal strivings: his obsessions and expression of regression and fixation at the anal-sadistic stage, with defence mechanisms such as isolation, reaction formation, undoing, and displacement. His extreme passivity and subservience towards father figures may be interpreted as what has been termed a 'negative Oedipus complex' (from Freud, 1923), his psyche as punitive and narcissistic, adopting a passive homosexual attitude to his father, or psychically castrating himself in order to win paternal goodwill (Spratt 1966). Numerous psychoanalytical authors have proposed either the non-existence of the classical Oedipus complex in Indian society or else this sort of negative complex in which the son identifies early with the mother and avoids aggression towards his father (Johnson and Price-Williams 1997); and similarly in Japan (Doi, 1973). Contesting this view, Goldman (1978) argues that Indian epics are rich with examples of a range of classical Oedipal conflicts, albeit often in displaced forms, between pupils and gurus, and between *ksatriyas* (of the former warrior caste) and *brahmins* (priests). He outlines three major variants of Oedipal conflict in the classical Indian epics (Mahabharata, Ramayana, and Puranas).

1. A son, almost always a surrogate son, successfully challenges a father figure and through this attack achieves maturity and temporal power (as we find in European folk narratives: Bettelheim, 1976).

2. The son attacks a surrogate father and/or surrogate mother. He may succeed in actually killing the father but whether he does or not, here he is punished with symbolic castration. This pattern, recalling the Andhaka myth, says Goldman, is more popular in India than in Europe.

3. A heroic son anticipates and avoids overt Oedipal conflict and paternal aggression by freely submitting to the father's will, in effect castrating himself. Heroes of this type are never punished but on the contrary rewarded in various ways; however, these rewards are generally compensatory, for the major Indian heroes of this type are commonly excluded from the pleasures and privileges of sexuality and temporal power.

Goldman argues that in view of the strict proscriptions against sons challenging their fathers or entertaining sexual thoughts about their mothers, Oedipal aggression *as a rule* must be displaced on to father and mother surrogates, including siblings and parents' siblings. Concluding that the third variant is the most dominant conflict in Indian mythology, he considers this understanding valuable for looking at a number of poorly explained phenomena, such as the subservience to authority, the long tolerance of foreign rule, the sanctity of the cow, sentiments of passive non-violence yet not infrequent real communal violence, and the highly placed value on renunciation (compare Ramanujan, 1983).

In rejoinders to this reading of the Hindu epics, both Obeyesekere (1990) and Kakar (1997) suggest Goldman's argument still represents a western 'category error'. Following on from Spiro's (1992) psychoanalytical rebuttal of Malinowski's well-known thesis on the absence of father-directed Oedipal conflicts amongst matrilineal societies, together with clinical and ethnographic observations from Italy (Parson, 1964), India (Kakar, 1981, 1989; Kurtz 1992), and Japan (Roland, 1988), Obeyesekere proposes that such arguments over the existence of hidden Oedipal complexes must be clarified through 'intelligent' (that is, strongly revisionist) psychoanalytical formulations. Mechanisms such as displacement and symbolic reversal, he suggests, could well be applied in the reverse direction, taking the Indian 'negative' Oedipus complex as central and the European complex as the variant, thus each pathologizing in turn excessive independence or repressed dependency needs with their pathologically aggressive stance towards father figures. In his generally supportive defence of psychoanalysis, Obeyesekere argues that rather than accepting the universality of a eurocentric Oedipus complex and measuring its goodness-of-fit with other cultures, it may perhaps be more appropriate to conceptualize 'circles of desire' in which several erotic and/or antagonistic relationships between various family members exist, and that certain segments of these relationships are privileged over others at varying sociopolitical periods in different cultures:

> . . . the Indian Oedipus is not a variant form of a universal complex: it *is* the segment of Oedipal relations that is culturally significant and also determinative of a great many neuroses. A myth then can be paradigmatic of the complex, for it is indeed likely that the set of significant relationships isolated by the analyst [or the patient] may also be the culturally significant one and is consequently represented in myth. But on the other hand, this might *not* be the case; it may well be that some cultures do not organise psychic conflicts in the family into a complex or a myth or both, in which case these conflicts can exist as more or less free-floating deep motivations that may or may not be represented in symbolic forms.
> (*Obeyesekere, 1990, p. 99.*)

Somewhat more generous to the classical psychoanalytical position than Obeyesekere, Johnson and Price-Williams (1997) propose the term 'family complex' to include Freud's Oedipus complex, its feminine counterpart, and the negative Oedipus complex, along with the possibility of Oedipal displacements on to siblings.

Returning to the myth of Andhaka, there remain issues that demand further comment. First, the published story is a modern interpretation by contemporary writers involved in producing popular educational materials: actions of divinities are frequently expressed in this comic strip, not as cosmic events but rather as human pragmatic decisions. Oral and Puranic versions of the myth do not accord with the one popularized here, although there are considerable parallels.* The mythical Andhaka may be represented as a demon. We do not consider it necessary to delve too far into this matter, but rather agree with Lévi-Strauss that all the variants of a myth together comprise its meaning. This contemporary depiction is one amongst several. Its resonance with the local culture and with our patient's biography do serve as evidence to consider its 'healing potential' in this particular instance. In contrast to Oedipus, the reversal in this myth, with the mythical Andhaka choosing his destiny at the very outset, his blindness from birth, his austerities in the forest, and his restitution by both Shiva and Parvati followed by Andhaka's spiritual and psychological transformation, are at odds with Oedipus' fated killing of his father Laius, marriage to Jocasta, and then putting out his eyes in guilt that drives him into the forest as a penitent outlaw. Although the psychoanalyst and anthropologist Georges Devereux (1983) provides us with several variants of the Oedipal myth in classical Greek and Hellenistic literature, the myth as depicted by Sophocles and thence by Freud did not incorporate such alternatives. Obeyesekere (1990) considers this to support his thesis that Freud's own choice of one

---

* For variations of the Andhaka myth, see Kramrisch (1988), pp. 374–87. These extend to include Andhaka's son, the demon Adi, who attempts to seek revenge for his father's humiliation at the hand of Shiva. He disguises himself as a snake to enter Shiva's quarters and then takes the form of Parvati (Shiva's wife) with sharp teeth in her vagina, hoping to castrate Shiva. However, Shiva is able to see through his disguise and kills Adi with a thunderbolt fired from his *lingam* (phallus). In other versions, Andhaka is impaled on Shiva's trident for a thousand years until his lower half is dried up by the rays of the sun and his upper half drenched by the downpour of the clouds.

version may itself be considered as a cultural choice constrained by its own late Victorian popularity; and similarly for the theory Freud then developed around it (Deleuze and Guattari, 1984).

Popular narratives in India exist in both written and oral forms. Their stories are told and re-told several times across generations and indeed, like that of Oedipus, across cultures (Rank, 1992; Johnson and Price-Williams, 1997). In the process, they are likely to be aligned to local realities and to be *contextualized* at particular times by the narrators for a specific purpose (Guzder and Krishna, 1991). Thus Ramanujan's (1983) rendering of an Oedipal narrative by an illiterate Kannada woman from the female protagonist's point of view, a story told invariably to girls and with the men actors depicted simply as pawns in a story primarily about women's fate, exemplifies the diverse meanings available in narrative folklore as a cultural resource. Given the rapid changes in contemporary Indian political and economic structures, such stories may well be recontextualised to represent new cultural dilemmas and their psychological experience in the future. As families fragment from their joint and extended social functions into nuclear parent-based households, as the individualism of so-called 'globalization' takes hold, the notion of the Indian self as embedded in the larger communal self (Bharati, 1985) may no longer re-main tenable, and such shifts in family structures may well lead to the dominance of latent or frankly novel erotic alliances within the family.

Our use of psychodynamic therapy, contextualized in the wider setting of the practice of psychological therapy in India, also raises some questions.

First, the nature of the therapeutic setting: compared with the privacy of a Western psycho-therapist's office and couch, sessions with Andhaka took place in a wide variety of settings that cut through the cultural landscape: in open, public, and often overcrowded clinics, multiple bio-graphies condensed into a singular narrative, with their dramatic characteristics, in which both therapist and patient are actors, decoding and recoding deeper and wider cultural texts, in closed wards, through interventions on the highway, and in ECT queues, propositions of mar-riage, and endearing farewells. Therapy then necessarily works through, or at least acquires, the flavour of wider cultural activities which if screened out would hardly be locally valid. This seems in striking contrast to our North London psychotherapist's office: a tense waiting room, a ritualized entry into a quiet office with its professionalized cultural symbols such as, say, the hanging rorschach chart, Greek figurines, a clock that establishes linear therapy time, and the 'invisible' therapist sitting behind the couch. Such a setting, as ritualized as its Indian counter-part, is designed to facilitate free associations and introspective tasks punctuated with silences. This cultural milieu moulds and structures the very experience of therapy for both therapist and patient but follows very different directions when seen across cultures (Lévi-Strauss, 1968). Both spaces are exclusive yet professionalized extensions of the local cultural spaces in which they are rooted. To attempt stamping or substituting one for the other therefore violates the basic premises of providing culturally appropriate (i.e. possible) methods, and, indeed, the very direction of 'conflict' resolution. Therapy with Andhaka offered an opportunity to reflect upon the pressing need to move away from a formulation resting on intrapsychic tensions and indi-vidual dynamic enquiry to a world peopled by demons and spirits that engage with family and communal concerns and conflicts. How is it possible to relate the linear time that structures Western therapy to an Indian astrological (circular) time for felicitous meeting with the doctor/therapist and one that, as here, appears controlled more by the patient than the therapist? How does one reconcile a Western preference for talking with a knowledgeable stranger with an Indian choice of a wise elderly friend or relative?

In contrast to the rigours of personal analysis, seminars, and training over extended periods that characterize Western psychotherapeutic training, psychiatric training in India continues within the framework of a *guru–chela* apprenticeship but has, over the years added, to it a watered down version of western psychotherapy. The process of deliberately filtering off cultural components of patients' narratives to yield symptoms and signs, including defence mechanisms that devalue projections on to mythical characters, is considered credible and meritorious. We argue that this relates to an effort on the part of alienated health professionals attempting to approximate their patients' stories as stories to Western therapeutic narratives, to arrive at some sort of goodness-of-fit with the latter. This appears to be the only way they can resolve their dilemma: being accepted by their Western counterparts, which in turn translates into merit amongst local colleagues. Once a cultural cleansing is achieved, therapy, or for that matter any other health intervention, can proceed as outlined in the eagerly awaited journals and books that arrive by post or through the philanthropic gesture of western colleagues.

From translation to creolization

Current post-colonial theorizing, however, now highlights the power of local narratives to provide a counter-language that offers space for alternative stories and epistemologies. What has got culturally translated and by whom and for what purpose? Who selects certain voices, views, and texts? The stakes are higher when the narrator is both politically and psychologically subordinate to the translator: as in doctors' recasting of their patients' stories. Translations of theory and therapy in a wider sense are then similar to retelling of the same story adapted each time in each unique setting for a particular purpose. Indeed, translation is one of the primary means by which 'cultures travel' (Dingwaney and Maier, 1996); and post-colonial theorists have argued that the 'bankruptcy of available [western] categories' have led to a 'distorted' translation of non-Western texts (and cultures) to suit the needs of the new dominant classes (Nandy, 1983).

Within the discipline of psychiatry and psychotherapy, there has been little effort in both Indian and Western academic worlds to utilize the language of the 'other'. At best, both attempt translations into standard English that homogenize the 'other'. At worst, we render difference irrelevant by seeking deeper universal structures (Steiner, 1975). But these issues are not merely confined to apparently distinct First and Third Worlds, for they take place in intercultural, creolized settings, and indeed in the 'interdialectical transations of everyday life, in the reading of virtually every human utterance that the texts we make about other texts represent imperfectly' (White, 1996).

Andhaka, by introducing the cosmic myth, unknowingly succeeds in taking the dominant language (psychoanalysis) and turns it against itself, in order to express his own suffering. In the process, a chain of translations are set up: the 'original' Sanskrit myth in its multiple versions; the publishers of the cosmic myth choosing to privilege a particular English version to comply with cosmopolitan taste; our patient then interpreting this myth to cope with and reconfigure his own distress; our subsequent professional translation through a clinical formulation of his narrative that then results in this chapter. Have we then violated fidelity to the original text? To the extent that a 'deeper' multifaceted texture interweaving Bangalore, Kannada, local mythology, and medical culture remains untranslated, silent, and unknown, this resonates with Robert Frost's characterization of 'poetry' ('what gets lost in translation'). On the other hand, we might compare this with a cited local instance that argues the significant gains to be had from translation: in White's (1996) retelling, the furniture store cheats you, the law provides a place to tell that story, and its language in which to do so, that may give you the power to get your money back. In our story, Andhaka bestows his power on us, both literally, through his relationship with SJ at the hospital, and symbolically, as in the Shiva myth, and in allowing that we become mediators of his story. In the process, Andhaka is able to restructure his own script by incorporating both mythical and psychological elements. And we, as mediators, have developed some awareness of the local cultural and moral worlds and their effect on the theories of our discipline. This change within the translator's 'self' as 'new author', turns all actors (including publisher, patient, and ourselves) into 'translated' men (Rushdie, 1983). However, this *collective* ability to use (and misuse) this power to translate cultural worlds and render them meaningful to the outsider remains problematic. Unlike White's Westernized example, where judicial power is supposedly fair to all, current clinical academic theories of the mind on other cultures continue to represent 'them' on 'our', not 'their', terms. It is difficult to propose hysteria as a type of spirit possession: compare the reverse (Littlewood, 1996a).

Post-colonial critical theory (in India now known as 'subaltern theory') on literature and history has been influential in that set of positions generally classed as 'post-modern'. In place of the 'grand meta-narratives' derived from the western englightenment, which promised us faithful representations of natural and social life, post-modernism prefers a loose assortment of complementary yet conflicting narratives, fragmented, partial, iterative, creolized, and interpenetrating, expressing the pragmatics of experience and identity over a truth to reality 'out there': discursive practices rather than hegemonic texts privileged by professional authority (their 'official', hence true, meaning). Yet personal experience, although central, is not to be considered primary, for human experience is always enacted through our production and transmission of signs (Derrida, 1973). And such signs have no invariable given meaning as immediate referrants to reality, but rather, through the endless deferred displacement of meaning from signifier to signifier (Derrida's famous *différence*). Cultures mediate reality by, in effect, creating it: individual perception, consciousness, and experience being the very cross-referencing of our systems of representation. And in all of this, the deconstructed human loses their primacy as the idealized subject.

Where does this then leave the compelling urgency of human 'illness' and 'suffering'? We might perhaps propose that both public and private illness may be seen as an aporia (*ibid.*) or lacuna between what a story attempts to say and what it is constrained to say: crises of contradiction when experience as narrated betrays the tension between experiential rhetoric and social logic, between what it manifestly means to convey and what it is none the less constrained to mean: an absolute indeterminacy (Turner, 1981; p. 153). We have previously approximated to this resistance of interpretation in more traditional idioms which do not altogether discard an independent natural world—as the contradiction between the naturalistic and personalistic modes of thought: an ironic simultaneity (Littlewood, 1996b). And the promise of 'healing' is thence a mediated reconciliation. Is Andhaka Oedipus? Or Oedipus Andhaka? Both and neither.

Acknowledgements

We are grateful for comments on an earlier draft by Yoram Bilu, Begum Maitra, Glenn Roberts, and Mitchell Weiss.

References

Ayyangar, T. S. R. (1952). *The yoga upanishads*, (trans. into English on the basis of the commentary of Sri Upanisadbrahmayogin). The Adyar Library, Madras.

Barthes, R. (1974). An introduction to the structural analysis of narrative. *New Literary History*, **6**, 237–72.

Bharati, A. (1985). The self in Hindu thought and action. In *Culture and self: Asian and Western perspectives*, (ed. A. J. Marsella, G. Devos, and F. L. K. Hsu) Tavistock, London.

Bilu, Y. and Witztum, E. (1995). The transmigration of Emperor Titus: religious idioms in the construction and alleviation of distress in a Jewish ultra-orthodox patient. *British Medical Anthropology Review* (n.s.), **3**, 16–26.

Bracero, W. (1996). Ancestral voices: narrative and multicultural perspective with an Asian schizophrenic. *Psychotherapy*, **33**, 48–67.

Deleuze, G. and Guattari, F. (1984). *Anti-Oedipus: capitalism and schizophrenia*. Athlone, London.

Derrida, J. (1973). *Speech and phenomen and other essays on Husserl's theory of signs*. Northwestern University Press, Evanston.

Devereux, G. (1983). Why Oedipus killed Laius: a note on the complementary Oedipus complex in Greek drama. In *Oedipus: A Folklore casebook*, (ed. L. Edmunds and A. Dundes) University of Wisconsin Press, Madison.

Dingwaney, A. and Maier, C. (ed.) (1996). *Between languages and cultures: translation and cross-cultural texts*. Oxford University Press, Delhi.

Doi, T. (1973). The anatomy of dependence. Kudansha, Tokyo.

Dow, J. (1968). Universal aspects of symbolic healing: a theoretical synthesis. *American Anthropologist*, **88**, 56–69.

Edmunds, L. and Dundes, A. (ed.) (1983). *Oedipus: a folklore casebook*. University of Wisconsin Press, Madison.

Erndi, K. M. (1993). *Victory to the mother: the Hindu goddesses of north western India in myth*. Oxford University Press, Oxford.

Freedman, J. and Coombs, G. (1996). *Narrative therapy: the social construction of preferred realities*. Norton, New York.

Freud, S. (1923). The Ego and the Id. *Standard Edition*, **19**, 12–66.

Gersie, A. (1996). *Reflections on therapeutic storymaking*. Jessica Kingsley, London.

Goldman, R. P. (1978). Fathers, sons and gurus: Oedipal conflict in the Sanskrit epics. *Journal of Indian Philosophy*, **6**, 325–92.

Guzder, J. and Krishna, M. (1991). Sita-Shakti: cultural paradigms for Indian women. *Transcultural Psychiatric Research Review*, **28**, 257–301.

Jadhav, S. (1994). Folk appropriation of ECT in South India. *Psychiatric Bulletin*, **128**, 180.

Johnson, A. W. and Price-Williams, D. (1997). Oedipus ubiquitous: the family complex in world folk literature. Stanford University Press, Stanford.

Kakar, S. (1981). *The inner world: a psycho-analytic study of childhood and society in India*. Oxford University Press, Delhi.

Kakar, S. (1989). *Intimate relations: exploring Indian sexuality*. Penguin, Harmondsworth.

Kakar, S. (1997). *Culture and psyche*. Oxford University Press, Delhi.

Kleinman, A. (1988). *The illness narratives: suffering, healing and the human condition*. Basic Books, New York.

Kramrisch, S. (1988). The presence of Śiva. Motilal Banarsidass, Varanasi.

Kurtz, S. M. (1992). *All the mothers are one*. Columbia University Press, New York.

Le Page, R. B. and Tabouret-Keller, A. (1985). *Acts of identity: creole based approaches to language and ethnicity*. Cambridge University Press, Cambridge.

Lévi-Strauss, C. (1968). The effectiveness of symbols. In *Structural anthropology*, (ed. C. Lévi-Strauss). Penguin, Harmondsworth.

Littlewood, R. (1996a). Psychiatry's culture. *International Journal of Social Psychiatry*, **42**, 245–68.

Littlewood, R. (1996b). *Reason and necessity in the specification of the multiple self*. Royal Anthropological Institute, London.

Mishara, A. (1995). Narrative and psychotherapy. *American Journal of Psychotherapy*, **49**, 180–95.

Nandy, A. (1983). *The intimate enemy: loss and recovery of self under colonization*. Oxford University Press, Delhi.

Obeyesekere, G. (1990). *The work of culture*. University of Chicago Press, Chicago.

Pai, A. (1985). Andhaka: the demon son of Shiva. In *Amar Chitra Katha: stories of Shiva*, Navaratna No. 8. India Book House, Bombay.

Parsons, A. (1964). Is the Oedipus complex universal? *The psychoanalytic study of society*. **3**, 278–328.

Ramanujan, A. K. (1983). *The Indian Oedipus*. In Oedipus: a folklore casebook, (ed. L. Edmunds and A. Dundes). University of Wisconsin Press, Madison.

Rank, O. (1992). *The incest theme in literature and legend: fundamentals of a psychology of literary creation*. Johns Hopkins University Press, Baltimore.

Roland, A. (1988). *In search of self in India and Japan: towards a cross-cultural psychology*. Princeton University Press, Princeton.

Rushdie, S. (1983). *Shame*. Aventura, London.

Sarbin, E. (ed.) (1986). *Narrative psychology*. Praeger, New York.

Spratt, P. (1966). Hindu culture and personality: a psychoanalytic study. Manaktala, Bombay.

Steiner, G. (1975). After Babel: aspects of language and translation. Oxford University Press.

Turner, V. (1980). Social dramas and stories about them. *Critical Inquiry*, **7** (1), 141–68.

Verma, V. (1988). Culture, personality and psychotherapy. *International Journal of Social Psychiatry*, **34** (2), 142–149.

White, J. B. (1996). On the virtues of not understanding, in Dingwaney and Maier, *op. cit.*

White, H. (1987). The content of the form narrative discourse and historical representation. John Hopkins University Press, Baltimore.

White, M. and Epston, D. (1990). Narrative means to therapeutic ends. Norton, New York.

6   Sacred tales

Andrew Sims

In the first draft of this chapter the word *sacred* became *scared*. Perhaps it is only when the subject of the story is very frightening indeed, affecting our health and our lives, that it can become truly sacred.

Tales and tails

In this chapter we will look at some of the stories behind the sources of energy in modern British health care. I see us, like the observers at an old-fashioned battle, standing on a hillside looking at and recognizing the prominent individuals as they approach us. We have difficulty identifying them as they leap into our view, and we may only be able to recognize them by their tails as they disappear once again. So, as the new National Health Service was unveiled before us in the early 1990s, we knew that we were to be confronted with *purchasers* and *providers* but it was not so easy to see at that stage how *market forces* would come to distort certain services. We have come to realize that it is 'only by their tails that ye shall know them'.

We have tried to follow a thread, or a tail, that runs through the tales of medicine, and, more specifically, of psychiatry. It is not only the beliefs and expectations of patients that affect the outcome of the therapeutic interaction. The values, the life agenda, and the guiding story of the psychiatrist also have overriding significance. It is 'only by their tales that ye shall know them'.

Where do the stories accepted by psychiatrists lead them? In the 19th century, the background belief and assumptions of Dr W. Crochley S. Clapham, a *protopsychiatrist* in Wakefield, Yorkshire, resulted in his weighing the brains of 'Roman Catholic', 'Protestant Dissent', and 'Church of England' patients at post-mortem, and coming to conclusions on the differences between them (Clapham, 1876): 'In the three great divisions of Christianity as professed in this country . . . it is curious to find that not only have the Roman Catholics heavier brains than the Protestant Dissenters, and these again than those of the Church party, but also that the Cerebellum, Pons, and Medulla, as compared with the entire brain, are proportionately larger in the Church of England cases than in the Roman Catholics . . .' In the 20th century, Kay Redfield Jamison (1993) has extensively studied the relationship between manic depressive illness and the artistic, especially poetic, temperament. Both these studies, one that seems so bizarre to us and one that seems so reasonable, could only be undertaken because of the background structures of the authors' very different worlds, and thus over what they were prepared to allow their enquiring eye to wander; their guiding myths.

People are not necessarily rational in the way they lead their lives. They work from background ideas and supposed certainties that have been handed down to them by their parents, more distant ancestors, their culture and society, and their professional teachers. Human beings are adept at living quite comfortably with inconsistencies, and perhaps the more rational they appear to others the greater is their tolerance for conflict and incompatibility.

In order to maintain the momentum of living and endeavouring, we need to have something or someone to believe in, some sort of allegiance. What a person declares publicly as their *belief* or *goal in life* may not necessarily be that individual's true aim and direction. This is true of the medical profession as well as of patients: twin stories of the caring, committed doctor and the avaricious, arrogant one run in parallel through the centuries.

Priests and doctors appear to have some characteristics in common. However, there are more features that distinguish the two professions, and it is as harmful for the recipient of their ministrations to have a doctor officiating as a priest as to have a priest prescribing as a doctor.

Some of the more specific myths of medicine surround the areas of training, science, putting experience into practice, and health care as a commercial commodity. A wonderful web of strong but filigree threads has been woven by and about doctors over the centuries. Sacred tales abound in all these apparently objective descriptions of the work of doctors and the concerns of their patients. At first sight medical treatment is a rational interaction involving the provision of a closely specified intervention by a doctor to (or sometimes into) a patient who knows exactly what he or she wants and is getting. Behind this superficial level of explanation there are many complicated and often unexpressed messages and meanings on both sides.

The end of our being: gold standards for psychiatric practice

Sacred, in our language as in others that are Latin based, started its existence as a past participle, and passively so—*dedicated, consecrated, set apart, has been made holy*. That emphasis from the original meaning of sacred is what holds the rather disparate parts of this chapter together. They are all stories about what someone at some time has made holy, and this holiness has been thrust upon them, sometimes against their will: the young professor wears an open-necked shirt and asks his students to call him 'Mike'—but it doesn't really work. Even the most egalitarian societies cannot function comfortably without pedestals, and the title *professor* inevitably becomes the podium for a pedestal.

Another skein that draws the separate threads together is the idea encapsulated within the phrase, 'the end of our being'. As used on solemn, proper, even sacred occasions, *end* is ambiguous. It describes both purpose and ultimate destiny, which for sober, serious people amounts to the same thing. The chief *end* or purpose of humans, for the early Puritans, was not their head end but 'worshipping God and enjoying Him for ever'. The ultimate end, in the destiny sense, would be to go on doing this for ever more.

These *stories*, then, are about ends as aims and goals, both the gold standard that I aspire to achieve now and the ultimate objective to which this leads; they are hopelessly idealistic and difficult of attainment: goals to be aimed at, not minimal standards to be surpassed. They are also about who I am, where I am, and what I am doing: my *being*. This is a serious story, proceeding with due gravitas and, as in Kierkegaard's 'being in the world lovingly', a very good maxim for psychiatrists. This theme of acting lovingly is surely the essence of what Leonard Stein has described as 'assertive community therapy' for helping severely mentally ill people who live outside hospital (Stein and Test, 1980): 'A supportive system that *assertively* helps the patient with . . . material resources such as food . . . coping skills to meet the demands of community life . . . motivation to persevere and remain involved with life . . . freedom from pathologically dependent relationships' and 'support and education of community members who are involved with patients'. This story of total care is both idealistic, in that it establishes an almost impossibly high standard, and realistic, in that we expect ourselves to be able to carry it out.

'Sacred tales' involve psychiatric patients and their treatment, psychiatrists, and others who undertake that treatment. These are humans living and acting, not just carrying out problem-solving behaviour according to stimulus and response principles. The basic tool of the psychiatrist, like the geologist's hammer or the builder's spirit level, is her shared humanity with the patient and the capacity this gives for empathy. It makes possible Jaspersian *understanding* by the psychiatrist who can hypothesize: 'if I had gone through that series of internal and external events, my present subjective experience would be just as my patient is now describing', and also, through this shared humanity, by the patient realizing that his sufferings are appreciated and understood (Jaspers, 1959). The psychiatrist will be referred to as 'she' and the patient as 'he' to give credence to current realities. Female doctors are rapidly approaching half the work force in psychiatry whilst male distress is also increasing, with indicators such as relatively higher rates of suicide for males (and with this increasing), and males experiencing more symptoms than females from unemployment and divorce.

There has often been a mismatch between what patients regard as important and hold sacred, and what psychiatrists look for in their assessment. Nowhere is this more apparent than in what patients regard as spiritual problems and psychiatrists consider either to be evidence of mental illness or, alternatively, ignore altogether. Spiritual problems and religious beliefs are quite frequent in the material presented to psychiatrists by their patients. In the same way that psychiatrists are sometimes critical of Cartesian dichotomy resulting in 'mindless' or 'brainless' psychiatry (Eisenberg, 1986), so we should legitimately be critical of the doctor who ignores the important religious or spiritual dimension of the patient's distress (Sims, 1994). Practising religious beliefs has been shown to have a beneficial effect upon recovery from both physical and psychiatric disorder (Craigie *et al.*, 1990; Larson *et al.*, 1992). Religious belief may be involved in the delusions of psychotic patients and be a factor in disturbed and dangerous behaviour. It is essential that psychiatrists know what their patients hold sacred, understand the implications of this for his equanimity, treat his beliefs and even prejudices with due sensitivity, and communicate to him that religious beliefs and practices are fully respected.

Lack of appreciation of religious beliefs by psychiatrists follows a long tradition of mutual mistrust between the Church and what subsequently became the psychiatric establishment. It was a brave, even heroic, act to wrest the treatment of mental illness out of ecclesiastical grip and place it unequivocally within medicine. Even though this was carried out by orthodox believers, such as Vives in the 16th century, it was adjudged by the monolithic, clerical establishment as suspect and iconoclastic. Subsequently, many of the roots of modern day psychiatry have been atheistic: Freud, although developing a comprehensive psychological explanation that has been considered to be religious in nature (Webster, 1995), regarded religion as a form of neurosis; Pavlov's theories on conditioning were essentially materialist in their philosophical underpinning; Skinner's operant conditioning was reductionist and left no room for super-natural belief; the very word *pharmacology*, so prominent in modern psychiatry, is derived from the Greek word for a sorcerer. Not surprisingly, there is scope for misunderstanding: devout members of religious organizations of many different creeds have been warned that psychiatry is opposed to religion, and psychiatrists have sometimes considered that religious practice damages the health and well-being of their patients.

These misunderstandings between individuals with sincerely held grounds for action, which appear to follow rationally from underlying assumptions, are deeply ingrained. They are recognized by those aspiring to transcultural psychiatry but often the differences in springs for action that arise from different narratives are ignored by psychiatrists who think that because they share ethnic origin with their patient, and were born in the same city, they will necessarily have the same attitudes. The different explanatory stories of patient and psychiatrist may dominate their behaviour and prevent communication with the other. We will return to this theme again later, but to simplify: the patient with a dominant religious or other belief system recognizes that the psychiatrist not only offers treatment but also an apparently conflicting world view of how he, the patient, arrived in his current predicament. The psychiatrist does indeed believe that she has a story that will be both helpful for the future and explanatory for the past. She does not see this as secular religion, but that is how the patient may perceive it.

Travellers tales: how patients and doctors are influenced by stories rather than 'facts'

It is surprising how widespread belief is in 'behemoth' and 'leviathan'—imaginary monsters half-recalled by visitors to the frontier of Hell. Scratch the surface of a rational medical practitioner and one finds a superstitious witch doctor. Even the Domus Medica of the Royal Society of Medicine substitutes Room No. 12A for 13! Myths abound concerning all powerful structures; for example, concerning the General Medical Council (GMC), perhaps the most awe-inspiring organization in British medicine to the individual doctor, it has been ascribed that 'they' are planting spurious patients in general practitioners' waiting rooms to catch out the unwary doctor in unprofessional practice. This was never true, but it accurately represents doctors' fears of the GMC's omnipotence; a myth is not necessarily factually accurate but contains within it the essence of the truth. Not only patients but also doctors are dominated and limited by stories that go beyond the truth.

Metapsychology describes those untested and probably untestable hypotheses upon which so much of our practice is based. The word, and the notion, is derived from *metaphysics* which means 'philosophical speculation beyond the current or even seemingly possible limits of science . . .' (Gregory, 1987). It is probable that there is no such thing as a theory-free observation in science or a value-free decision in clinical practice. We are at the mercy not only of what we have experienced, but also of the interpretation we put upon it.

Physics, a metaphor for living solely by scientific principles, is a sparsely furnished house where very few of us live. Usually we are just 'beyond physics', like Aristotle's *Metaphysics*, trying to give reasons for the things we do, but hard put to explain every attitude and item of behaviour rationally. We live by a conceptual framework which proscribes certain things we must not do until a supervening explanatory story replaces it and makes these things permissible. A middle-aged woman stops eating beef because her father had died 10 years previously of an unexplained illness, 'and it might have been BSE'. Our hypothetical formulations, like any other archaic structure such as a Roman temple, have multiple origins from different periods of time. They are immensely powerful and mould our everyday behaviour; 'ideas have legs and they march in other people's armies'. This is equally true for those with conventional religious beliefs and for those trying to base their lives on scientific rationalism. Doctors are influenced by *wondrous* travellers' tales.

When, as psychiatrists, we interview a new patient, we start by 'taking the history'. The history is *his story*: that is, not just an account of all the happenings of our patient's life, it is an interpretation through his eyes, and is presented to us in the way he intends us to receive it. Not only are the facts described, but also the guiding myths of this particular person throughout his life. For his own subjective appreciation, these must be coherent and explanatory, but it is not necessary for them to be fair in their assessment of other people, or accurate.

Important for assessment in psychiatry is measurement of change. Is the patient getting better or worse in his general condition? What changes have there been and in which of the symptoms that were originally presented? The account the patient gives about his condition is a useful marker: a widening gulf between the patient's description of how it is and how it should be, or a widening divergence between how he explains his world compared with others' assessment is perhaps the clearest indication of deterioration in the mental state. This is demonstrated in the elaboration of more and more complex delusions in a psychotic illness, or in the progressive loss of control of circumstances in the story of how other people are making *my* life so difficult in a deteriorating neurotic disorder.

Living with apparent inconsistencies is a normal experience of everyday life. Some of the most successful and creative thinkers and innovators, in all areas of life, have survived fairly comfortably with huge discrepancies between their guiding myths. They have retired from their professional careers, and subsequently died, without ever resolving these conflicts. Perhaps an overarching formulation or background religious or philosophical belief allowed them to use both stories in different segments of activity, and yet keep them apart. For our patients this has often not been possible. The final breakdown, the point at which they seek help may well come when, fully recognizing the inconsistencies in their life, they can no longer tolerate them. The development of mental symptoms produces increasing contradiction between their conflicting conceptual frameworks and, eventually, this is no longer containable. The gulf between how it is and how it should be, or between how I see it and how it really is, has become unbridgeable. Of course, the words 'gulf', 'bridge', and 'see', without which it is impossible to make this point, are all images from a travel narrative.

'This story shall the good man teach his son': one can only live by 'good' stories

The tales by which people live, and even die, may be elaborately embroidered. In fact, when Henry V spoke the above about Agincourt, he assumed that a certain amount of embellishment would take place. Action demanded as a result of the story is of extreme importance; when a father tells his son about his military exploits he is exhorting his son to do likewise. It is not only the father who lives by this story, but also his son, and perhaps many subsequent generations.

As far as our patients are concerned, the major problem with their story is that they can no longer live by it as an unfailing code for the conduct of daily life. It has broken down. In terms of literary criticism, according to Frye (1957), it is *pathos*: 'The best word for low mimetic or domestic tragedy is, perhaps, pathos, and pathos has a close relation to the sensational reflex of tears. Pathos presents its hero as isolated by a weakness which appeals to our sympathy because it is on our own level of experience. I speak of a hero, but the central figure of pathos is often a woman or a child (or both, as in the death-scenes of Little Eva and Little Nell), and we have a whole procession of pathetic female sacrifices in English low mimetic fiction from Clarissa Harlow to Hardy's Tess and James's Daisy Miller. We note that while tragedy may massacre a whole cast, pathos is usually concentrated on a single character, partly because low mimetic society is more strongly individualised'. More than half of psychiatric patients are female; a recurrent feature of their story is how they alone are miserable, experience failure, have tragedies, are ignored by others, are treated with disrespect and discriminated against, while the rest of the world enjoys itself. Often these impressions are justified.

The doctor also has a story, sometimes called a *diagnostic formulation*, which has consequences for the patient and, to a lesser extent, for the doctor. For no other condition in psychiatry has this been more dramatic than for dissociative fugue, the ultimate in 'Travellers tales'. Originally regarded as a distinct psychiatric illness in 1887, in Bordeaux, these people were referred to as 'les aliénés voyageurs'. The term was often used to describe vagrants, a common social problem 100 years ago, as now. However, military doctors defined it as an illness in order to protect army deserters from summary execution (Hacking, 1996). This particular tall story was clearly life-saving!

The story told by the patient and the story heard by the doctor depend upon the overt and covert relationship between them. When the patient talks to the doctor, the doctor has certain expectations which may differ from those the patient expects the doctor to expect. Hopefully, this difference between observed and expected will evoke the doctor's careful concentration, but sometimes, unfortunately, the doctor only listens to what fulfils professional preconceptions. Ritualizing the process of diagnosis can exacerbate this particular problem. A patient, who was also a physician, sought out a particular psychiatrist because of the psychiatrist's reputation for minimal drug intervention. The psychiatrist, knowing the patient to come from a biologically oriented speciality, used more drug treatment than was his custom. Fortunately, doctor and patient talked to each other concerning their expectations at this point and prevented what could otherwise have become a therapeutic impasse.

Beliefs and allegiances can lead to distortion and misunderstanding in the therapeutic alliance. A patient with anxiety and depressive symptoms insists, when the general practitioner wishes to make a referral, on seeing a 'Christian psychiatrist'. When the referral is made and the psychiatric intervention is taking place with someone regarded as an appropriate psychiatrist, it transpires that the patient's agenda for psychiatric management only permits the patient and the chosen psychiatrist to discuss what are regarded as 'spiritual' issues and the unpleasant effects upon the patient's sensitive soul of figures from her past, including her parents, whom she has labelled non-Christian. When the psychiatrist states that her professional formulation would indicate cognitive behavioural therapy and an SSRI (Selective Serotonin Reuptake Inhibitor) antidepressant, the consultation is promptly terminated and the search for 'someone who really understands me' begins all over again. If patient and doctor, however similar they may have appeared to be, are actually working to different narratives, the therapeutic alliance will not function.

A well-meaning but somewhat doctrinaire local politician gets involved with the provision of mental health services to a community, many members of which came originally from a small village in Kashmir. He insists that only a psychiatrist from overseas can provide services to these patients. Fortunately, this story has a happy ending as the Chinese psychiatrist, with no South Asian languages and no rural experience, is culturally aware and provides an excellent service to this particular patient group. There was no need for the psychiatrist to share cultural background with these patients but it was important to understand their stories.

Sometimes, because of the doctor's own background and preconceptions, he (and in this situation it is more often he) is not able to hear and respond to the patient's description of misery. This can be likened to a figurative knot in the stethoscope (Sims, 1996). The doctor may cope with professional pressures by habitually suppressing his own emotional expression, hence tying the knot. Doctors have a reputation for being poor at communication. This may be explained by their predominant age, sex, social class, and background. It may also be learned, finding that the mechanism of denial is self-preservative in coping with emotions created by the extreme suffering and sometimes inexplicable death of the patient. The training of doctors is arduous and extremely competitive; some suspect that any sign of weakness might jeopardize their career and raise questions of suitability for the most prestigious jobs. Not hearing the patient's anguish may be a desperate attempt to defend oneself against overwhelming emotional demands. The 'knot in the stethoscope' is within the physician's responsibility in communication. It prevents the physician from hearing the heart beat and the life breath of the patient. When emotional receptivity is blocked it does not just result in communication being as limited as if the stethoscope, the professional symbol of listening, was not used at all; it forms a total barrier to communication. Our professional role and status can prevent us hearing any of the emotional expression of our patients.

'Thomas Sydenham is dead and I am not feeling too good myself': lessons from medical history, 'good' and 'bad' doctors

There are ambivalent attitudes towards the practice of medicine, how it is conducted, and how others regard that practice; medical history clearly shows this. On the one hand, there is some veneration for the heroes of the past—a quotation from Thomas Sydenham would make an excellent way with which to begin a medical lecture. On the other hand, it is fashionable to show that medicine is progressive and scientific, continually abandoning the prejudices of the past. A bright young medical researcher is calling upon a seconder with gravitas in the debate if he can demonstrate that his innovation reinforces the sustaining values of the medical profession. The ambivalence lies in that both tradition and the pursuit of progress are accepted by doctors and patients as stereotypes for medical practice: do these stereotypes enable or disable?

Throughout history there has been a massive polarization of doctors, as seen by their patients, into 'good' and 'bad': doctors make you worse and are avaricious, versus the caring, committed doctor devoted to the needs of the poorest patients and seeking no other reward than seeing the patient get better. This lofty view of medical practice is gratifyingly still held by a considerable number of medical students and practising doctors.

Let us review some of these tales about doctors. Matthew Prior, in the early 18th century, takes up the first of our themes:

> Cur'd yesterday of my disease,
> I died last night of my physician
> (*Prior, 1704.*)

This recurring myth is not actually true of doctors, nor ever has been. Doctors very rarely kill their patients, largely because they do not have that amount of power. Dying of medical neglect is much less common than many patients think. The myth contained in the story is that doctors are amazingly powerful and if only they had used their knowledge and skill on our behalf then the deceased could have been saved. The reality is that in most instances medical intervention neither prolongs nor accelerates either recovery or death.

Next is a longer quotation from later in the 18th century in which George Crabbe mocks many of these medical stereotypes:

> Anon, a figure enters, quaintly neat,
> All pride and business, bustle and conceit,
> With looks unalter'd by these scenes of woe,
> With speed that, entering, speaks his haste to go
> He bids the gazing throng around him fly
> And carries fate and physic in his eye:
> A potent quack, long versed in human ills,
> Who first insults the victim whom he kills;
> Whose invidious hand a drowsy Bench protect,
> And whose most tender mercy is neglect,
> Paid by the parish for attendance here,
> He wears contempt upon his sapient sneer;
> In haste he seeks the bed where misery lies,
> Impatience marked in his averted eyes;
> And, some habitual queries o'er,
> Without reply, he rushes to the door.
> (*Crabbe, 1783.*)

This description contains many of the demonizing characteristics of the much feared doctor. He, and it is more often he and not she, is proud and pompous. He treats his non-paying patients with unconcealed disdain. He is in a hurry, he avoids ordinary conversation and human contact. He is protected by the legal authorities and the established order. Above all else he is incredibly powerful; that bit is shared by both 'good' and 'bad' doctor myths.

Now let us look at the other side of the coin. I do not know if it is significant that my next two quotations come from the late 19th century; after the Medical Act had cleansed the profession of its worse abusers, and before the era of effective remedies. Rudyard Kipling emphasizes the commitment of the doctor to his work, especially in the number of hours of anxious endeavour, in 'A doctor's work':

> In all time of flood, fire, famine, plague, pestilence, battle, murder and sudden death it will be required of you that you report for duty at once, and go on duty at once, and that you stay on duty until your strength fails you or your conscience relieves you; whichever may be the longer period . . . have you heard of any Bill for an eight hours day for doctors?

You belong to the privileged classes. May I remind you of some of your privileges? You and Kings are the only people whose explanation the police will accept if you exceed the legal limit in your car. On presentation of your visiting card you can pass through the most turbulent crowd unmolested and even with applause. If you fly a yellow flag over a centre of the population you can turn it into a desert. If you choose to fly a Red Cross flag over a desert you can turn it into a centre of population towards which, as I have seen, men will crawl on hands and knees. You can forbid any ship to enter any port in the world. If you think it necessary to the success of any operation in which you are interested you can stop a 20,000 ton liner with mail in mid-ocean till the operation is concluded.

(*Kipling, 1928.*)

Once again the force of the myth is the almost god-like, certainly regal, power of the doctor. The doctor can do almost anything when in role.

So much for the public health doctor in the thick of the crowd dealing with a rapidly fatal epidemic, but how about the doctor with one individual patient in the quietness of the sick room? W. E. Henley gives the patient's perspective of a caring physician:

His brow spreads large and placid, and his eye
Is deep and bright, with steady looks that still.
Soft lines of tranquil thought his face fulfil—
His face at once benign and proud and shy.
If envy scant, if ignorance deny
His faultless patience, his unyielding will,
Beautiful gentleness and splendid skill
Innumerable gratitudes reply.
His wise, rare smile is sweet with certainties,
And seems in all his patience to compel
Such love and faith as failure cannot quell.

(*Henley, 1873*)

If only . . . this patient is not so much describing a real doctor but a fervent wish, a physician the whole of whose powers and energies are devoted to looking after . . . *me*!

Hogarth and Fyldes portray these two differing physicians visually. Dickens, Trollope, and numerous other authors describe them. Despite the known and obvious limitations of medical practice, the belief in arcane knowledge and the image of incisive potency is repeated through successive generations. Clearly, all these patients cannot be ignorant about the very narrow range of medical efficacy. The only possible explanation must be that patients demand their doctors to live a lofty fiction: be omniscient, Olympian, both closely caring and objectively remote.

Within the medical profession itself this ambivalence is also significant. On the one hand, individual doctors and their trade union defending their rights, demonstrate the impossibility of the tasks thrust upon them and demand more resources in order to achieve a reasonable standard of care. At the same time, the profession, from the time of the Hippocratic Oath onwards, is unashamed in establishing for itself idealistic goals that are almost unattainable.

These goals demonstrate narrative at work in the practice of medicine; they are personalized and written in the language of epic. The Declaration of Geneva (World Medical Association, 1968) is a modern restatement of the Hippocratic Oath and it will be quoted in full since it gives the clearest indication of what are currently the aspirations of the medical profession in idealistic mode:

I solemnly pledge myself to consecrate my life to the service of humanity;
I will give to my teachers the respect and gratitude which is their due;

I will respect the secrets which are confided in me, even after the patient has died;
I will maintain by all the means in my power the honour and the noble traditions of the medical profession;
My colleagues will be my brothers;
I will not permit consideration of religion, nationality, race, party politics or social standing to intervene between my duty and my patients;
I will maintain the utmost respect for human life from the time of conception;
Even under threat, I will not use my medical knowledge contrary to the law of humanity.
I make these promises solemnly, freely and upon my honour.

Life and death, use of time, financial reward, and respect for humanity receive comment. The themes are recurrent. However, it is the medical profession itself making a statement; the element of potency is muted. We know that we can not really do that much in most situations.

In the United Kingdom, the General Medical Council has also produced what could be seen as a credal statement, that is a 'sacred tale', under the heading 'The duties of a doctor':

Patients must be able to trust doctors with their lives and well-being. To justify that trust, we as a profession have a duty to maintain a good standard of practice and care and to show respect for human life.

In particular, as a doctor, you must:

◆ Make the care of your patient your first concern;

◆ Treat every patient politely and considerately;

◆ Respect a patient's dignity and privacy;

◆ Listen to patients and respect their views;

◆ Give patients information in a way they can understand;

◆ Respect the rights of patients to be fully involved in decisions about their care;

◆ Keep all professional knowledge and skills up to date;

◆ Recognise the limits of your professional competence;

◆ Be honest and trustworthy;

◆ Respect and protect confidential information;

◆ Make sure that your personal beliefs do not prejudice your patient's care;

◆ Act quickly to protect patients from risk if you have good reason to believe that you or a colleague may not be fit to practice;

◆ Avoid abusing your position as a doctor; and,

◆ Work with colleagues in a way that best serve patients' interests.

In all these matters you must never discriminate unfairly against your patients or colleagues. And you must always be prepared to justify your actions to them.
(*Good medical practice, 1995.*)

The stated aims of the Royal College of Psychiatrists in its Royal Charter are as follows:

To advance the science and practice of psychiatry and related subjects;
To promote public knowledge of psychiatry;
To promote study and research in psychiatry and related subjects and to publish the results of all such studies and research.

Once again, the objectives are entirely lofty and set a standard for attainment. It is only by setting ideals that we are able to attain a reasonable level. These are all pious statements: 'religious' in the sense that this is what doctors *bind* themselves to carry out, 'sacred' in the sense that they *dedicate* their professional lives to these ideals, 'credal' in the sense that the doctor says: 'This is what *I believe*' about my professional practice.

There are, then, two radically different stories, but, like two different accounts from the scene of the crime, they are describing the same event. It is not the case that patients tell one story and doctors another. Although their emphases are different, the two conflicting stories come both from doctors and from patients. Doctors are sometimes avaricious, negligent, arrogant, crass, and unfeeling. They are also sometimes breathtakingly altruistic, caring to their own detriment, sympathetic, understanding, and sensitive. Not only are some doctors one and some the other, but the same doctor may show different characteristics at different times and even, such is the complexity of human nature, at the same time. Which story is true? The answer is neither and both. The stories carry the myth of medical practitioner attitudes, and patient hopes and expectations.

The priest as psychiatrist–the psychiatrist as priest: the importance of role in professional behaviour

There are interesting similarities and contrasts between the work of psychiatrists and ministers of religion: parishioners and patients place the different professionals in somewhat similar narratives, with comparable expectations. There are also very real differences that need to be given expression; the two professions function in very different settings. I wish to consider here some further aspects of the psychiatrist on the one hand espousing, or being forced into the role, and on the other avoiding any semblance of, the work of the priest.

The dilemma for the psychiatrist, acting as receptacle for the pain, suffering, and guilt of patients yet not entering into religious explanations, holding a world view as an individual, yet knowing that any hint of imposing this upon the patient will be harmful, highlights both the power and the potential for misunderstanding that can arise from patients' and doctors' differing narratives. Patient and doctor give differing accounts for describing the relationship that links them. The psychiatrist has an idea of her place in the world, how she relates to others, and, specifically, her relationship with this patient. She also has an idea of how she is viewed by the patient and how this view of the patient about herself differs from her own view of herself. In fact, the patient's view of the psychiatrist is probably different from both of these but involves how the psychiatrist considers her relationship with me, the patient, and how this view of me differs from my own view of myself as patient, and my place in the world both as patient and as an individual in society. The psychiatrist also has a self-image, which is radically altered by the different roles she takes up and puts down at different times through her life and on different occasions on any single day: as doctor with this individual patient, as manager of a multidisciplinary team, as consultant psychiatrist supervising a more junior doctor, as teacher with undergraduate medical students, and so on; as mother, as sister, as daughter, as the closest human being now alive on the planet to an isolated, extremely neurotic schoolfriend from 30 years ago; as an individual with religious beliefs who is also a member of a Church and sings in the choir. It is hardly surprising that there is scope for misunderstanding.

Some doctors are aware of dissonance between the sacred stories of their personal beliefs, religious or otherwise, and their professional practice. They realize that they must not jeopardize the patient's health or well-being because of their beliefs, but at the same time they know that the *ideal* psychiatrist (according to Jaspers, 1959) is 'the one who will combine scientific attitudes of the sceptic with a powerful impressive personality and a profound existential faith . . .' Harmonization comes from being sensitive to the existential or religious framework of the patient, using this for the patient's benefit, but at the same time fitting this new knowledge and experience into the doctor's own beliefs and guiding stories to integrate the out-working of her own faith.

In this particular dilemma, the two horns are the religious faith and world view of the patient and of the doctor; misunderstandings can arise even when trying to make allowances for the other's perspective. Sustained convictions are held with the force of a commandment and powerfully influence behaviour. This was exemplified by an 89-year-old woman who wrote to the newspaper saying that she was too frightened to claim her two million pound winnings on the National Lottery. Most readers were unable to understand her position and assumed that she must be of unsound mind, not knowing her story. She and her husband, out of religious conviction, had never gambled. Her husband had recently been admitted to hospital and died there. Whilst in hospital, without her knowing it he had bought a lottery ticket and this had been the winner. Far from being delighted with her success, she saw his subsequent death as retribution, and so the money had become tainted, threatening, and evil.

How does a doctor work with the patient's religious conviction and the effect this has upon his behaviour and life-style? Certainly not by ignoring those beliefs, nor by imposing the doctor's own beliefs upon the patient. A middle-aged woman living with her family develops a moderately severe depressive illness. She becomes convinced that she has committed the unforgivable sin: 'the blasphemy against the Spirit will not be forgiven' (Matthew 13.31). She has worried a lot about the Holy Spirit and wonders if her thoughts could have amounted to blasphemy. She has become convinced she has committed that sin although she does not really know what it is. Does the doctor tell her that she feels this way because of her depressive illness (which is probably true), or try to argue her out of her belief on the basis of what the doctor believes? Neither; but this doctor acted in the role of psychiatrist, using the attitudes, belief, understanding, and knowledge of the patient. She, the patient, also believed that 'if we confess our sins, He (Jesus Christ) is faithful and just and will forgive us our sins and purify us from all unrighteousness' (I. John I.9). The psychiatrist, without imposing upon her anything that she herself did not accept, was able to set up a situation in which she was 'arguing' with herself and hence changing her attitudes through her own cognitive set. She was helped to argue in her head: 'if every sin confessed before God can be forgiven, then the reason an individual sin cannot be forgiven must be because it is not and cannot be confessed before God. That implies denying the existence or potency of God and His Spirit in the world from now into perpetuity. I am not and have never done that, and therefore I have not committed the unforgivable sin.' This is an over-simplification of a complex process.

Psychiatric treatment of patients with religious symptoms has been described by Bishay and Ormston (1996), using cognitive therapy, and by Beck *et al.* (1979) for depression. The patient's mood is dependent upon his cognitions and hence on the narrative of his life. Treatment implies helping him to become aware of his cognitive distortions and dysfunctional constructs in order for him to be able to challenge these and replace them from his own background perspectives and world view. When dealing with religious symptoms the therapist must know about the patient's religious beliefs, without necessarily sharing them. The beliefs of patients should form an important part of the knowledge base for a psychiatrist, but this is often neglected during medical training.

Patients, and especially those with powerful religious convictions, have expectations, and often apprehensions, before psychiatric interview, such as whether the psychiatrist will accept, reject, or ignore the patient's beliefs and their association with psychic pain; with each of these approaches there is a potential problem. If the psychiatrist appears to accept the patient's belief wholesale, there are two areas of danger. First, the psychiatrist may be seen by the patient not only to accept the constructs of the religious belief but also the patient's views concerning himself within those beliefs: for example, that he, the patient is guilty, sinful, deserving of punishment, and that the painful emotion is entirely justifiable and appropriate. Secondly, there is a strong tendency for the psychiatrist to be drawn out of the role of therapist and into the role of priest, thus being propelled into moral comment upon the actions of the patient.

If the psychiatrist is considered by the patient to be rejecting his religion then, faith being so central in its effects upon the whole of life, dialogue at all levels between patient and doctor may become blocked, and the patient may not be able to hear any of the doctor's recommendations about his health; the psychiatrist's opinion has become invalidated. If the psychiatrist ignores the patient's beliefs and how they affect his everyday behaviour, the patient will become highly selective as to what information is volunteered, and the psychiatrist may get a false impression of his life situation. The psychiatrist needs to convey to the patient that the patient's religious beliefs will be respected and understood, and that the world view of the doctor will not be intruded into the interview.

Psychiatrists from different countries, cultures, and religions are agreed that they do not make moral judgements based upon the patient's past behaviour, but deal with the here and now. The method of working of the psychiatrist is 'pragmatic, empirical and limited; the world view of the eye down the microscope, or the gastroscope; the ear which listens intently for bowel sounds or the description of hallucinatory voices . . . there are many psychiatrists who appear to work quite confidently without any world view at all, whose view of illness is the conglomerate of the complaints their patients present to them; and of health, freedom from these nuisances' (Sims, 1992).

It is not quite as simple as this, however, as the doctor is a human being. Like the patient, the doctor also has a world view, holds spiritual values, may even have religious beliefs; and, of course, atheism as explanatory of the world situation is a religion. The doctor should acknowledge her own beliefs and values and use these to improve her understanding of patients with differing beliefs and faith.

Will it never end?: medical education as a continuing process

There is a guiding myth that has moulded the behaviour of generations in the medical profession: medicine as a *learned profession*. Of course, *doctor* means teacher, and implies that every doctor is a teacher and every teacher is a perpetual student. Medical education starts on the day of entering medical school, and continues until that doctor retires from all medical practice. Many do not consider that their studying is over even then, as a visit to the library of the Royal

Society of Medicine on any week day will amply prove. Within medicine, an entrenched value system of knowledge establishes experiment and experimental evidence as the most highly regarded in the hierarchy, information from an acknowledged authority is next, and general, unattributed knowledge last. The medical expert seeks to replace knowledge based upon authority by knowledge from research findings, whilst less prestigious doctors are seeking to base their practice upon the authority of these experts. Medicine thinks of itself as the model for a scientific profession.

This is an era of increasing specialization. In the past, medical students were taught by doctors who knew a great deal about their subject but nothing about the process of education. Within recent years medical education has become a specialism in its own right and is perhaps one of the most rapidly developing subjects within medicine in the last five years. With increasing specialization has come a vocabulary of educational terms and a raft of new medical educational concepts. Each of *knowledge*, *skills*, and *attitudes* requires a different method of teaching medical students. With the enormous increase in the *knowledge* base of medicine, medical students can no longer be exposed to all the available information, far less can they learn it, and from this has developed the need to define the *core curriculum*. Whereas in the past the *skills* that a junior doctor needed for practice were ignored in formal training and acquired by imitating those a little more senior, it is now accepted that clinical skills can be learnt without hurting patients and that they need to be practised and rehearsed thoroughly before the individual is safe for clinical work. It is now recognized that communication with patients, with relatives, and between doctors is a skill that also has to be learned. Although it has always been part of the task of the medical student to acquire the *attitudes* of the profession, it is only relatively recently that medical teachers have tried to find out how to inculcate attitudes that benefit patients.

Significant in postgraduate medical education is the programme of promotion, which is attained by achieving specific educational objectives. Current progression in the United Kingdom is from preregistration house officer to senior house officer, specialist registrar, and, ultimately, the accolade of consultant in the chosen specialty, with similar progression through the grades to professor on the academic side. Along whichever pathway the aspiring junior doctor proceeds, each change of job title is seen as a major achievement, a significant rite of passage. The learning experiences which have to be undertaken before the individual can be a candidate for promotion are more or less clearly laid out, but the informal requirements such as having the 'right' attitude and having published 'enough' papers are often more demanding than the formal requirements of examinations passed, and require time spent in each designated post. Not only does this process allow the individual to obtain the knowledge and learn the skills relevant to her chosen specialty, it also gives time and exposure to acquire the *persona* of the profession.

An interesting concept for the process of enabling an individual to join the medical profession, or a new specialty within it, is the term *induction*, which elsewhere in medicine has a technical meaning with significant parallels. Induction of labour describes the intervention, when, at full-term pregnancy, a woman does not go into labour spontaneously. The image is of the infant's carefully controlled entry into the world. Let us look briefly at this process at two specific points in medical training: first, on starting as a medical student, and secondly, at the beginning of specialist psychiatric training. Traditionally, and for most doctors who are currently in practice, the greatest effect upon us of our new status in our first week as a medical student was entering the dissecting room. Medical students talked about little else; there was a frisson of excitement and horror associated with their initiation which promoted bonding with the peer group and a certain distance from all others. Some of the 'nothing but' attitudes prevalent later on are inculcated at that first experience. It is easy to acquire notions that human beings are 'nothing but' dead mammals when one's first experience of humans, after years of dissection of amphibians and other mammals, is the atmosphere of mass mortality in the dissecting room.

Having chosen as my career to specialize in psychiatry and having obtained a suitable training post, my first day in psychiatry was formative. After about two hours in the specialty I was sent, as 'the psychiatrist', to the Accident and Emergency Department to see 'an overdose'. The patient concerned was suffering from chronic alcohol misuse, he had swallowed a number of tablets, and was not sure how much of what. He was still somewhat drunk, he had no permanent home, and no relatives with whom he was in contact. I was baffled, and my education, in learning attitudes and to some extent skills although not knowledge, started from that point. This new world into which I was being delivered from the womb of my previous innocence was hard, cold, and not particularly welcoming.

The word usually used for the postgraduate education in medicine is *training*. This also creates an evocative image, for example, the training of fruit-bearing shoots, which implies controlling the growth into what is considered to be an appropriate direction. Encouraging some aspects of growth, discouraging others, and lopping off unwanted developments with the secateurs' peremptory cut, in the medical idiom might well be examinations and their frequently unfortunate results, but also suggests the admonitions of senior consultants. Most doctors can remember being harshly treated by their training consultants, and they may reveal the mental scars to prove it! This metaphor, as well as evoking appropriate professional fruitfulness, also suggests possible distortions of development and permanent callous formation.

The terms continuing medical education (CME) and continuing professional development (CPD) have been introduced to cover the process that takes place once the doctor has become a trained specialist, which may last for 32 years out of a professional career of 40 years. Continuing medical education implies acquiring new and maintaining existing medical knowledge and skills. Continuing professional development, the preferred term of the Royal College of Psychiatrists, is more comprehensive and includes both this and also learning to manage a service, working with a multidisciplinary team, and developing one's own professional potential. The varying goals of this educational process will require different educational methods. The detail will not be worked through here, but the point, as far as narrative is concerned, is that CME depicts the senior doctor going back to medical school, eyes down the microscope. CPD portrays learning new professional approaches for working harmoniously with other professions, new methods of treatment that are more acceptable to patients, new attitudes for leadership and for maintaining professional interest and appropriate concern for patients, and learning good management skills and cost efficiency. The answer to the question with which this section started, 'Will it never end?', comes with continuing professional development. The education of the doctor only ends with retirement. This challenges the notion of the omniscient consultant: the doctor is just a student and by no means God.

We could not look at medical education from the ironical perspective of the story-teller without glancing at examinations. The examination, and especially the medical postgraduate examination, is the most sacred rite performed by the high priests of the medical profession. It is how we learn, word perfect, the tribe's story, by presenting it before the elders. Like other initiation rites it may be excruciatingly painful. Examinations have a special aura in medical mythology and the stories of those who have aspired to succeed. The first plan formed after a newly qualified doctor chooses their medical specialty is how to embark upon and pass the postgraduate examination; often, the first act in establishing a new medical specialty has been to establish a specialist examination with all its relevant paraphernalia. Whereas machismo conversation amongst rugby players may concentrate upon the severity of their injuries, amongst medical trainees it compares the failure rates for different specialist examinations. Kudos is attached to passing an examination with only a 20% pass rate, and for some strange reason that admiration is transferred to the examination itself! This prodigal failure rate comes at the same time as the current serious need for more trained specialists. There seems to be little wrong with the academic component of the training given to junior doctors so why have we chosen to use examinations to control the numbers coming into specialties? Unfortunately, the ordeal of the postgraduate examination has become embroiled with perverse incentives such as 'I had to pass it, why shouldn't they' and 'a high fail rate ensures a high quality of candidate'.

There is, surely, an element of tribal ritual about the MRCPsych examination for psychiatrists. The motto of the Royal College of Psychiatrists is 'let wisdom guide', but, too easily, conformity with current norms of clinical practice and the medium-term retention of a trunk-full of facts determines success. The exclusion of any reference to the spiritual state of patients, to value systems, from the examination indicates to novices that the psychiatric establishment will endorse their ignoring it also in their subsequent practice. How can we so glibly deny patients the right of taking seriously what they believe to be important?

This concentration upon the examination as a means to promotion within the profession has resulted in a complete industry of examination aids, training courses, manuals, software, and so on. The individual's future is dependent upon the highly arbitrary yet quantifiable nature of competitive examination. There are parallels with the elaborate systems of examinations developed in ancient China, success in which controlled entry to all senior, bureaucratic positions in government. No professional progress was possible without passing, and there were many levels of examination up to the most prestigious and difficult. In that culture also there was concern about training the examiners, about avoiding political interference with the examination process, and 'by the 1740's the examinations as a whole were coming under attack as sterile exercises that failed to select the finest scholars for office' (Spence, 1990). Much work has been done in training examiners for postgraduate medical examinations and monitoring and auditing the assessments carried out, and an arcane science has developed in the writing, setting, and marking of multiple choice questionnaires. Medical examinations have been an opportunity for doctors to demonstrate one of their abiding passions—playfulness with number.

The stories the experts would have us believe: science and scientism

It is very important to the self-image of doctors that theirs should be considered a scientific discipline; in academic circles it is regarded as applied science. For training in a medical specialty, including psychiatry, one studies first the basic sciences that underpin factual knowledge in that specialty. What are the basic sciences for psychiatry? In what way are they fundamental to practice, and do they need to be narrowly scientific to be acceptable as bases? Highest status is usually given to the biological sciences—neuroanatomy, neurochemistry, and neurophysiology, and the applications of these sciences in neuroimaging and neuropharmacology. Perhaps this is because they are closest to the fundamentals of other areas of medicine. The second level of acceptability is given to the social sciences—psychology, sociology, social anthropology, and so on. Their relevance for psychiatry is obvious, but the interpretation of research findings is less clear-cut and there are many important areas where it has not been possible, so far, to construct adequate, valid, and reliable experiments. Much of the data is essentially naturalistic and subject to methodological error. Lowest credibility resides in such subjects as philosophy and ethics, which, although fundamental to the study of psychiatry and the development of treatment strategies, are regarded as unscientific and therefore essentially unreliable in both a technical (consistent on repetition) and popular sense. The humanities come in, then, as a very poor fourth. In the strange hagiography of medicine, the spiritual element of our profession and our patient's experience, ironically, has the lowest value, and is held to be the least sacred.

The real bases to psychiatric practice are descriptive psychopathology, that is observing and categorizing the description of self-experience and the behaviour of patients, and clinical epidemiology, the distribution of abnormal phenomena and the people experiencing them within defined populations. The other sciences and humanities mentioned above are essential additions to these fundamental methods for studying our patients.

Observations initially made objectively on a few occasions pass into the knowledge base or folklore of the subject. One example is the long-held belief that it takes at least two weeks for effective antidepressant medication to start benefiting severely depressed patients. From many studies of treatment for depression with different antidepressant drugs this has become accepted by psychiatrists. Parker (1996), regards this as myth and has given the following reasons for it being transmitted to generations of psychiatric trainees: failure to recognize that improvement trajectories are different for responders and non-responders; ratings and clinical assessments too infrequent in the first fortnight; failure to concede separate clinical subtypes; failure to distinguish between response and improvement; artefactual influences; treatment dose inefficiency. He has made a convincing case that onset of action occurs soon after administration of antidepressant medication. The interesting feature from looking at this as narrative is that once the belief, apparently based upon research evidence, is firmly established, it is very difficult to change the collective view of the profession.

There is a strong belief in medicine that no stone should be left unturned in order to make a diagnosis, but physical 'stones' are more highly rated than psychological or psychodynamic, and it would be seen as a more heinous omission to fail to identify an untreatable brain tumour by neglecting to arrange the appropriate brain scan than to fail to pick up a treatable disturbance in family relationships by not asking the appropriate questions. Many cautionary tales are recounted of finding an organic lesion in a patient in whom someone else had said that the problems were entirely psychological, neurotic, or hysterical. Such findings are supported with physical images such as brain scan or laboratory investigations, unlike missed family dynamics, where there will be no such pictorial abnormality to demonstrate one's diagnostic acumen, or lack of it. There is much emphasis on the technical applications of our practice: neuroimaging is indeed wonderful but it does not make a substantial difference to treatment in most cases. Others, such as lawyers, may also collude with us in regarding physical findings more highly, for example, in this statement of defensive medicine: 'We need psychometry and a CT scan for medico-legal purposes.'

There are many sacred tales in medicine but undoubtedly the most sacred, amounting to sacramental, are the research tales. Take, for instance, *nosology*, the study of psychiatric classification, a subject of considerable interest to both British and American researchers. It is helpful to remember that diagnoses are stories, pictures of reality, but that their content has a marked effect upon how we treat people. Classification has an unending fascination for research psychiatrists, perhaps once again, because it allows us expression of that passionate love affair between medicine and numeracy.

There are two major nosological systems extant in psychiatry: ICD 10 (World Health Organization, 1992) and DSM IV (American Psychiatric Association, 1994); they are not dissimilar. A man in his early 60s abuses his professional position by making sexual advances towards a boy, aged 17. He has a long history of changing his jobs, he has entered and left many relationships, both hetero- and homosexual, he has abused alcohol and other drugs, he is a talented artist, an excellent musician, and an entertaining companion. He dislikes himself, varies in mood from confident irascibility to profound self-doubt. He has always been unsure whether his preferred life-style is for wife and family or homosexual promiscuity, and he has experienced both and now ended up with neither. He feels profoundly unfulfilled and has emotionally blackmailed his attempted boyfriend with threats of suicide. Moralists and sensible parents would regard him and label him in one light and the law in another. However, the above description conforms very closely with ICD 10, F60.31: 'Emotionally unstable personality disorder, Borderline type'. If one places his personal story within the context of the ICD rubric, he can be 'medicalized', a subject suitable for treatment, and his future narrative proceeds from there. Nosology spawns upon an immensely powerful story.

Old wives' tales: one sort of evidence to the exclusion of all others

Considering research in medicine and how doctors regard it, leads on to discussion of practice behaviour, which is partly based upon the traditions in which the doctor trained. There has been a strong trend in recent years to diminish the influence of tradition and challenge established practice. Bursting on to the scene in every medical discipline, including psychiatry, and spotlighted from the balcony of the Department of Health is a talkative newcomer—'evidence-based medicine'. It is to the medical profession what prose was to the French epigrammatist, who discovered that he had been writing it all his life! Despite this element of dressing up a well-tried notion in new terminology, it has been very influential in the last few years. No political speech about health is complete without it, no learned review of a topic of treatment can afford to ignore it.

Why has this become suddenly fashionable? Evaluating the available evidence before embarking upon treatment has always been respected in medicine, with some practitioners even trying to carry it out! The latest wave of interest was provoked by the duo of developments in research method and current attention to the costs of health care. These are dependent upon the growth of information technology and health economics resulting in more sophisticated epidemiology, which not only defines specific populations and their characteristics, but is also able to link this to health and financial gains. Research initiatives previously of interest only to academics are now driven by managers, and this will escalate with the research and development initiatives of individual trusts in the National Health Service in the United Kingdom.

Because measurement and the evaluation of outcome is complex in psychiatry it is only with the more recent development of sophisticated techniques that it has become possible to come to evidence-based conclusions on the relative effectiveness of different methods of treatment: for instance, for psychotherapy and counselling, evidence has been expensive to collect and difficult to evaluate. However, the first level of questions have now been answered; psychotherapy, type not specified, *is* more effective than no treatment at all. We are now at the stage of answering second-level questions, such as what type of psychotherapy is most cost effective and for how long should treatment be carried out? It will be interesting to see to what extent research findings mould future practice, influence management strategy, and direct future policy. As an example, a recent study has evaluated the use of practice counsellors in general practice and shown them to be largely ineffective therapeutically (Fahy and Wessely, 1993). If this does not modify usage one can only assume that general practitioners themselves were not using counsellors for their therapeutic effectiveness but for some other purpose.

A development from evidence-based medicine has been the preparation and publication of practice guidelines for various topics of medical treatment. These are based upon critical review, with meta-analysis of all relevant and methodologically sound research studies. Interestingly, good practice guidelines produced nationally are more likely to be evidence-based but have less effect in moulding practice; locally produced guidelines are less likely to be based upon research findings but are much more likely to be acted upon.

At risk, because of the current enthusiasm for evidence-based medicine, are those areas of clinical practice that cannot be, or so far have not been, investigated using these techniques. This may be because the methodology is too difficult to apply, or it would be unethical to research the topic in a naturalistic and therefore valid way, or simply because it is not currently fashionable and does not obtain research support from grant givers. Areas of practice for which the research findings are unequivocal receive a high profile and are likely to be supported with personnel and other resources; for example, demonstrating that psychosocial interventions for the relatives of schizophrenic patients had proved beneficial to the long-term management of the patients themselves, using meta-analysis in a topical review (Mari and Streiner, 1994), has already, and will continue to, result in funds being provided for research and the training of personnel in this area. This is entirely laudable but it would be unfortunate if it were followed by withdrawal of resources from other important topics. Evidence-based medicine is no excuse for abandoning good clinical practice.

Although the apprenticeship style of training for individual therapists has great advantages for learning clinical skills, such teaching does contain the danger of transmitting old wives' tales within the somewhat idiosyncratic relationship between an experienced psychotherapist and an idealistic neophyte. Unless the trainer is both responsible and self-disciplined, the gold of proof is alloyed with the dross of unsupported personal prejudice. For example, at a banal level, a trainee psychotherapist was told that the room where she regularly saw patients was too big. This was an individual whim of her supervisor but it had harmful consequences for the hospital where she worked, as she received this advice and acted upon it with all the veneration of a commandment written on stone. In another training situation, an experienced psychodynamic psychotherapist, with a degree in French and no education in science, tried to convince medically qualified trainees concerning biological notions of child development that Galen might have found old-fashioned. Educational supervisors (senior doctors responsible for the work of a specialist trainee) are in a position of considerable responsibility and trust. The ideas that they communicate, sometimes unconsciously, may influence, for good or ill, the future clinical practice of their trainees.

Those working in professional isolation tend to rely excessively upon old wives' tales. Their isolation may be geographical, intellectual, or self-imposed. Geographical isolation is the easiest to deal with; there are always books and other forms of distance learning, and it is especially important for those who are remote from regular, frequent professional contact to attend conferences and other events. Such an individual is a psychiatrist working in a remote town in Pakistan who is much better informed than many consultant psychiatrists working in teaching hospitals in Britain. Intellectual isolation is a potential hazard arising from the move towards community psychiatry. Colleagues from the same profession may rarely meet, and members of the multidisciplinary team may work mostly as individuals remote from other team members. Trainees may have less access to libraries, teaching facilities, and discussion with their peers. Again, if this problem is recognized as being a serious hindrance to maintaining good clinical standards, it can be dealt with effectively in adequate provision of continuing professional development. Self-imposed isolation is the most hazardous of all. A person who sets up barriers to horizontal communication with professional colleagues may become increasingly idiosyncratic in their practice, and eventually they become a menace to their patients. An acceptable form of mentoring is probably the most effective prophylactic.

The market place: forcing an inappropriate model upon an unreceptive constituency

The National Health Service was established in 1948, and in its first 50 years it can claim to have become a 'living legend', easily the most popular of British institutions, outstripping the royal family and others such as the police, universal education, and parliament. With its pre-eminence in public estimation it was thought unassailable until the 'economic reform' of the early 1990s. The then prevalent political ideology, often described as 'Thatcherism', demanded that market forces be introduced into the Health Service, that local NHS Trusts should compete with their neighbours, that the output and cost efficiency of doctors should be measured and results published and that the market should be extended throughout the Health Service. Nobody was listening when it was whispered that real markets do not function like that; far from cut-throat competition being the order of the day, in an oriental market the individual traders work together to their own benefit and to the occasional exploitation of their customers! It was also ignored that living markets have developed over generations, establishing sophisticated interactions and subtle interdependencies. Most of those working directly with patients never believed the market story.

The language of the market place has, however, permeated every corner of the National Health Service, including mental health services: 'moneytalk' and 'managementspeak' can be heard in any National Health Service Trust or Health Authority. The so-called 'NHS reforms' divided those employed into two separate forces, theoretically in perpetual confrontation and not in dialogue with each other: the purchasers and the providers. Like the 'blues' and 'greens' factions of ancient Constantinople (Norwich, 1988), there was nothing intrinsically different about the individuals comprising these groups, but once again like the 'blues' and 'greens', the division into purchaser or provider has permeated the whole of the NHS, with one important exception: general practice has been set up as the gatekeeper to specialist health services and therefore is a purchaser, perhaps the most significant of all purchasers; yet, primary care is, in terms of patient contact, the largest provider. Thus at the heart of the new market economy governing the NHS there was a conflict of interest.

In mental health services, those responsible for provision have become much more aware of the costs of what they do. Less appropriately, making profits and budget savings have become ends in their own right. Whereas in the past it might have been established that a new post was required to serve patients' needs in a particular population, now it is not at all unlikely that a doctor or manager will produce a remark such as, 'let us buy a cognitive therapist' or 'a treatment package for post-traumatic stress disorder should sell well'. Human beings, members of staff, are not infrequently seen as commodities that need to be fitted into the economic equation. Services are sometimes initiated, not for the degree of human suffering that might be alleviated, but because of the business plan of the trust. Such approaches should not necessarily be the recipient of sometimes nostalgic moral opprobrium, but we do need insight into what we are doing. Certainly, we should consider economic costs and benefits and not be reluctant to take economic advantage when it is to the benefit of the population served, but it is also important to keep to our original script and to remember that the primary task is creating a service for individual patients and not building a successful business where these two are in competition.

It is appropriate to end with these stories of the market place because, of all the monolithic medical myths that have been visited, this is the one that is most likely to prove ephemeral. It was a powerful and dominating narrative when this chapter was first drafted, but it was already heresy by the time it was proof-read. Will it still be remembered, let alone sacred, when published?

References

American Psychiatric Association (1994). *Diagnostic and statistical manual of mental disorers* (4th edn), DSM-IV. American Psychiatric Association, Washington, D.C.

Beck, A. T., Rush, A. J., Shaw, D. F., and Embery, G. (1979). *Cognitive therapy of depression.* The Guildford Press, New York.

Bishay, N. R. and Ormston, J. (1996). Cognitive disorders of religious concepts and their treatment. *Behavioural Cognitive Bulletin from the Psychotherapy Section of the Royal College of Psychiatrists*, **4**, 20–8.

Clapham, C. (1876). The weight of the brain in the insane. *The West Riding Lunatic Asylum Medical Reprots*, **VI**, 11–26.

Crabbe, G. (1783). *The village* in *The complete poetical works of George Crabbe* (ed. N. Dalrymple-Champneys & A. Pollard, 1988). Clarendon Press, Oxford.

Craigie, F. C., Larson, D. B., and Liu, I. Y. (1990). References to religion in the Journal of Family Practice: dimensions and valence of spirituality. *Journal of Family Practice*, **30**, 477–80.

Eisenberg, I. (1986). Mindlessness and brainlessness in psychiatry. *British Journal of Psychiatry*, **148**, 497–508.

Fahy, T. and Wessely, S. (1993). Should purchasers pay for psychotherapy? *British Medical Journal*, **307**, 576–7.

Frye, N. (1957). *Anatomy of criticism*. Princeton University Press, Princeton.

General Medical Council (1995) *Good Medical Practice*. General Medical Council, London.

Gregory, R. L. (1987). *The Oxford companion to the mind*. Oxford University Press, Oxford.

Hacking, I. (1996). Les alienes voyageurs: how fugue became a medical entity. *History of Psychiatry*, **VII**, 425–49.

Henley, W. E. (1873). *In hospital: rhymes & rhythms*. 3rd Edn (1921). Mosher, Portland.

Jamison, K. R. (1993). *Touched with fire: manic-depressive illness and the artistic temperament*. The Free Press, New York.

Jaspers, K. (1959). *General psychopathology* (7th edn), (trans. J. Hoenig and M. W. Hamilton 1963). Manchester University Press, Manchester.

Kierkegaard, S. A. (1940). *Stages on Life's Way*. Translated by W. Lowrie. Oxford Univesity Press, London.

Kipling, R. (1928). *A book of words*. MacMillan, London.

Larson, D. B., Sherrill, K. A., Lyons, J. S. Craigie F. C., Thielman S. B., Greenwold M. A. & Larson S. A. (1992). Association between dimensions of religious commitment and mental health reported in the American Journal of Psychiatry and the Archives of General Psychiatry: 1978–1989. *American Journal of Psychiatry*, **149**, 557–9.

Mari, J. E. D. J. and Streiner, D. L. (1994). An overview of family interventions and relapse in schizophrenia: meta-analysis of research findings. *Psychological Medicine*, **24**, 565–79.

Norwich, J. J. (1988). *Byzantium: the early centuries*. Guild Publishing, London.

Parker, G. (1996). On lightening up: improvement trajectories in recovery from depression. *Advances in Psychiatric Treatment*, 2187–93.

Prior, M. (1704). *The remedy worse than the disease*. In *The literary works of Mathew Prior* (Ed. H. Bunker Wright and M. K. Spears, 1959). Clarendon Press, Oxford.

Royal College of Psychiatrists (1971) Royal Charter. Royal College of Psychiatrists, London.

Sims, A. (1992). Symptoms and beliefs. *Journal of the Royal Society of Health*, **112**, 42–6.

Sims, A. (1994). 'Psyche'—spirit as well as mind? *British Journal of Psychiatry*, **165**, 441–6.

Sims, A. (1996). *The knotted stethoscope*. Churches Council for Health and Healing, London.

Spence, J. D. (1990). *The search for modern China*. Hutchinson, London.

Stein, L. J. and Test, M. A. (1980). Alternative to mental hospital treatment—I. Conceptual model, treatment program and clinical evaluation. *Archives of General Psychiatry*, **37**, 392–7.

Webster, R. (1995). *Why Freud was wrong*. Harper Collins, London.

World Health Organization (1992). *The ICD-10 classification of mental and behavioural disorders: Clinical descriptions and diagnostic guidelines*. World Health Organization, Geneva.

World Medical Association (1968). Declaration of Geneva. *World Medical Association*, Geneva.

III   Ends

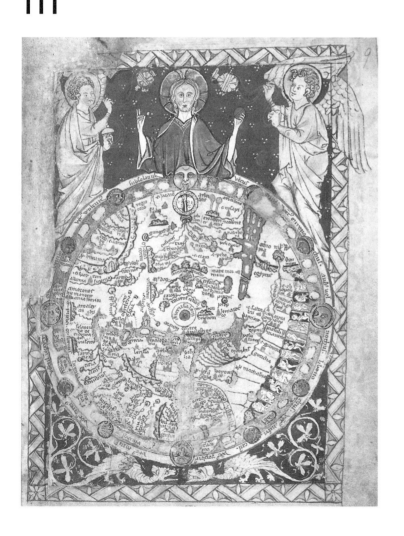

7   Creating a coherent story in family therapy

John Byng-Hall

In the first session Sara, aged six, was the first to speak. She sat up very straight, looked me in the eye, and said 'I killed my brother'. The 'A' family, who had originated from South America, had been referred after a second cot death. Sara had been sleeping between her parents, and was found lying on top of her dead brother. It was the ultimate dreaded catastrophe—another dead baby. Lightning does strike twice after all. Since then, the mother, Anna, had become reluctant to let the family out of her sight, and was largely housebound. Carlos aged eight was feeling very constrained and was running off, and father, Mario, had been coming in late at night, much to mother's dismay. In addition there was a new baby, Zeta, aged four months, who everyone was watching like a hawk day and night.

I asked the parents what Sara had been told. It had apparently been explained many times that it had not been her fault. I wondered whether despite their disavowals each member of the family may secretly believe that Sara's version might be right. This is one common reason why a belief is maintained by one person despite overt denials by other members of the family; if so Sara is likely to go on seeing herself as a killer. A thorough investigation of whether the second baby had been killed had been undertaken. (Munchausen by proxy for instance had to be excluded.) The idea of a family killer had thus been around for a while. I said that in my experience everyone feels responsible for a cot death however silly that may seem. Each then came out with their own version of what they did or did not do that contributed to what happened. Sara was surprised to hear these other stories, but did not give up her own version.

Later in the session I asked about the first cot death. Father and Carlos, immediately looked at mother's face. Each took a piece of tissue and went to sit either side of her, staring intently at her face. As the tears started to roll down her cheeks they wiped them dry. This told a story without words; one that contradicted another view that both males can run away from mother in her hour of need. This silent enactment of a counter plot to the main plot gained in meaning, and was eventually put into words.

From the referral letter I also knew that the mother had been held up at gun point in armed robberies in two unrelated episodes in the last year. Lightning can strike more than twice.

The 'A' family story will be used to illustrate aspects of narrative and ways of working with stories in family therapy throughout the chapter.

Introduction

So-called narrative approaches in family therapy have become fashionable recently (White and Epston, 1990). I do not see myself as a narrative therapist. This term is, in my view, a mistake in logical typing; all talking cures are narrative therapies. I see my understanding of narrative, and how it can enhance my work as being an integral part of my practice of family therapy. Context is crucial in narrative. A story is told in the context of listening. The way a family story is heard and responded to moulds the story itself. A family discussion provides a context in which everyone is both narrator and listener, and meaning unfolds over time. Where did the topic come from? How does it relate to the current situation? Where is it leading? The context of theory influences the way that family therapists tell their story about narrative. There have been two main strands to recent theorizing. One starts from outside the individual, focusing on social perspectives, the other from inside the individual and how he or she creates a story. A systems theory perspective must, of course, address how these two domains mutually influence one another.

Social constructionism explores the effect of social factors on narrative, which is thought of as being co-constructed (in their jargon) between people, and how therapy is co-constructed by family and therapist (McNamee and Gergan, 1992). The power dimension has frequently been emphasized, especially by Michael White who is the most influential narrative therapist. He uses Foucault's philosophical analysis of how discourse is used in society; dominant discourses ousting other discourses in the power struggle (White and Epston, 1990). Therapy is thus seen as a political act in which the therapist attempts to help the clients to use their preferred discourse and escape the dominant discourse. I find that theorizing can be limited; it is often rather abstract—evidence that philosophy rather than knowledge about how people feel and think is being used in the theory—although descriptions of what Michael White does are often moving. He is a powerful and innovative therapist. Parry (1991), using a post-modern perspective, explores how we are all characters in each other's stories and how our own stories only go forward as we act in a way that also helps others' stories to go forward. Other narrative approaches focus more on the symbolic and personal nature of stories (Roberts, 1994). My approach to theory is to attempt to link personal and social aspects of narrative into a mutually influencing, coherent whole, and, where possible, to put this within a research frame.

This chapter will focus on how to help families to share their stories with each other and thus improve how they communicate. This helps them to collaborate and to resolve their own difficulties. They can take these skills home with them. The therapy itself provides a setting in which the family can create a richer story for itself; one that gives meaning to its struggles, and, most importantly, includes the family members as authors of their stories rather than featuring as victims of other people's mistakes, or of a malign fate. Their story of the therapy itself becomes one of being the place where they found ways of solving their own problems, as opposed to the therapist 'fixing' it for them.

The format of the chapter will involve two interweaving stories. First, that of my own journey—both professional and personal—in theorizing about myths and stories since 1973, and how these articulate with other ideas. The second story is that of the therapy with the 'A' family. This double level text is congruent with the idea that the therapy story is co-constructed between family and therapist. For this reason I use the first person in this chapter. This recognizes that the therapist's theory is also a story, albeit with attempts to link it, where possible, to research data.

I will use the attachment research finding that coherent narrative is more likely to be associated with secure attachments than is incoherent narrative, and that those with secure attachments function better and are less likely to have problems. The aim of the work is to increase the coherence of family discussion. I explore contradictions, and where these come from, and try to make some sense of why they should have arisen in the first place. The therapy should provide a secure base that allows family members to feel secure enough to explore difficult, and potentially conflictual, thoughts and experiences. They need to feel safe enough to share issues that otherwise would remain taboo.

The capacity to share experiences, ideas, and memories within the family—the stuff of family narrative—can be thought of as being on a continuum from: (i) hidden from one's self; to (ii) hidden from the other family members; to (iii) hidden from some of the others, as in family secrets; to (iv) open appropriate sharing; to (v) over exposed, including intrusive attempts to find out what others are thinking, or flooding each other with inappropriate personal experience.

Intrapsychic mechanisms interplay with interpersonal processes to hide or share experiences, thus influencing the level and quality of the emotions that the content engenders. For instance, an individual can more easily repress or forget a certain experience in a family that does not ever talk about that experience. If someone were to do so, the subject would be changed, or the children may create a distraction so that the topic never gets an open airing. In different contexts the balance can change. A setting in which pain and distress can be empathized with, and tolerated, will allow for greater sharing. Family therapy offers an opportunity to widen the issues that are permissible and fruitful to discuss.

As I am advocating helping families to tell their stories as coherently and clearly as possible, it is beholden on me to attempt to do the same in my writing, and to use clear ideas with as little jargon as possible. In the midst of the complexity of a family session the therapist needs theories that he or she can easily translate into words that are understandable even by the children. I also believe that if an idea about families cannot be put in plain words it is probably muddled. Clever, convoluted theories can obscure, while giving the illusion of knowing; therapists can deceive themselves.

Family mythology and narrative in family therapy

From problem-saturated stories to competence

One thing a therapist should never do to a family is undermine members in front of each other, especially the parents in front of their children. On referral to therapy the family's stories are, however, frequently saturated with problems and a sense of failure (White and Epston, 1990). Their stories, nevertheless, can often be heard to tell of moments in which the family managed to stem the tide. Family therapists can elicit and emphasize any moments of success, however minor, and go on to highlight the creative aspects of the family's struggle to succeed. This can help the family to feel respected and safer from being exposed, or publicly criticized as they frequently anticipate they will be. Looking for positive features can also open up new possibilities and validates new identities for its members. Unfortunately, it is not that simple. Family therapists need to hear the family's worst fears, and to acknowledge the seriousness of what they are doing to each other, otherwise they will not feel that the therapist can tackle their problems. Also, they may escalate the problems because they do not feel the therapist has heard how bad it is. If these difficulties are discussed, even if only briefly in the first session, I have found that also quickly recognizing the strengths of family members can then help them to feel secure enough to tell me about their less satisfactory behaviour. This is one of the reasons that family therapists have found ways of positively labelling those aspects of family life that are functional. It is not a sign of superficiality, or mere reassurance, but of building secure foundations for tackling more difficult issues. The 'A' family are a good example as it was very important to identify and support their strengths, which they needed in order to survive and overcome their difficulties.

A journey through theory

Family myths: mutual support through shared role images

A good way of maintaining one's self image is to surround one self with people who will validate it. Families can do this for their members. When I started working with families in 1969 I was struck by how some families, even those who could not cope with their children and who were admitted to Hill End Adolescent Unit (Byng-Hall and Bruggen, 1974), often still managed to see themselves in a better light than others saw them. Outsiders might see these views as mythical in the sense of having a false quality to them. In 1973, I conceptualized family myths as being the consensus within the family of what sort of family it was, and what each member's characteristic role was within the family. These images are not irrevocably challenged even if there are other, possibly less kind, views held privately (Byng-Hall, 1973). Put another way, the family myth is preserved by a tacit agreement not to tell certain home truths, or to dismiss jointly these observations if they are made. This provides a context in which members can maintain their own acceptable self-images, or identities. It also allows for collusive idealization in some families in the face of contradictory evidence; the phenomenon I originally noticed at Hill End.

If someone in the family, such as an adolescent, steps outside these beliefs and persistently challenges their validity through words or behaviour, he or she risks being scapegoated, and seen as the source of all the problems, or is thrown out of the home, as at Hill End. This neatly maintains the family myth intact; 'we are nice—he is horrible.' In other families, some of the new perspectives stemming from a challenge to the consensus may be incorporated, thus enriching the family mythology. For instance, a family may share a role image of a father as being sturdy, who, at another level, is vulnerable. Everyone may feel better with the image of strength and so the myth is bolstered, especially, perhaps, when the father seems at the point of cracking. In the case of the 'A' family the problem was that their consensus threatened to break down. Although the father, Mario, was, in practice, doing most of the caring, he was near breaking point. Nevertheless, the survival of the family demanded that he did remain coping and available to everyone. Interestingly, as soon as he knew I was going to be available to see the family he was able to let go and became realistically depressed.

I conceptualized these ideas (Byng-Hall, 1973) in terms of object relations theory which I was studying at the time, and saw the family myth as a family defence, similar to a psychoanalytical defence. I likened it to a dream in which the manifest and acceptable account disguises the repudiated images underneath, for instance, overzealous support for father whenever he is criticized suggests the presence of an Achilles's heel. Ferriera (1963) considered that all families needed these family myths.

Family stories and legends

The term myth can either refer to a commonly held belief that is untrue, or to a traditional story that offers an explanation of some phenomenon. Thus, a myth can either hide, or, in story form, reveal the essence of a situation. When exploring the family's history I began to ask families for stories about their past instead of asking about what sort of people their ancestors were (Byng-Hall, 1979). In this I moved from issues of identity to those of plot and narrative. Of course the stories told provided a much more graphic picture of the characters in the plot; in other words they also more vividly illustrated the identities that I had been seeking in consensus family myths. I came to see family mythology as being a mixture of perceived identities and family stories that supported those identities. It followed naturally that I started to re-edit the family mythology by returning to key stories for a retelling later in therapy—to see if they have been reshaped and reinterpreted through fresh ways of thinking about relationships. It was also an opportunity to add fresh meaning, thus offering further ways of enriching family life (Byng-Hall, 1979).

Stories told about the past are often evoked by the particular situation in which the family now finds itself. One example of this occurred in work with the 'A' family. A fire alarm went off during one of the sessions. While standing outside the clinic they recalled hearing an IRA bomb going off in the vicinity of their home. Once they were back in the consulting room, father described how he had been a hostage in an aircraft hijacking, with a gun held to his head. He had been the last to be released after many hours of fearing for his life. He described this in vivid detail. This resonance with past experience, of course, also makes it possible to link the story to what is happening in therapy. In this case it lead to a discussion about the feelings of helplessness evoked by dangerous events outside the control of the family.

It was later in therapy, when the family was beginning to feel that they might be able to influence future events, that the baby, Zeta, had climbed and fell out of her cot, but was unharmed. Later in the session mother told me about the civil war that had led to her family's emigration. She described how an uncle had been killed by a mine, and then how, as a child, she had been playing with her siblings in the garden when her mother, hearing a suspicious noise, suddenly scooped up the children and took then indoors just prior to the garden being strafed with gunfire. The story line had moved from disaster arriving out of the blue to one in which something can be done and fate does not necessarily deal out fatal cards; children may be protected after all.

The therapist's own legends

Family legends are stories that are told again and again down the generations, and may act like parables about how the family should behave. I explored some of my own legends to see what influence they exerted on my view of myself and how other members of my family saw themselves. I then attempted to re-edit them. First, I explored a story that had been told to me as a child about Admiral Byng who was my great-great-etc.-uncle who had been shot for failing to win a sea battle in the Mediterranean in 1756, but returned instead to harbour for refitting following an indecisive engagement (Byng-Hall, 1982). This episode had been discussed over the years in literature because it became seen as a classical piece of scapegoating for political blundering. Admiral Byng had been sent too late to be effective. Voltaire had written in

Candide about how the English shot admirals from time to time 'pour encourager les autres'. This documentation enabled me to trace how the story had been re-edited throughout history to fit the circumstances of the nation at the time of writing. For instance, Winston Churchill in the *History of English speaking peoples* used it as a cautionary tale about what might happen if you left the battlefield too soon, something the British had to avoid in the Second World War.

When I was told the story in childhood it had been in a similar form to Churchill's version, and also served as a cautionary tale against 'running away' from a potentially dangerous isolated situation in Kenya, where I had been brought up. Later, as a way of re-editing the legend, I researched the episode in the British Library and found that virtually nothing in this version of the story had been true except that he had been shot. I had found it surprisingly hard to accept that all the evidence pointed to Byng being brave rather than cowardly in the face of the enemy. The legend had evidently influenced my belief system more than I thought. I then explored how the legend had affected other members of the family, finding that it had had a surprising impact. I shared my new information with them, in an attempt to re-edit the legend I had told them. I came to the conclusion that family therapists could usefully explore their own stories and legends.

Legends do not have to be about the distant past, the more recent past is just as effective, perhaps more so. I explored my family stories about security in my childhood as manifested in a number of stories about leopards that lived in the bush near our house (Byng-Hall, 1995a, p. 150). I sat down and wrote down as many stories as I could remember about danger and security during my early childhood that I had either been told, or told myself. In both these publications I describe ways to explore one's own family legends. It is important to know how one is influenced by one's own family mythology. This is one avenue, open to everyone, of achieving greater appreciation of the richness of family stories and how their influence can be felt in the present. It is important to recognize that the remembered past is in each telling. We sometimes learn more about ourselves and our current context from the way we weave and elaborate the stories than we do from the content of the story.

Family scripts: and rewriting them

What matters more is what families and individuals do about their beliefs, rather than the beliefs themselves. It is possible, after all, to have many private versions of reality, which might seem strange to others, but do not necessarily impinge on the family, or outsiders, in unfortunate ways. The concept of family scripts provides a way of thinking about what is prescribed in family relationships (Byng-Hall, 1985). A family script can be defined as 'the family's shared expectation of how family roles are to be performed in various contexts' (Byng-Hall 1995a, p. 4). These expectations are based on what has been done, or is perceived to have been done in the past, and they then act as self-fulfilling prophesies for the future, each member coming in on cue to play their expected role in the task at hand. The term 'expectations' often conveys the prescriptive 'ought to be done'. Normally, scripts provide an efficient way of collaborating in particular family functions or relationships. Family scripts can either be restrictive, confining members rigidly to particular roles played in a designated way, or, in contrast, they can provide general guidelines within which a rich repertoire of roles can be played in various contexts, and improvization can extend their range even further. In this case the family script can readily be rewritten in the face of changing circumstances.

Stories play an important role in rewriting family scripts. As each typical family's scenario is enacted it is played with some variation in form and outcome. Any variations beyond the norm are likely to become the focus of attention, and are thus rather more likely to be remembered than a routine performance. These varied episodes may then become the subject of family stories that are likely to be told in a way that suggests that either the particular innovation was to be encouraged to be repeated, or to be avoided in future. If innovative moves are then repeated they become part of what can be expected and thus join the repertoire of the family script.

These new moves may be merely variations on old themes. Sometimes, however, the implications of the new behaviour may potentially change the nature of the relationship itself. Often, however, these new scenarios are quickly forgotten, unless the significance of what happened is heightened, so that the implications are understood and acknowledged by all those involved. Cronen and Pearce (1985) point out that social meanings are hierarchically organized so that one level is the context for construing the meaning at a lower level in the hierarchy. The hierarchy is usually organized on the basis that meanings emanating from a wider arena—in terms of the number of people involved and/or a longer time span—are likely to be more pervasive than those with a narrower base. Family mythology usually provides a meaningful context for family scripts, which in turn provide the context for interpreting the meaning of a particular episode of family interaction (Byng-Hall 1995a, p. 58). It is more difficult, however, but still possible, for the implications of events lower in the hierarchy to change the meaning of those above them. For instance, what happened in a family row might occasionally alter the way the whole relationship is seen, and so rewrite the family script. A less dramatic episode can, however, do the same, and therapists can play an important role in establishing the significance of a particular turn of events, which might not otherwise have seemed important.

Changes during therapy, occurring either in between or during sessions, can be woven into a powerful story of change, which becomes part of the story of therapy itself. As a routine I usually ask at the beginning of each session; 'What has been happening?' This often elicits descriptions of events, some of which were clearly difficult. I then ask what was usual about the way it went, this I call the old script, and what was new. As there is always something fresh in each episode it is, surprisingly, often possible to identify what that new move was, and why and how it lead to a different outcome. By asking how each member was involved in the scenario a systemic picture of family interaction emerges, in which all contribute in what they did or did not do to what happened. This leads to a fresh systemic co-constructed story based on how they changed the course of an event.

The nature of the episode itself is frequently less important than the emerging belief that the family can change what they do with each other, and that that change can produce results. They can gain a sense of being able to influence their own destiny. The family then expects that it can rewrite its own script: that, indeed, it is their new family script.

This was the issue for the 'A' family. They had developed a tragic script in which it was expected that catastrophe would automatically strike again however hard they had tried to avoid it, as in a Greek tragedy in which a particular fate is predicted, and duly comes to pass what ever is done. During therapy the 'A' family eventually came to see themselves differently, as having a heavy burden with which they could struggle, sometimes successfully, sometimes not.

Attachments and security

Coherence of narrative

Attachment theory research provides some important data about narrative and how it influences relationships. Mary Main and her associates (Main *et al.* 1985) explored the narrative style that adults used when interviewed about their childhood in the adult attachment interview (AAI). This is also discussed in Chapter 3. Parents whose children are securely attached to them are likely to have a coherent story to tell about their own childhood attachments. Those whose children have an insecure attachment have an incoherent narrative. This is clinically significant because children who have had secure attachments to a parent do better on a whole range of functioning and in relationships, such as with peers, than do those who have had insecure attachments, who in addition are more likely to develop problems (Belsky and Nezworski, 1988). This suggests alterations in narrative style that can be achieved during family therapy which might benefit the current family. If children also learn to tell a coherent story about their family they are more likely to develop a secure attachment with their children in the next generation, thus breaking a cycle of insecurity that is otherwise likely to be transmitted down the generations.

The concept of coherence has two main components (Main, 1991, p. 144); first, internal consistency in which elements of the narrative do not contradict each other, and, secondly, whether or not it is plausible—does the story fit with what is likely to happen in real life? In the adult attachment interview (AAI) the individual is asked about his or her childhood. At first the interviewee is asked for five adjectives to describe each parent, and then he or she is asked to illustrate each adjective by describing an episode. This may reveal an internal inconsistency, for instance a parent may be described as wonderful but the episode illustrates neglect. Further questions may also reveal inconsistencies, such as an inquiry about a time that he or she had been in distress, or ill, and how parents responded and why.

The transcript of the interview is rated as secure if it is internally consistent and plausible, and the rater feels satisfied that the assessment was close to what the interviewee had experienced. In other words, the rater felt he or she could empathize fairly accurately with the narrator throughout the story. The story would convey appropriate emotions to fit the episodes described, and include his or her own behaviour to help to explain why parents responded as they did. Fonagy *et al.* (1991) devised an additional scale for rating the transcript; this was aimed at gauging peoples' motives for doing what they did, and was called self reflective function. This scale also predicted that the interviewee who scored highly would have a securely attached child. This suggests that understanding motives enables one to tell a meaningful story to oneself and others about relationships, and this helps to make it possible to tune into children's attachment cues and to respond appropriately.

When coherence is rated highly the rater is also likely to feel that the story conveys one consistent model of relationships. An individual is, however, likely to have many mental representations of attachments stemming from many experiences. He or she must then have a way of assessing whether any two representations are incompatible with one another. One way of doing this is to use metacognitive monitoring (Main, 1991), which is thinking about thinking. Children can develop this capacity between three and six years old. After that they can step back and ponder on their own thoughts and assess whether one set of ideas would exclude another. In this way they can dismiss some ideas while integrating others into a more comprehensive but consistent model of what happens in relationships. To do this they are also likely to need a parent who also has a consistent and coherent view about relationships. The data about intergenerational patterns fit this idea, since parents who tell a coherent story are more likely to have a securely attached child, who is in turn more likely to be able tell a coherent story about their own earlier childhood by the age of 10. The coherence is thus likely to become part of the attachment relationship itself, and is manifest in its conversations. Listening that searches for clear meanings helps to encourage coherent stories being told, just as the narrator can show the listener how to make sense of the way people treat each other.

Family legends told within such a relationship are realistic about what people achieve; good and bad behaviour is seen as part of everyday life. The tales can also be moving accounts of what happened and so are worth listening to.

Incoherent narrative: multiple models and metacognitive monitoring

Mary Main (1991) discusses how incoherent narrative could be based on multiple models of attachment relationships that are contradictory to each other, an idea first introduced by Bowlby (1973). Bowlby discussed how children that are told one thing but observe something very different are prone to develop incompatible models: he described a study in which children who were very disturbed had witnessed the suicide of a parent but were told something quite different, for instance one child found a parent hanging, but was told that the parent had died in a car accident. Main (1991) argues that young children who have not developed a capacity for metacognitions are prone to development of multiple models of the same situation; they cannot discard incompatible models. Metacognitive monitoring is also more difficult if the information is distorted. Many defensive or self-deceiving processes that parents use are compartmentalizing processes that act to separate feeling, attention, perception, and memory, which inherently limits metacognitive monitoring (Main, 1991, p. 146). Not surprisingly, securely attached children have greater metacognitive capacity than insecurely attached children.

Family stories and legends can be classified along lines similar to AAI categories. These classifications are clinical and descriptive rather than research based. They are based on overall attachment style. Some families do have similar attachments, although the research shows that the form of one attachment to one parent does not correlate with that with the other parent, so there is probably some variation within most families.

Incoherent/dismissive style: shared denial of importance of involvement

Parents who are categorized as dismissive on the AAI show that they defensively exclude information that is hurtful to remember. They forget large parts of their childhood. They idealize their own parents while giving accounts of neglectful or rejecting parents, thus they have incompatible models of attachment. By failing to see the discrepancy between the nice belief and the hurtful memory they are saved from facing some very uncomfortable conclusions. They also avoid actions that will revive those memories, so that when their children make emotional demands on them they reject the child; just as they were rejected as children. In turn, their children learn not to be exposed to so much pain by switching off their attachment behaviour when they most need comfort. This leads to, for instance, avoiding rather than greeting a parent on reunion following a separation, turning away, and focusing on toys instead. Interaction becomes detached and emotionally cool. This is adaptive, as emotional demands often lead to rejection. The motto about feelings is 'Don't care. Then you can't be hurt', which may be the core message of family legends.

The family stories that are told are dismissive of the importance of attachments. Narrators often idealize themselves, and their parents, but may denigrate individual family members. Their stories cannot be taken at face value because of the distortions involved. The legends are often brief and limited in emotional range. They are often stark and mythical; full of heroes and villains (for examples, see Byng-Hall, 1995a, p. 146). It is hard to 'feel' oneself into the story. Rejection and throwing family members out is a common theme in family stories.

Incoherent/preoccupied style: 'ghosts from the past'

Parents who are categorized as preoccupied on the AAI spend much time being preoccupied with unresolved issues from the past. Children learn that if they work hard enough at getting attention, say by being demanding, the parent may suddenly come back into the present and be temporarily warm and loving. This of course reinforces the demanding and clinging behaviour. Generational boundaries become blurred both in the parent's recalling of the past—they may suddenly slip into their own parent's voice—but also in the present, when role reversal occurs. Children become parents to their parents, thus becoming their own grandparents. Children do not recognize the privacy of other people's thoughts and mind reading occurs. These families have an enmeshed style of relating in which there are intrusive attempts to find out what is in other people's minds, and lengthy imposition of one's own preoccupations on others.

The family stories are often preoccupied with the rights and wrongs of what happened, which is often described in rambling detail. It is as if the teller has disappeared into the past, which lives on, and ghosts of ancestors flit across the stage. Legends are few because no one story is clear and repeated in a similar form. What may become legendary is the fact that the parent went on and on and on about the vagaries of the past.

Contradictory stories: 'too close/too far' dilemmas

Enmeshed as well as distant relationships can exist within the same family. Relationships are 'too close/too far' (Byng-Hall, 1980). Distant members hide their feelings and retreat, while clinging ones demand to know what the more distant members are thinking. Interaction patterns often include pursuer/pursued sequences, with one trying to escape and the other trying to pull them back. They criticize each other's distance as being either too close or too far.

Their stories may reflect these episodes, and the narrator conveys his or her characteristic attitude to closeness and distance. Although the two underlying models of self-protection are contradictory in terms of strategy, it is still possible to see that they have the same overall aim— that of trying to maintain the relationship and increase a sense of security.

Unresolved mourning or trauma

Some transcripts on the AAI are coherent until a traumatic attachment-related event, such as loss, is mentioned. The coherence then goes to pieces and the lost person may be talked about as if he or she were both alive and dead. These parents are more likely to have children who are insecurely attached in a disorganized/disorientated way. They had no clear strategy for managing attachment behaviour. One possible model for this is that a process of dissociation unlinks the contradictory images of the parent, and the child finds this frightening, and also dissociates his or her responses, thus breaking up the normal organization of attachment behaviour, leaving the infant disorientated. It is unclear how this might influence legends, except that clear descriptions of an unmourned figure may not be handed on to the next generation.

The family as a secure base

Ainsworth (1967) used the concept of a 'secure base' that a parent provides a child, so that he or she can feel secure enough to explore, safe in the knowledge that the parent is there if needed. This concept can be extended to the family, which can provide a sense of being there for its members (Byng-Hall, 1995b). The secure family can provide a setting in which ideas can be explored and disputed. This is possible because absolute priority is given to provide care when it is really needed. This provides the freedom to argue and disagree—even have rows—without the fear that care will be threatened. This then provides a social context in which incongruities can be explored; what might be called an exercise in family metacognition. Any totally contradictory ideas are likely to be exposed in the discussion and the nature of the difference aired. Some different views can be accepted—an agreement to disagree, which is also a coherent view of family life. To hold the view that everyone thinks the same would be both implausible and inconsistent: some enmeshed families nevertheless try to foster that mistaken notion. Logical inconsistencies may be exposed and children learn how to differentiate between a difference of opinion and holding on to two incompatible ways of thinking.

In my practice the goal of family therapy is to provide a temporary secure therapeutic base for the family, so that they then can explore ways in which they can increase the security of their own base. They can then go on solving problems after therapy. Work will then focus on the many factors in the family that undermine the security felt in the family (Byng-Hall, 1995a, p. 106). These include, among other things: anything that takes carers out of the family, either physically or emotionally, or parental conflicts that are so threatening that they take precedence over caring and children are brought in to be on one or other parents's side. Family therapy techniques can help to resolve some of these issues, which frees family members to feel secure enough to explore ideas more easily. In addition, techniques to make a more coherent story out of current interaction, and intergenerational patterns, can be used.

Interactional awareness

How can family therapists enable family members to perceive interaction in a coherent way? I attempt to help members to improve their interactional awareness (Byng-Hall, 1995a, p. 39). This involves helping individuals to: (i) become more aware of the likely implications for each person of what is currently happening; (ii) remain empathic with each person and their motives as they become involved in the plot; and (iii) be aware of their own contributions to what is going on. These capacities would enable each to be able to tell a meaningful story about an episode that includes him or herself in the plot. Some capacity for interactional awareness is also required of family therapists. The therapist can then be a narrator to the family process. When something is transacted in a family session the therapist describes what he or she has just witnessed and then asks whether that is how others saw it, and inquires how each felt about what was going on. This can lead to an exploration of why the scenario unfolded as it did. If this is done often throughout the therapy, family members can start to learn how to narrate internally, or sometimes out loud, during interaction. It is interesting that secure children are more likely to narrate to themselves about what they are doing. A potential story is thus born every time the family interacts, and can so be used to tell the story of what happened between sessions. Each time this happens wider and wider contextual issues can be explored: What led up to it? Where was everyone at the time? What was the influence of father's absence? Would they chose to do differently next time? Families start looking at the context rather than at individuals' culpability, for explanations and a plan for the future.

Making sense of transgenerational scripts

Some phenomena in families make little sense unless the transgenerational context is taken into account. In the 'A' family, for instance, when mother went into inexplicable levels of controlling behaviour when Carlos rode a bicycle it could be understood when learning that her grandmother allowed an uncle so much freedom he had a serious accident on a bicycle.

When comparing what goes on now with what happened when the parents were similar ages to their children it is common to find three main patterns. The first is that of repeating the same form of parenting, what I call following replicative scripts (Byng-Hall, 1985). If the therapist points out that the parent is being loyal to his or her own parent in doing it the same way it can, in my experience, release them from having to carry on doing so, especially if they are already unhappy about behaving that way. Not infrequently he or she has not previously spotted the connection, perhaps because identification with a parent happens largely outside awareness. Secondly, parents may try hard not to do certain things to their own children that had been done to them as children. These I call corrective scripts. It is easy to label this positively, defining it as the parent's struggle to do better for his or her children than it had been possible for his or her own parents to do for them. Some parents readily recognize this as they had often been all too aware of the discomfort of that aspect of their childhood experience. Not infrequently, they can even remember vowing never to do the same thing to their own children. The third pattern is of parenting in a completely fresh way—an innovative script.

It is important, if possible, to explore the history back to the children's great grandparents in order to understand how current parenting styles were influenced by the grandparents, who in their turn were struggling to do better within their own historical context. If this is not done, blaming parents can be merely switched to blaming grandparents. The story of parenting styles also becomes a more coherent story; one of maintaining aspects of family tradition in changing circumstances, while also struggling to do better in each generation, but of course never getting it exactly right. This allows for some forgiveness across generations, and between partners who can come to understand the other's dilemmas better. The use of the family tree, or geno-gram, to structure the historical review is described below (p. 146).

The story of therapy: from a tragic to a coping script

Hearing their story; what killed Ben?

It is useful to hear the current stories first. It reveals how many contradictory versions exist. I let families tell it in their own way before co-constructing an edited version.

Mrs A started the beginning of the second session by saying that Sara had come to the clinic to find out if she killed her brother. This set the scene for the parents to tell the children the story as they understood it. Father took on the task of talking to Sara about cot deaths. He knew Sara thought she had killed her brother by stopping his breathing by lying on him. This was a heroic task for the father, especially as he tried to explain how the pathologists had not found any signs of suffocating at post-mortem. Can this story be told to a six-year-old whose cognitive capacity is still limited, and keeping in mind that Carlos had been five and Sara nearly three when it had happened?

> FATHER (to Sara): What did Ben die of?
>
> SARA: Cot death. But he wasn't in his cot.
>
> FATHER: You were right he wasn't in his cot. Babies can die in beds. He died of something. Doctors don't know exactly what it is. If a baby dies of suffocation. Do you know what suffocation is? If I put my hand right over my mouth I can't breathe can I? That is suffocation. If you were to lie on Ben and stop him breathing it would mean that he had died of suffocation.
>
> SARA (sits up, sighs and looks up at her father clearly taking this as confirmation of her own story): Oh yes.
>
> FATHER: When someone dies . . .
>
> SARA (interrupts, nodding): They stop breathing.
>
> FATHER: They stop breathing you are right.
>
> SARA (lies back in her chair and is very still): I've stopped breathing.
>
> FATHER: But you are still alive. (He goes on to try to explain how the doctors had looked at Ben's lungs, pointing at her chest.) If a baby dies through not breathing they find things in those lungs.
>
> SARA: Behind your nipples.
>
> FATHER: Yes but in Ben's case they did not find anything. So that is why they know he did not die because you were lying on top of him . . . So do you still think you did kill him? (Sara shakes her head slowly). How did he die?
>
> SARA: By a cot death.
>
> FATHER: What is a cot death. (long silence)
>
> MOTHER: Doctors don't even know, so how can Sara?

I was left aware just how much of a muddle everyone is in about this, including the doctors. I judged that a clearer explanation of the muddle was unlikely to leave Sara less likely to stick to her clear version of Ben's death caused by lying on top of him and stopping him breathing. In the meantime Sara is left with a frightening confusion of images: lying on top, nipples/lungs, cots, beds, stopping breathing, things found in lungs, things not found in lungs, dying if you stop breathing, stopping breathing and being alive, suffocating/hands over faces, etc. I knew that she had already had many such explanations so it was not worth trying to clarify her father's version at this point. I decided to wait until the family had established a more coherent view of what happened and then have them tell her again.

Mother then blamed herself. She explained that she used to go secretly to Sara's cot and take her out and bring her into the marital bed because she was so worried about her. (Sara was born after the first cot death so had been the replacement baby for that baby, and so of course had been monitored very closely at night. Mother was concerned that this was the reason that Sara had come into the marital bed.) She also had a clear idea of what caused the death. Ben had overheated as a result of being between the parents (plus Sara on top of him—although she did not spell this out in front of Sara in this session). Overheating she said would not have shown on an autopsy. It is now clear that Sara and her mother shared an overlapping scenario that led to the death, although the final cause of death was different for each, while each claimed responsibility for different aspects of the same drama.

The two males seemed less articulate about self-blame for the death. Father said he did not feel guilty all the time. He had become numb after Ben's death and very forgetful. I pointed out that he seemed to have tried to forget the pain but forgotten lots of other things as well in the process. He told me he had had a near breakdown while on holiday in South America, getting very irritable and upset. His current guilt was about not giving his children enough attention. The two males, father and Carlos, seemed to have been allocated the caring roles in the aftermath of the tragedies. That was where their propensity for guilt now lay.

Mutual protection; keeping everyone breathing

I asked how each showed their sadness. Carlos, when pressed, admitted he had been crying at night. He would pull his bed clothes over his head to hide his tears from the others. Sara would notice, however, and come and pull the clothing back again. She said that she worried that the clothes might stop him breathing. No-one had known, let alone understood, this before. A general discussion ensued about how everyone now worried about the others dying. I asked who now worried most about the baby Zeta's breathing. There was a race to put up hands and much laughter. Each of them could now make some reparation for past negligence through their concern about Zeta.

In this session the family was able to share their views about what caused the cot deaths, and how they felt guilty about not preventing them. The double tragedy left them thinking they had to protect each other. If lightning can strike twice, why not three times? Sara had also revealed how she could imagine herself dying. Fear of death was pervasive.

Actions can tell a story

One of the delights of working with children is that they can tell their story so vividly through action, or symbolically in play and drawing. In the fourth session the 'A' family discussed how Ben had been amazingly fit, which meant that they were doubly careful in the way they watched Zeta. 'Once you have let your guard down and it was a disaster you can never let your guard down again.' Even while this was being discussed, however, Carlos went over to the mother and took Zeta off her lap and carried her to his seat and put her on his lap. After a few minutes of preoccupied discussion the mother suddenly noticed that the baby had gone. She was shocked that she had been doing the very thing that she had been telling me she would never do: fail to monitor Zeta. (On examining the videotape later, it was clear that she had noticed Carlos doing this but remained preoccupied with her story.) While old terrifying scenarios are being remembered they may muddle perceptions of what is happening now, making it more difficult to respond appropriately, especially to less dramatic current cues. This may indeed be one mechanism by which a self-fulfilling prophesy of tragedy could be fulfilled.

Later in the same session Sara had taken the baby and sat her on her own lap, facing away. I noticed that Sara had her arms round Zeta's chest and was jerking her chest repeatedly, while watching whether her parents noticed. They did not. As this jerking looked quite vicious I commented that Sara seemed to be asking the parents to make sure that she was safe with the baby.

Telling and retelling the stories

The first retelling of Ben's death was undertaken on the eighth session. I asked them to recount in detail what each had seen and done. Carlos told the story first. He had come to the parent's bedroom in the morning and seen Ben's face under Sara. Carlos had woken his parents who tried to make Ben breathe. I asked how they had done this. Sara immediately demonstrated how this was done, first by banging on her own chest, and then went over to the baby, and pushed on her chest in the same rhythm and intensity as she had done when squeezing Zeta on her lap previously. Now I knew what she had been conveying to me in jerking Zeta's chest during the fourth session. Mother told me that Sara sometimes banged the baby on the chest in a similar way, and that at times this seemed too hard.

This led to a lengthy discussion about how the two children had witnessed the failed resuscitation attempts, and how totally nightmarish it had been for the parents. Mother had tried first but was too hysterical, so father took over. He also found that he could not do it properly. It must, however, have looked to the children as if their parents were damaging Ben not helping him, just as I had previously mistaken Sara's jerking as intending to hurt not help.

When Zeta reached the age of one year the apnoea pad, (which sounded an alarm if her breathing stopped) broke down and it was suggested that they now gave it up. This created a crisis in which the family could not sleep and they had many flashbacks to the cot deaths. At one point I noticed that Carlos was kissing Zeta in a way that seemed strange. He had been very affectionate to his baby sister, including showering her with a lot of kisses, but this time he was covering her mouth with his mouth while she was lying on her back and he was on all fours and at right angles to her. I suddenly realized that it was exactly like giving a kiss of life to a baby lying on the floor. I pointed this out. This was Carlos' enacted 'flashback'.

This provided another opportunity to revisit the story. This time it was possible to go through the description in greater detail. The kiss of life was given first by mother and then by father, who put Ben on the hall floor. Both children were watching. Sara told me that her father had been lying on top of Ben. There was a discussion about how hard it was for Sara as a three-year-old to know what was happening. It was also interesting that the two frightening images overlapped; Sara and father lying on top of Ben. Father talked about how awful he felt about having not given the kiss of life as he should have done. He only put his mouth over Ben's mouth and not over his nose as well. It was agreed, however, that Ben had probably been dead for several hours by then. This knowledge did not, unfortunately, lessen the anguish.

The story had been re-edited once again. What was important was that the story was beginning to enlarge and to have an agreed sequence of events, which, if linked together, created a meaningful scenario, and that the children's images could be added to this in a way that allowed the grown-ups to appreciate the way that it had been perceived by the children. The story was no longer broken up into fragments, dissociated from each other, so that each fragment could only be contemplated one at a time.

History of past traumas; drawing the family tree

A family tree, or genogram (McGoldrick and Gerson, 1985) was drawn. Mother had had a very disrupted and traumatic upbringing in South America before the family emigrated to England. There had been a civil war in which gunfire had killed members of the family, and she had narrowly escaped herself. It was then possible to understand why she responded as she did to being held up in the building society in an armed raid, and later being told to lie down in a supermarket by an armed man who raided the till. It made even more sense of why she thought every strange man might be about to attack her. When the family moved home, later on in therapy, she became strangely preoccupied with how the new neighbourhood were persecuting her because she was not English. When I asked about the time that her family first arrived in England when she was six, Sara's age, this response made sense. It was a great relief to mother, who was assuming she was becoming paranoid.

One of the other advantages of drawing a family tree is that it requires a systematic listing of family births and deaths. One of my routine questions to each family is whether or not there were any pregnancies other than those that led to the children in the tree. This can uncover miscarriages, abortions, and stillbirths; those events that include both new life and death and which are often not talked about, can carry powerful legacies for the family script. The main modification to drawing the family tree with the 'A' family was that I put the parents in the tree before the children, leaving blank spaces for them to be filled in later. I knew that there had been eight pregnancies and only three live children, so I felt that I needed to know the family better before taking them through the emotional trauma of talking about each failed pregnancy and then re-discussing the cot deaths. By starting with the first pregnancies, it was possible to understand the response to subsequent pregnancies. This again makes for a more coherent story. I spun out the drawing of the pregnancies over many months so that each death or loss of pregnancy would have adequate time to be worked through, something that had not been possible to do at the time.

After all the pregnancies had been covered mother was able to tell a more general story. After loosing several babies, mother felt that she just had to make up for them all by going on having more. This is a quite understandable and quite common replacement phenomenon. Carlos came after two failed pregnancies and was followed by a sister. Carlos was much loved, but when Carlos was 18 months his little sister died. Mother described how she then shut down her emotions, but recognized that she also cut out Carlos at that time, much to her dismay. Sara had been the replacement for the first dead baby. However, this did not work and she was left aching for the lost baby and so had another one, Ben. The whole family then began to come out of their depression slowly. Ben was very lively and mother found that she could relate to him as himself and not the shadow of the dead baby girl. The relief of normality returning was enormous for everyone. This set the scene for the enormity of what happened when Ben died.

Mother became suicidally depressed and was advised to go to hospital, but refused because she would not leave her other two children. She was treated in a day hospital instead. Father became her 'community mental nurse' and Carlos his 'assistant nurse'. Mother became pregnant again but was advised to have a termination because of her mental state. Zeta was planned later. Mother found herself cutting off from Zeta as well, especially when she went through the ages at which the other two babies died. She could not risk getting too close, in case Zeta died as well. I did some work on their attachment, as Zeta was beginning to develop an avoidant attachment to her mother, while appearing to be securely attached to her father. Slowly it became clear that at about eight months after starting work with me, and when Zeta had reached the age of one and so was less at risk of dying of cot death, mother started to enjoy her baby daughter. She told me that she now saw Zeta as an individual not as a ghost of the other two. Mother had started by leaving all the childcare in the sessions to her husband, but steadily took more and more of a central role in looking after all three children. It remained characteristic, however, that father returned to playing with the children whenever a difficult topic arose.

Parents' different narrative styles

> MOTHER: We grieved in a different fashion. I talked about it all the time. Mario wouldn't. (He nods.)
> THERAPIST (to father): You talk about it here.
> FATHER: When you are at home, where it happened, it is difficult. There are so many things to do. (Busily helping the children to draw.)
> MOTHER: I get really wound up about you not talking.

Mother would focus, and ruminate, on difficult emotional issues; father would at times escape from them. This difference was a source of considerable tension. She would be desperate to know what was in her husband's mind. He would feel trapped and exposed and wanted to escape; as he indeed had done by coming in late before referral. In short, they had a 'too close/too far' relationship. They told me that they had decided to split up because of this tension just before the first cot death, but the tragedy had brought them together again. Caring for the children or for mother's depression kept father at home. This form of distance regulation, triangulating others in, or using a symptom that needs to be cared for are common ways of stabilizing pursuer/ pursued escalations (Byng-Hall, 1980).

Later, when the discussion was focused on remembering and forgetting, following a retelling of the cot death story:

> MOTHER: It is as if it is all bits and pieces, and new bits come back. But it's beginning to come together. It takes a long time.
> FATHER: I just could not remember anything at first. My mind went numb.

She tended to dissociate fragments of memory as a way of avoiding the implications of the whole story: he damped down the full realization by pushing it out of his awareness.

The couple's stories or legend-telling style were also very different. She would tell long and often convoluted stories about the past. These stories would often dwell on the injustices of the situation. She also became very preoccupied while telling them, disappearing into the story and loosing touch with events around her during the story. An example of this was given above when she was describing how she could never let her guard down, while not noticing Carlos taking the baby. Later in therapy she told this story, but was also able to make a comment about herself. It followed a long story about how she saw 'ghosts' as a little girl:

> My mother came round to our house after the deaths and sprinkled some holy water. (Laughed.) It was to get the evil out. Her father had once seen a ghost that had told him that if he dug in a particular place he would find some holy water. That was how he became famous for his holy well. I cannot believe in all that stuff. It's a pity as I always see the worst possibilities.

This led to a discussion about their tragic script and how they might begin to expect some better things to happen.

Father told few stories, and those tended to be in response to questions. The only long story told spontaneously was about the hijacking episode, during a session with the couple on their own. When the topic of the hijack came up in a family session Carlos said that he did not know about it. This is the way to find out whether a story is a family legend or not, to ask if the children have heard it before. They may have been told, as father claimed here, but the story was not told in a way that was remembered, or repeated. A family legend only becomes a legend when others hear, remember, and can, and often do, repeat it. The family tree showed few stories on his side of the tree, whereas his wife's side was overcrowded with them.

The parents communications started to improve as mother's sense of humour returned and they were able, at times, to banter and tease each other, and even laugh about their situation. The family story-telling was of the contradictory variety, mother's style being definitely preoccupied/'ghosts from the past'. Father had some features of the avoidant and forgetting style, but he was not dismissive of the importance of relationships. He took them very seriously. The unresolved mourning showed up whenever the topic of the cot deaths came up and the story started to break up into pieces.

The stories about their relationship were often about different ways of wanting to be close.

Carlos and Sara become ordinary children

Carlos had been a parentified child, like a little old man, on constant look out for his parents' depression, and caring for his sister as well. His own tears were kept hidden under the bedclothes except when Sara lifted the covers off. He was easily left out in the sessions. I had to focus deliberately on how to reconnect him to his mother's care. On one occasion she hugged him, which was a breakthrough. Progress came when he started to become naughty. He was no longer 'on duty' as assistant nurse now that his parents were coping better. His parents, however, were very upset and angry with him as they had built up expectations of him as a little adult helper. They needed help to see that this new mischievous little boy was to be welcomed.

At the beginning of therapy Sara had been very restless and distracted. Her school were very worried about her and she had special teaching because she was not learning. She was very active in the therapy and drew colourful pictures. After about three months of work she started to settle down. At school she quickly became the best pupil in the class and was clearly very bright. She also started to become naughty. On one occasion she was very angry with me at the beginning of the session because she had drawn a heart with a pencil, but had then wanted a rubber to erase it, but I did not have one. She furiously scribbled over the top of the heart. Later in the session she drew a beautiful heart in bright colours and wrote 'I LOVE MUMMY, CARLOS, ZETA AND DADDY.' I asked to see both pictures and commented that at times she was very

very angry when she wanted something that was not given to her, at others she could feel very loving and that it was difficult when she felt both feelings at the same time. She was beginning to integrate conflictual feelings, and find that she was not rejected for expressing anger.

On one occasion her parents had been allowing her to hold the baby so I commented on the fact that her parents saw her as someone who was safe with babies. At this point she crawled under the table which was in the middle of the room and came over to my side of the table so that I could have a conversation with her that her parents could not see. I asked her whether she still felt that she killed her brother, she nodded. I think it was easier for her to express her continuing doubts, which went counter to what her parents were telling her, out of her parents' sight. Her mother, hearing, was surprised said 'You still do not believe the grown-ups when they tell you did not kill Ben?' Again she nodded. After standing up Sara got out some gold stars from school that she had earned for good behaviour and showed them to me. I said that she knew she could be good as well as worrying that she was bad. She was beginning to accept that she could have both good and bad behaviour. The long past act of lying on top of her brother was no longer defining her as merely a killer; she was now a good, but at times a mischievous, little girl, just like everyone else.

Zeta quite simply had had the role of keeping everyone alive. She was the source of all hope and enjoyment. This role for babies in depressed families puts their development at risk. I was relieved to see her becoming demanding and upset. The best news was seeing her cuddling with her mother.

Sudden adversity: a move from the tragic script to 'we can manage'

As the situation was finally improving the family heard that their flat was about to be repossessed because their mortgage payment had fallen behind. Despair and a sense of helplessness returned. The tragic script ruled once again. In this case the self-fulfilling prophesy could be seen to have played a part. Mother was astounded that the finances had got into such a bad way. Father had not kept her informed, or been able to avert the disaster. Nothing he did seemed to have any effect anyway, and everything seemed destined to go wrong, so why try?

This new situation, however, had to be faced. The image of being made homeless seemed to be looming and catastrophic. I had a session with the parents on their own to discuss tactics. My position was to get them to explore what good they could get out of this. I asked whether they wanted to stay in their flat or not? They thought not, it had so many awful memories as well as being the place that mother had retreated to, away from the world with curtains drawn. I offered to write a report to use as they wished. This report just told their story without any flourishes, and then spelt out what I feared might happen if they were made homeless. This included the possibility of a further mental breakdown and possibly even suicide. I also spelt out that if this crisis was handled well, the family could complete their recovery and flourish. Everything in the report was what I believed, and presented without jargon, allowing the reader to empathize with the family in all its tribulations. The family told me that it had a powerful effect. The power to move was in their story, not vested in my authority. What was important, however, was that my authority would help to make sure that their story was heard. Using the report as one of his tools, father handled all the negotiations around the repossession himself. He took charge of the situation. Eventually, after many scares they were rehoused in a much more suitable setting.

My worry was that the report might act as yet another part of the tragic script: 'if this happens then disaster will strike'. But unless I spelled out the dangers it might not have led to the appropriate action. The community, including myself, as well as the family, might have allowed the tragic script to be fulfilled by doing nothing. By spelling out the strengths of the family I had hoped that that could add to a new emerging script, that this was a normal family slowly emerging from abnormal difficulties. The family also responded to the challenge. They told me that reading the report was moving to them as well, and so became a part of their story also.

The future

At the time of writing telling Sara in a family session that she did not kill her brother, postponed from earlier, still has not taken place. She is now seven. It now seems almost irrelevant as she is coming top of her class and seems not to be preoccupied with the cot deaths any more. The family has moved on to thinking more about the future. This, paradoxically, is probably a sign that the family is ready for this retelling as some of the emotional barriers to hearing another story have been removed. The whole family may be ready to hear something new. Hopefully a more coherent, re-edited family story will become part of the family mythology.

In the second month of therapy I had made a prediction, which is one way of influencing a co-constructed family story or belief.

> Therapist: In time you will make some sort of sense of this. The story might go something like this. Each of you may have the thought that you could have done something to prevent it (the second cot death), but each of you will know that you could not have done so. Also each of you thought that you hurt him (the dead baby) but will know that he died from something which was not anything to do with the the family.

We shall see. All family stories are like this. Waiting for the next retelling; always on the move.

References

Ainsworth, M. D. S. (1967). *Infancy in Uganda: infant care and growth of attachment*. The John Hopkins Press, Baltimore.

Belsky, J. and Nezworsky, T. (1988). *Clinical implications of attachment*. Lawrence Erlbaum Associates, New Jersey and London.

Bowlby, J. (1973). *Attachment and loss; Vol. 2 separation; anxiety and anger*. Hogarth, London.

Byng-Hall, J. (1973). Family myths used as defence in conjoint family therapy. *British Journal of Medical Psychology*, **46**, 239–50.

Byng-Hall, J. and Bruggen, P. (1974). Family admission decisions as a therapeutic tool. *Family Process*, **13**, 443–59.

Byng-Hall, J. (1979). Re-editing family mythology during family therapy. *Journal of Family Therapy*, **1**, 103–16.

Byng-Hall, J. (1980). The symptom bearer as marital distance regulator: clinical implications. *Family Process*, **19**, 355–65.

Byng-Hall, J. (1982). Family legends: their significance for the family therapist. In *Family therapy: complementary frameworks of theory and practice*, Vol. 2. (ed. A. Bentovim, A. Cooklin, and G. Gorell Barnes). Academic Press: London.

Byng-Hall, J. (1985). The family script: a useful bridge between theory and practice. *Journal of Family Therapy*, **7**, 301–05.

Byng-Hall, J. (1995a). *Rewriting family scripts: improvisation and systems change*. Guilford Press, New York and London.

Byng-Hall, J. (1995b). Creating a secure family base: some implications of attachment theory for family therapy. *Family Process*, **34**, 45–58.

Cronen, V. E. and Pearce, W. B. (1985). Toward an explanation of how the Milan method works: an invitation to a systemic epistemology and the evolution of family systems. In *Applications of systemic family therapy: the Milan approach*, (ed. D. Campbell and R. Draper). Grune and Stratton, London and New York.

Ferreira, A. (1963). Family myth and homeostasis. *Archives of General Psychiatry*, **9**, 457–63.

Fonagy, P., Steele, M., Steele, H., Moran, G. S., and Higgitt, A. C. (1991). The capacity for understanding mental states: the reflective self/parent in mother and child and its significance for security of attachment. *Infant Mental Health Journal*, **12**, 201–18.

Main, M. (1991). Metacognitive knowledge, metacognitive monitoring, and singular (incoherent) vs. multiple (incoherent) models of attachment: findings and directions for future research. In *Attachment across the life cycle*, (ed. C. M. Parkes, J. Stevenson-Hinde, and P. Marris). Tavistock/Routledge, London, New York.

Main, M., Kaplan, N., and Cassidy, J. (1985). Security in infancy, childhood, and adulthood: a move to the level of representation. In *Monograph of the Society for Research in Child Development*, Serial No. 209. 50: Nos. 1–2, (ed. I. Bretherton and E. Waters). The University of Chicago Press, Chicago.

McGoldrick, M. and Gerson, R. (1985). *Genograms in family assessment*. Norton, New York and London.

McNamee, S. and Gergen, K. J. (1992). *Therapy as social construction*. Sage, London.

Parry, A. (1991). A universe of stories. *Family Process*, **30**, 37–54.

Roberts, J. (1994). *Tales and transformations: stories in families and family therapy*. Norton, New York and London.

White, M. and Epston, D. (1990). *Narrative means to therapeutic ends*. Norton, New York and London.

8 The rehabilitation of rehabilitation: a narrative approach to psychosis*

Glenn Roberts

When, on 21 May 1972, a man leapt upon the pedestal of Michelangelo's Vatican Pieta and hit the Virgin Mary on the head with a hammer, he was clearly committing an act of gross and spectacular vandalism, probably iconoclasm, and possibly apostasy. His personal details were widely reported but I have chosen to omit them, for why should his name be forever linked to this disgrace? His behaviour, in attempting to destroy an art treasure conservatively valued at £100 million, brought him instant fame and infamy such that 25 years later we remain aware of all these details. His assertion at the time, 'I am Jesus Christ risen from the dead,' was similarly reported, as was his statement to the congregation of St Peter's that he was ready to be crucified.

It is a common view that where an action is incomprehensible or peculiarly destructive, whether publicly or privately, the person must be mad—and sometimes they are. As a result of being found thus, the distressed man described above was deported to Austria instead of being charged for his actions. Where, the story continues, 'as far as anyone knows he is still at large never having been heard of or see again' (Gamboni, 1997).

This way of telling a story about madness, which sets an insane act at the centre of the account and leaves the person, his life, his problems, his suffering, and his fate, unknown, is one of the central problems in making sense of psychosis and drawing alongside those suffering from it. It may be possible to offer a humane and compassionate response without understanding the person or his predicament, but it is extremely difficult to make or maintain a relationship with someone who cannot be understood.

Contemporary rehabilitation of the long-term mentally ill has been described as ideally based on, 'an individualised assessment of need and a sensitive understanding of the person's inner world' (Holloway, 1988). However, it is by no means clear how this 'sensitive understanding' may be achieved, and patients continue to criticize the impersonality of psychiatric approaches which are referred to as, 'mechanistic and dismissive of individuality' (Rogers *et al.*, 1993). Scientific psychiatry and psychology, driven by logical positivism (Murray, 1997), have become progressively preoccupied with a pursuit of objective and measurable dimensions, with a corresponding neglect of the subjective and personal. Strauss (1994) has commented on psychiatry's own problem with depersonalization; 'Our field, reeling from the previous excesses of

* This chapter is adapted from a paper originally presented at the annual residential conference of the Psychotherapy Section of the Royal College of Psychiatrists and the Association of University Teachers in Psychiatry, York University, 1994.

subjective reports and impressions, has now swung far to the other side, all but discounting subjectivity in scientific and academic work. . . . how little the psychiatric format—present illness, past history, family history, allows for noticing or recording the persons' experience. From such a format, it is fact almost impossible for the person to be discoverable.'

He illustrates this difficulty with an account of a young man with a lengthy history of schizophrenia who had participated in successive research interviews over 10 years. When asked which was the worst year of his life he unexpectedly identified a period when the objective ratings of his psychopathology and social functioning were rather favourable but, unknown to the researchers, he was traumatically rejected by his family and although relatively well, felt abandoned. Strauss suggests that rediscovering an emphasis on the personal story may provide a means of overcoming 'the gross inadequacy, in the mental health field, of our attention to the subjective side of a person's, experience.' Story may thus provide a vehicle for integrating objective and subjective dimensions of experience and provide a scientific centre for understanding the course of mental disorders without ignoring huge amounts of data. Story can also carry the ambition of progressing beyond the biopsychosocial model, a transition from focusing on 'disordered persons', their disability, and psychopathology, to a 'life context model' (Davidson and Strauss, 1995) with an emphasis on intentionality, temporality, meaning, and the coexistence of competence and dysfunction. It represents a re-entering of theoretical and therapeutic approaches on the person, his individuality, experience, and strengths, rather than solely on diagnosis and dysfunction.

Issues of engagement and disengagement, of the struggle to understand and the limits of understanding remain central to contemporary effort in rehabilitation. This chapter is primarily concerned with the narrative approach to psychopathology and treatment, and the restoration of meaning to madness.

Psychosis, madness, and the problem of meaning

It may at first seem that with psychosis we have reached the limits of a narrative approach. We appear to face a break, a discontinuity so wide that the whole notion of narrative appears to have collapsed. Schizophrenia is the only illness defined by inexplicability and includes 'bizarrness' in its definition. Hogarth describes the perplexity and fear that madness has always evoked.

> Madness, Thou chaos of ye brain,
> What art? That Pleasure givest and pain?
> Mechanic Fancy that can build,
> Vast labyrinths and Mazes wild,
> With Rule disjointed, shapeless measure,
> Fill'd with Horror, filled with Pleasure
> (*William Hogarth, Bedlam, 1735.*)

We can of course make stories *about* madness and thereby give shape to this 'shapeless measure'. Connoly (1830) describes meeting a tall, portly, and good-looking gentleman on the long gallery of a lunatic asylum and offers a picture of what anyone would take to be a madman.

> On his breast he wore a piece of list arranged like the ribbon of the Order of the Bath, and had on a leather apron, indicative of his being a free mason . . . he knew Bonapart very well himself. He and the Emperor had in fact been at the end of that gallery not long ago, surrounded by men with fixed bayonets, and if they had touched Napoleon, he should have been first to draw a sword. With dignified earnestness he assured us, that he had received a particular commission from the

Almighty; and he invited us to enter his apartment that he might show us the holy angels, the Virgin and the Venus . . . the walls, which had been white, were written upon in almost every part, with black letters, chiefly the never ending titles of his greatness and power.'

Connoly thus illustrates how, from our first encounter with a person suffering from psychosis, we are brought into confrontation with the problem of meaning. We can describe the person and his strange beliefs, odd emotional reactions, and behaviour, but how are we to understand him, and what may be the implications of whether we can understand him or not for forming a relationship?

Some may be satisfied with recognizing a pattern of symptoms and making a diagnosis, of schizophrenia or an affective psychosis, as if that disposed of this extraordinary transformation. How is it that someone comes to believe and tell such stories? If we seek any deeper sense of connection, if we try to understand what the person is saying or doing, we may find ourselves bewildered and confused. It is as though we, the supposedly sane, are guided by different lights and journey by different maps; we struggle to find common ground and easily give up. We appear to have come to the limits of rationality and are liable to accept our failure to form an empathic bridge. This is what we expect in madness.

There is much that conspires against building understanding and finding meaning in madness. But before we travel any further into this peculiar world I would like to set out some terms of reference and offer at least a preliminary sketch of the direction I shall take. Psychoses are principally associated with five sets of phenomena: delusions, hallucinations, disordered patterns of thinking and emotion, and the behaviour that may arise from any or all of these. I shall be narrowing our exploration to a discussion of delusions and follow Jaspers (1963) view that, 'since time immemorial delusion has been taken as the basic characteristic of madness.' Even if we are not taking in the whole territory it is reasonable to claim that we are somewhere near the centre ground.

It is not often that the terms psychosis and madness are used together, for they belong to different discourses, medicine and literature, and yet they are complementary. *I propose to use the term psychosis when speaking of the illness process and madness as its experiential and expressive consequences.*

It has been argued throughout this volume that narrative is a fundamental way of creating meaning and organizing understanding in sickness and in health, and that the dialogue between the resulting illness and healing narratives is the essence of therapy.

The central premise I wish to explore is that delusions are creative attributions of meaning to the experience of psychotic disintegration and that their formation, elaboration, and persistence is in some significant way mediated by narrative processes, i.e. *that 'madness' is an understandable response to 'psychosis' achieved by narrative means*, and, most importantly, we shall be able to better care for these patients if we are able to understand them. The distinction between illness and the mediating mechanisms mobilized to cope with it is extremely important because, 'it becomes possible to isolate the characteristics of the illness itself and the antecedents. By differentiating coping from illness, it also becomes possible to understand the person's efforts at healing and prevention, and which of these processes may be effective and thus relevant to treatment' (Strauss, 1989).

I shall argue that a narrative approach provides the materials with which the divided discourses of psychiatry and psychotherapy may be drawn into closer relationship, and in accepting

Satre's criticism (in Sims, 1988) that, 'psychiatry is too quickly satisfied when it throws light on the general structures of delusions and does not seek to comprehend the individual, concrete content of the psychosis,' I shall explore the potential of narrative to contain a duel emphasis on form and content and thereby contextualize symptoms in the biographical experience of the individual.

But, these are almost my conclusions. Our first steps need to be based on a review of the problems encountered in looking for meaning and understanding in madness.

Sense and nonsense

The 'split mind' of schizophrenia finds a reflection in all kinds of splits and separations which have characterized society's response to those suffering from psychosis, largely to their detriment. Returning to our beginning we find Connoly (1830) arguing the point with his contemporaries: 'They have sought for, and imagined, a strong definable boundary between sanity and insanity which has not only been imaginary, and arbitrarily placed but, by being supposed to separate all who were of unsound mind from the rest of men, has unfortunately been considered a justification of certain measures against the portion condemned which were for the majority unnecessary and afflicting.'

This was written in an era that built the asylums and defined their psychiatrists as 'alienists', whose patients were by implication 'aliens', the implications of which emerge from its definition: 'strange, foreign, not one of our own, of a nature repugnant adverse or opposed, one separated or excluded from citizenship and the privileges of a nation' (*Oxford English Dictionary*).

A major theme in the ascendancy of the anti-psychiatry movement since the 1960s has been a reaction to what was regarded as the stigmatizing reductionism of conventional psychiatric approaches. Laing's (1964) 'Divided Self', not only sought to articulate meaningfully the inner world of those suffering from psychosis, but also demonstrated that there are major divisions between mental health professionals, who themselves constituted a divided self. Ciompi (1989) has warned of the continuing tension between psychiatric and psychotherapeutic approaches resulting in, 'a disastrous splitting of our understanding and treatment of schizophrenia into either biological or psychological reductionism.'

There are also limits on what may be understood. Laing's (1964) exposition of meaning in madness makes his blunt assertion that there is something fundamentally elusive to understanding at the centre of schizophrenia all the more striking:

> What is required of us?
> Understand him?
> The kernel of the schizophrenic's experience of himself must remain incomprehensible to us. As long as we are sane and he is insane, it will remain so . . . one of the greatest barriers against getting to know a schizophrenic is his sheer incomprehensibility.

Alongside this we have Freud's (1939) hope that, 'recognition of its [the delusion's] kernel of truth would afford common ground upon which the therapeutic work could develop . . . the essence of it is that there is not only meaning in madness, as the poet has already perceived, but a fragment of historical truth.'

Scharfetter (1980) has also laid claim to the significance of delusional talk and the risks of disregarding the meaning of its content:

Through his delusion the patient is speaking of the threat to his existence, the disintegration of his existence, the destruction of his self-being and his world; he is telling us how he has been overwhelmed by people and things which are persecuting and poisoning his threatened, vulnerable, restricted existence. He is describing to us the reality of his life. We cannot do the patient justice without recognising that this is his life's reality, by taking it seriously, never if we treat it as delusion or fantasy. To do this is to push the patient aside, to push him further into his isolation.'

Garety and Hemsley (1994) have confidently contradicted the view that people with delusions are 'irretrievably lost in untruth' by reviewing the accumulating evidence for a cognitive approach to understanding the processes by which delusions may arise and be maintained. However, their description of reasoning bias and cognitive distortion places little emphasis on what the delusional patient is actually saying, and whilst they make a case for modifying delusional beliefs with cognitive interventions, they conclude that, 'the significance of the content of delusions remains unclear.'

Those who are working to help people suffering from psychosis are confronted with a major and uncomfortable dilemma, between seeking to understand and risk making links that are not there, or expecting not to make such links and failing to connect with what the person is saying, deepening his alienation.

Jenner *et al.* (1986) have described this tension as: 'a psychiatrist is doomed to bring his self and his Wetanschauung to his interviews. If he struggles to understand he may be acting analogously to those who similarly approach a man with a cerebral tumour. If he doesn't but instead medicates and feels content with a crippled readjustment, he may be unconsciously contributing to a Brave New World in which men are conveniently manipulated pharmacologically.'

His suggested approach to this seemingly unresolvable dilemma is, 'humility in the face of reality.' Which is a fine sentiment, but gives little guidance in practice. The potential of a narrative approach is in offering a bridge across the dilemma, drawing hermeneutic and biomedical perspectives together, for even the person with the tumour needs understanding if the complexities and significance of his illness experience are to be accounted for in his care and treatment (Murray, 1997).

The implications of meaninglessness

The costs of failing to find understanding may be considerable, for as Jaspers (1963) commented, 'everything understandable has a constituent potentiality of worth. In contrast we do not value the un-understandable.' People suffering from chronic psychotic illnesses, as some of the least understandable, are also some of the least valued members of society:

Chronic schizophrenic patients spend their lives in a world of public institutions and poverty . . . chronic patients often are to a lesser or greater degree homeless, familyless, jobless, penniless and marginally employable. Their world is often one of insecurity, lack of privacy, prejudice, impersonality and occasional violence.'
(*Josephs and Josephs, 1986.*)

Roadblocks on the path to meaning

The Jasperian tautology

Until recent developments in cognitive therapy, Jaspers' (1963) well-known assertion that psychosis was fundamentally un-understandable, and therefore psychologically unapproachable, has dominated psychiatric approaches to psychosis. It has carried pervasive implications of separateness and alienation. It follows that there is no point in seeking to understand delusions and if they do prove understandable they cannot have been delusions. However, the inclusion of un-understandability as a defining characteristic of delusion may have been applied far more broadly than Jaspers intended. For he limits the notion of un-understandability to the core of the psychotic process, i.e. to the primary delusion where 'content seems immediately present, vividly clear', or the prodromal delusional atmosphere consisting of 'certain primary sensations, vital feelings, moods, awareness: something is going on . . .', and which do not appear to have psychological antecedents. Whereas he clearly states that, 'we can understand and empathise with the content but cannot understand the occurrence of the delusion itself . . . this un-understandability is the essence of the psychotic experience.' Thus, he points to opportunities as well as limitations for understanding, and when commenting on elaborate delusional systems he states: 'A delusional system is constructed which in its own context is comprehensible, sometimes extremely closely argued and unintelligible only in its ultimate origins, these delusional systems are objectively meaningful structures and methodologically we can assign them to the psychology of creativity.' (Jaspers, 1963, p.106.)

Uncertainty over truth

The characteristic conviction of the psychotic presents another barrier to comprehension. Their model of truth (Wallace, 1988) is overwhelmingly subjective and needs neither objective verification nor consensual validation to carry an assurance of conviction. The deluded are fundamentalists who defend and protect their beliefs from any intrusion, including the intrusion of being understood, but they do so at considerable cost:

> the evidence of 'I know' (the truth) gives him an autistic, private, restricted and therefore privative view of the world and makes it impossible to reach a common understanding with others . . . it goes against both their reason and their capacity for empathy . . . delusion means isolation. The delusional patient is alone.'
> (*Scharfetter, 1980.*)

We are also faced with puzzling and overwhelming reversals such as Woodley (1947) describes from his own experience: 'Reality to the lunatic is your equivalent to sanity. To you insanity is a sad state, to be deplored. To the insane, reality is not only to be deplored, but avoided at all costs.'

The symptoms of psychosis continue not only to challenge our credulity and capacity for empathy but also invite us to consider the basic principles by which we negotiate the complexities of truth and reality.

> Extreme psychotic states offer a human parable . . . patients see into depths which do not belong so much to their illness as themselves as individuals with their historical truth . . . in psychotic reality we find an abundance of content representing fundamental problems of philosophy.'
> (*Jaspers, 1963, p.309.*)

Meaningless training

It may still be that psychiatric and other mental health professionals are poorly prepared to understand their patients. York (1988) has cogently argued that there is a widespread 'defect in training', which denies trainees the confidence that can come from understanding their patients from a psychological point of view, whether those patients are psychologically treatable or not. Roth (1970) emphasized that the structures of professional training, with its rapid changes of post and emphasis on resolution of acute symptoms, may result in the trainee failing to consider the meaning of the illness and losing sight of the longitudinal perspective of the person presenting his problems.

Klienman (1988) has commented on the implications of modern medicine in that, although unintended, the contemporary health care system, 'does just about everything to drive the practitioner's attention away from the experience of illness. The system thereby contributes importantly to the alienation of the chronically ill from their professional care givers and paradoxically to the relinquishment by the practitioners of that aspect of the healer's art that is most ancient, most powerful and most existentially rewarding.'

The life and work of Eugen Bleuler offer a vivid illustration of the benefits of harnessing together the art and science of medicine. Bleuler's observations, leading to the modern concept of schizophrenia, arose from intimate and continuous contact with his patients. He was 29 when appointed Chief of the Clinic Rheinou, a converted eighth century monastery, forming an island community in the Rhine. He lived there for 12 years, 'working with them (in agriculture) organising their free time (for instance, hiking with them, playing in the theatre with them, dancing with them). During his life with the patients, Bleuler had always a memo pad at hand, where he noted what touched and interested him in his patients behaviour. He frequently noted in shorthand what the patients actually said . . . he was eager to describe their symptoms in an objective scientific way and to suggest at the same time the importance of understanding the personal psychodynamic life of the individual' (Bleuler and Bleuler, 1986).

From this Bleuler (1951) drew confidence that whereas, 'at first all this may appear sheer nonsense', that, 'on closer scrutiny we find understandable connections in every one of these cases . . . the delusions of the paranoiac form a logical structure with only a few false premises and inferences in its foundation, or amongst its building stones; the delusions of the schizophrenic are not as systematic, yet they are not the chance heap of unruly chaos which they seem on superficial observation.' But the 'few false premises' must still be accounted for and constitute the limits of understanding, the psychosis to which the delusional structures are a narrative response.

Few psychiatrists today have a working practice that brings them into such frequent and close contact with their patients and we may similarly find Bleuler's conclusion inaccessible, that 'the schizophrenic is in not unintelligible and that we can develop empathy for him.' This assertion, that understanding delusional contents is a route into empathy, will be taken up later.

Although Strauss (1989) has been a persistent and persuasive advocate for a re-evaluation of individual longitudinal case studies as, 'an excellent, perhaps the best foundation for delineating complex causal processes in heterogeneous phenomena.' It has been and remains necessary to argue for the need to reinstate an intimate awareness of individuals alongside the generalizations of epidemiological studies and clinical trials in order to find meaning in madness. This appears as a specific example of a general concern raised about some consequences of medicine progress. For as Professor Roy Porter (1995) has observed: 'The rise of diagnostic technology, the religion of statistics, numbers and objectivity, the increasingly scientific self-image of the medical profession, and a powerful commitment to drug therapies . . . have all midwived the 'medical model', and its subsequent extension from general medicine to psychiatry . . . the patient as a person has been tending to 'disappear'.

Contagion: the fear of getting too close

A further obstacle to understanding is the commonly held fear of getting close to madness. For example, in an introductory text on *The art of psychotherapy*, Anthony Storr (1997) speaks of his choice, 'many years ago that I was not going to be one of those bold analysts who undertake therapy with psychotic patients,' and later honestly reveals that, 'I simply found that close encounters with schizophrenics seemed perilously upsetting' (but see his 'telling tale' later).

He helpfully sounds a warning for those who do choose to get close to psychosis for there is the same need for supervision and secure connection outside this disordered world as with any other mental health work, but the risks may be higher and the issues more complex.

Susan Estroff (1981) described her experiences as an anthropologist studying psychotic patients by joining them for long hours on an in-patient ward:

> The longer one attempts to enter the client's world without constant, active, outside reference points, the fuzzier becomes the distinction between crazy and un-crazy, self and other. The more time one spends amid confusion, fear, anxiety, and unhappiness, the more it is highlighted in oneself. Having lost and regained my perspective, objectivity, and confidence countless times during the past years, I would not attempt it alone again.'

This suggests that insanity is contagious and that there are dangers in getting too close. There is a risk of loss of perspective in holding the tension between illness and meaning, psychosis and madness. Fuller Torey (1995) has drawn attention to Balzac's heroine in *Louis Lambert*, a young woman dedicated to caring for her psychotic husband. He presents this as an illustration of the potential for understanding to enable compassion, but this is ambiguous for it also serves to underline the risks of becoming so immersed within the psychotic perspective that one loses objectivity altogether.

> No doubt Louis appears to be 'insane', she said, 'but he is not so . . . The equilibrium of my husband's mind is perfect. If he does not recognise you corporeally, do not think he has not seen you. He is able to disengage his body and see us under another form, I know not of what nature. When he speaks he says marvellous things. Only, in fact often, he completes in speech an idea begun in the silence of his mind, or else he begins a proposition in words and finishes it mentally. To other men he must appear insane; to me, who lives in his thought, all his ideas are lucid. I follow the path of his mind; and though I cannot understand many of its turns and digressions, I nevertheless reach the end with him . . . common minds to whom this quickness of mental vision is unknown, and who are ignorant of the inward travail of the soul, laugh at dreamers and call them madmen if they are given to such forgetfulness of connecting thoughts. Louis is always so; he wings his way through the spaces of thought with the agility of a swallow; yet I can follow him in all his circlings. That is the history of his so-called madness.'
>
> (*Fuller Torey, 1995.*)

Fuller Torey's assertion that 'such idealised understanding is only to be found in fiction' fails to notice that Louis Lambert's wife has not really 'understood' his madness at all, but has come to reject the concept of insanity altogether and replotted his disordered thoughts as 'quickness of mental vision' beyond the common mind. She may be illustrating one of the many ways in which intimacy may be preserved in the context of dissonant dialogues and one path of resolving the dreadful tension that many discover when seeking to understand madness.

Meaning and madness: a narrative approach

If understanding is desirable but difficult to access we can return to our theme with the reminder that 'understanding proceeds primarily by story' (Romanshyn, in Cox and Theilgaard, 1987) and as Kathryn Montgomery Hunter (1991) asks, 'and how else is the individual to be known but by a narrative account of his case?' Story is an ancient and ubiquitous carrier of meaning, but at first it may seems impossible to find an application in psychosis characterized by discontinuity, incomprehensibility, fracturing, and a rent in the narrative fabric.

John Donne's (1624) conviction, gained whilst seriously ill and contemplating the possibility of death, that, 'No man is an Iland, intire of it selfe; every man is a peece of the Continent, a part of the maine', may do well for the sane, but the mad appear to have taken some inexplicable journey that separates them from 'the maine' and defeats empathic contact and the possibility of fellow travelling.

However detached and alien psychotic states of mind appear to be, it is sometimes possible to build bridges across the turbulent and sometimes dangerous waters that separate these islanders from the mainland and that a narrative may offer some guidance in the construction of these causeways, to tell the story of how some have come to live on islands and to anticipate the difficulties of repatriation and reintegration with society.

So what are we to make of these mad stories? The search for meaning in madness can be considered at three overlapping levels:

(a) meaning *of* madness: narrative processes in the origins of delusion;

(b) meaning *in* madness: biographical associations with the contents of delusions; and

(c) meaning *through* madness: transformation of the perspectival world and the acquisition of purpose and meaning-in-life through delusional belief.

Meaning of madness

The origins of delusion are complex and cannot to be established with any certainty. However, if it is assumed that delusions, like other beliefs, arise in some temporal sequence, a simple schema can be constructed (Roberts, 1992), which allows suggested part models and established information to be assigned to three stages of development.

1. Prepsychotic: predisposing vulnerability factors and precipitants.

2. Acute: emergence of delusional beliefs and other features.

3. Chronic: consolidation and elaboration to produce systems of belief, a transformation of the life story.

The interface between each stage is governed by narrative processes.

The attribution of meaning to experience

The interaction of precipitating factors with predisposing conditions produces a state of unmanageable anxiety and inaugurates a prodromal state consisting of a loosening and disintegration of the previously held structures of meaning. This pre-delusional state is characterized by the appearance in consciousness of some unaccountable, unpredictable, anomalous experience.

There is an uncanny sense of strangeness, something of great importance but equally unfathomable going on. The transition into this state has been formulated by Cutting (1989) as 'a breakdown of gestalt perception', and there is general agreement that it is deeply perplexing and profoundly uncomfortable.

Many theorists have suggested that once this psychotic break has occurred the remaining healthy, cognitive, and intellectual capacities are used to make an imaginative jump, and construct rational explanations for anomalous experiences (Maher, 1974). More recently, there has been an accumulation of experimental studies that have demonstrated abnormal patterns of reasoning and attribution in delusional subjects.

These approaches suggest that delusions are initiated either by anomalous sensory or perceptual experiences or by a primary feeling of mysterious significance. When sensations are perplexing, painful, or unpleasant, it follows that concepts of invisible and powerful forces are drawn from the reservoirs of personal meaning, often derived from popular science and religion, to construct satisfying explanatory beliefs. Furthermore, the fact that others so not apparently share these beliefs introduces the possibility that either they are lying or that the individual is truly special (Maher and Ross, 1984). Research based on attribution theory has demonstrated that where unfamiliar events or behaviours are not readily explicable and social comparisons are unavailable, then there appears to be a universal tendency to view even the inanimate world anthropomorphically and attribute personal meanings to impersonal or depersonalized events (Johnson *et al.*, 1977). Tsuang *et al.* (1988) have pointed out the similarity between Maher's theory and the earlier formulation of De Clerambault, who proposed that delusions result from abnormal neurological events, which produce 'automatisms', unusual experiences that puzzle the patient and demand explanation.

Cognitive psychologists have found abnormalities in the attributional style of deluded subjects, characterized by a readiness to jump to conclusions on the basis of less data, a tendency to see coincidences as significant, and to make external attributions for unwelcome experiences (Bentall and Kany, 1989).

This process, of attributing meaning to experience, leading to the development of delusional beliefs, may act to resolve the anxiety generated by psychotic decompensation, for there is a basic human need to make sense of one's condition and the worse the conditions are the greater is this need (Bennet, 1983). Jaspers (1963) stated that 'this general delusional atmosphere with all its vagueness of content must be unbearable. Patients obviously suffer terribly under it and to reach some definite idea at last is like being relieved of some enormous burden.' Or, as a patient of mine once informed me, 'I have found the way to overcome paranoia—you have to believe it.'

The primary anguish of the psychotic is in just this dissolution of meaning and inability to make sense of his experience. He knows something of great significance is going on, but cannot say what it is. The formation of delusions can be seen as a narrative response to meaninglessness:- through which order and security are regained, the novel experience is incorporated within the individual's conceptual framework, and the occult potential of its mystery is defused.

Subjectively a delusion is simply a belief (Sims, 1988), and beliefs bind anxiety, justify social interaction, give support to defensive concerns, and serve as supports for cognitive activity in areas of uncertainty (Lansky, 1977). So, except in those rare cases of primary delusion, where content seems 'immediately present and vividly clear' (Jaspers, 1963) and without links to any obvious antecedents, *delusions emerge as new meanings attributed to anomalous experience*.

Arieti (1964) described this shift: 'indefinite feelings become finite, the imperceptible becomes perceptible, the vague menace is transformed into a definite threat . . . the sense of suspiciousness becomes the conviction . . . things that appear confusing and obscure have a meaning and purpose.'

These, delusional, beliefs then form the basis of a revised narrative, a telling primarily to oneself and later to others of a new and convincing explanation for what is going on. This has been described as a stage of 'explanatory insight' when the mystery is solved, the confusion and perplexity dispelled, and, even if the implications are threatening, at least they are known and action can be taken (Cameron, 1959; Maher and Ross, 1984). Conversely, '. . . no dread is worse than that of danger unknown' (Jaspers, 1963).

Consolidation and elaboration of delusional meanings

Meaning and purpose are often used simultaneously but carry different connotations. Meaning may be regarded as an approximate synonym for pattern and refers to sense or coherence, and therefore a search for meaning implies a search for coherence. Purpose refers to intention, aim, function, what something does and to what end. Thus, Yalom (1980) described the purpose of meaning as: 'an anxiety emollient: it comes into being to relieve the anxiety that comes from facing a life and a world without an ordained structure.'

This emphasizes the basic human need to have some superordinant sense of meaning, which is dislocated in psychotic breaks and remodelled within psychosis on delusional foundations (Bleuler's 'few false premises').

Wing and Brown's (1970, p.85) study of institutionalization in schizophrenia observed that, 'coherently expressed delusions stand out as having favourable implications on almost all counts. Patients with this symptom are less likely to show clinical poverty, less likely to be living in conditions of social understimulation, more likely to be short stay and are more likely to leave hospital (although their attitude may be unrealistic). . . . they are resistant to the ill effects of poverty of their social milieu.'

They make no comment on what the nature of this resistance may be and whether delusional elaboration is a cause or effect of good prognosis, but it may be restitutive and adaptive to find meaning within psychosis and to elaborate those meanings into coherent and comprehensive belief systems.

Penrose (1931) described in great detail the case of James R. who spent 50 years in Cardiff City Mental Hospital and evolved an extremely elaborate delusional system, a 'comprehensive imaginary world'. The author drew particular attention to his marked shyness, scrupulousness, and sensitivity, and his considerable sexual difficulties, venereal disease, and consequent moral conflict prior to the onset of psychosis. In conclusion, he said that, 'the mentality of the psychotic is not unlike the philosopher or abstract scientist . . . his activities have not merely succeeded in warding off reality. They have kept occupied his intellectual and emotional powers and kept them fresh all these years.'

In madness we see the paradoxical 'victory in defeat whereby those suffering from and struggling to cope with psychosis assert the inviolability of the self in the face of its complete fragility' (Josephs, 1988). However, as Sayer's (1989) illustrated, 'The Comforts of Madness' whilst representing a defensive adjustment to psychotic disintegration, remain exquisitely uncomfortable.

Thus, the delusional person has experienced a break, a fracturing, of the continuity of his lived narrative and responds to this dissolution of the self by the creation of new meanings, which are progressively elaborated to enable the construction or reconstruction of a life story such as to incorporate these otherwise disintegrative elements.

In this context it is interesting to note the view of Dupre (in Arthur, 1964) that some 'delusions of the imagination' are due to a pathological activity of creative imagination which he called 'mythomania'. And Norman (1899) noted long ago the similarity between a delusional system and the creation of a story with its resultant satisfactions: 'Among patients of the communicative type there are many who, while they proclaim the strongest opinions, restrict their actions always to declamation or writing; who are perfectly happy in the exercise of the chief function that seems to be left to them, pondering over their wonderful story and reasoning it out in the mode they deem convincingly logical.'

It seems characteristic of the chronically deluded that the more extensive the system of beliefs the more comprehensive a reconstruction of their life story is involved. Schilder's (1951) paper on the development of thought includes a description of a female patient with extensive delusions of procreation; he describes the way she, 'created a peculiar cosmology and even more peculiar fairy-tale world.'

Meaning in delusion: the relationship between delusional contents and life story

> Much madness is divinest sense to a discerning eye.
> (*Emily Dickinson, 1862*)

Hardy's poem, crafted around uncovering layers of meaning beneath a single strange and apparently senseless behaviour, describes how a trivial action can point to concealed issues of great importance and the depths of lost attachments, and illustrates something of the method of finding meaning in delusion:

The Whitewashed Wall

Why does she turn in that shy soft way,
Whenever she stirs the fire,
And kiss to the chimney corner wall,
As if entranced to admire its whitewashed bareness,
More than the sight of a rose of richest green?
I've known her long,
But this raptured rite I never before have seen.

Well once when her son cast his shadow there,
A friend took a pen and drew him upon that flame lit wall.
And the lines had a life-like semblance to him,
And there long stayed his familiar look.
But one day ere she knew,
The whitewasher came to cleanse the nook,
And covered the face from view.

Yes, he said, my brush goes on with a rush,
The draft is buried under.
When you have to whiten old cotts and brighten,
What else can you do I wonder.

But she knows he's there when she yearns for him,
Deep in the labouring night,
She sees him as close at hand and turns to him,
Under his sheet of white.
(*Hardy, 1918*)

The observer is confronted with something odd, inexplicable, and at first she may seem 'mad'. There would be no way of knowing or guessing that this grieving mother continues to long for her dead son and that her behaviour is related to her yearning for him. Her grief and the object of her grief are both concealed and yet her 'meaningless' behaviour provides access to both. However, in order to disinter this concealed meaning, as with seeking to understand psychotic behaviour and beliefs, there is a preliminary need to assume that her actions are meaningful, that there is something to discover, and that she may be best placed to reveal it, if an appropriate level of trust and confidence can be established. When understanding peels back 'the sheet of white' we are able to re-evaluate her odd behaviour as 'raptured' and repetitive because of the salience of its hidden meaning. Meaningful associations such as this can often be found between delusional contents and the life experience of the psychotic.

This perspective gains experimental support from the Vienna group (Berner *et al.*, 1986) who have presented a multiaxial classification of delusional states, including an axis recording the specific contents of the delusions. They concluded that, 'there seems to be no doubt that the specific circumstances of the personal history are frequently of great importance for the choice of "delusional theme".'

Forgus and De Wolfe (1974) offer further support in their study of the 'reality constructs' of 54 deluded subjects, which found that the dominant delusional themes matched the dominant categories used to conceptualize their perceptual and cognitive world.

It follows that not only may the deluded be saying something meaningful through their delusions, but what they say may be personally significant. Kaffman's (1984) study of 34 families where at least one member had developed a delusional system, concluded that there was always a basis in historical reality for the delusional beliefs and that this may support the incorrigibility of these 'false beliefs' because in some transformed and distorted way the individual is telling the truth. Similarly, the fact that delusional contents vary with social background make it clear that they are derived from acquired knowledge (Murphy, 1983) and the language in which a delusion is couched often indicates the patient's family background or culture, that is, the preferred channels of relatedness in his group (Weinstein, 1962).

Some stories

The radioactive lady

A middle aged Romanian woman was brought into hospital in a deeply distressed state claiming that she couldn't sleep and was visited at night by a radioactive lady, who injected her with lead. She was clearly depressed and there was a history of previous but lesser episodes. At first, and for some time, it was difficult to do anything but receive her distress and hear about her nightly torment. There was also a puzzling ambivalence in her attitude to the radioactive lady whom she was both pleased to be in contact with but who was also associated with great distress. The story behind this eventually emerged from her estranged daughters. She lived a somewhat isolated life, divorced and detached from her family, and ill at ease in her neighbourhood. Her closest friend had experienced a long illness with breast cancer, treated with intense radiotherapy and had died some weeks before she became depressed. It was then possible to understand the content of her depression as psychotic grief and talk with her about the radioactive lady, who stood for both her departed friend, now made radioactive, and the tormenting treaters whose painful and unsuccessful ministrations had led to her death. Having a pattern of understanding to make sense of her story also enabled the staff to empathize with her loneliness and grief and provided a route into establishing a therapeutic relationship.

Sometimes the inner story is completely inaccessible and only appears some time later and there may be good reasons for keeping it undisclosed.

I'm sorry doctor: I thought you were Herod

I had known Mary for some years and had been involved with several previous admissions with recurrences of her paranoid schizophrenic illness. I thought we got on fairly well. So, when it appeared that she was becoming ill again, although she had moved to an adjacent patch it seemed entirely appropriate that I go to see her, hoping that an established relationship would enable contact. She greeted me, by saying, 'Hullo Doctor, what is the time?' and was confused and frustrated when I looked at my watch and answered her. 'No, No!—What IS the time.' It took me a little while to realize she was preoccupied with the nature of time itself and was slipping rapidly into a state of psychotic confusion. She was admitted unwillingly in considerable anxiety and was initially very disturbed in her behaviour, needing physical restraint and at one point seclusion. But then everything went quiet, literally so, for although she became orderly and appropriate in her behaviour she also was mute, or at least she refused to speak to staff and completely ignored me, walking past and failing to acknowledge my greeting. Some weeks went by, during which she had the freedom of the general hospital and its grounds. She accepted a reinstatement of medication but still would not talk. And then one day she came into the ward round and said, 'I'm sorry Doctor, I thought you were Herod.'

She went on to explain that she had 'realized' whilst the staff were struggling with her that they were Gestapo and could reel off their ranks and attributions. She offered all this from the standpoint of sanity and with an air of benign amusement it was as though a fog between us had lifted. However, as we explored it further and I asked her for Jewish and wartime associations she spoke of her Jewish mother fleeing Germany for England and the hatred, fear, and tragedy she had grown up with. Many of her mother's family had been killed as children. Was this where Herod fitted in? The Biblical story rests upon the genocide of young children in an attempt to destroy the Christ child, the nation's hope.

If Mary did not have to contend with a psychotic illness I imagine she could have said how frightened she had become, and how our handling and containment of her reminded her of stories of persecution and captivity. But as it was we found ourselves caught in a reminiscent drama stretching from the Europe of her youth to ancient Palestine. Making these connections provided a means by which she could integrate some of her psychotic experiences and helped the ward staff who then felt they had at least some understanding of her and were touched by the tragedies she had within her, instead of her hostility and psychotic autism resulting in alienation.

But the dog couldn't hear them

Jean's severe schizophrenic illness is accompanied by many different hallucinations and delusions. Her brother has a similar illness and partly due to his long-term hospitalization, Jean has a great fear of psychiatric services. She was also greatly distrustful of men to begin with and was only able to say anything about her life after a prolonged period of out-patient attendance during which a measure of trust and predictability was established. She had suffered considerable deprivation and abuse as a child which she regarded as normal until she went to University. She was intelligent and devoted herself to study in literature and philosophy partly as an avenue of exploration, trying to make sense of her past. Although she presented with many delusions, there was a constant theme of persecution, hostility, intrusion, and attack—equivalent to her early life experience. She was puzzling over what was real and true and if her experience could be trusted. She accepted the possibility that although her experiences were true in the sense of a real experience they might also be true in some metaphoric way—pointing back to past realities.

Against this framework she noticed one day that her sensitive and alert dog did not apparently hear the loud screaming that she could hear. This allowed at least the possibility that it was different to a 'normal scream'. She was able to explore her associations to the scream and in doing so remembered it as her brother's scream when being beaten by their father. From this small beginning she was able to engage in a series of explorations looking for links between present symptomatic experience and past traumas. Many of these were written exercises that she took away from our sessions having negotiated a piece of reflective work. She gradually wrote about her past, and although many of the experiences continued, her fear diminished. Gradually she became able to bring her past life experience into a therapeutic relationship and place the form of many of her experiences within a diagnostic framework. The discovery of meaningfulness and of the great significance of meanings chosen provided the basis of relationship. She remained psychotic but became progressively less mad to the point where she was interested to read and discuss literature on schizophrenia and the content of our discussions spontaneously shifted from being engrossed with her delusional preoccupations to current relationships, hopes, and needs. The difference between a badge and a label may depend on whether a diagnosis, or some other defining meaning, is imposed or willingly adopted.

Laing observed (1964) that, 'the mad things said and done by the schizophrenic will remain essentially a closed book if one does not understand their existential context.' A narrative approach recontextualizes the mad things said and done in the life history of the individual, and in doing so at least partly opens the book to enable patient and therapist to read from the same text or texts, and find some common ground on which to meet (Davidson, 1993).

Meaning through delusion: the acquisition of meaning and purpose through delusional belief

Few authors have commented on what factors may contribute to the persistence, stability, and elaboration of delusions into systems of belief. Some have considered persistence as an indicator of the intractability of the underlying disorder, others that there may be advantages in persistence, and these 'satisfactions of psychosis' may be experienced as preferable to confronting reality again.

Meaninglessness is rarely mentioned as a clinical entity because it is generally considered to be a manifestation of some other 'primary' and more familiar syndrome such as depression or alcoholism (Yalom, 1980). Stafford-Clark (1970), writing as a psychiatrist to theologians, states that 'psychiatry has always had difficulty in accepting the need to believe as important and profound. Yet careful objective study of man's life reveals him in search not only of immediate satisfactions but beyond these in search of some point and purpose in living at all.' The corollary is that those things, ideas, relationships, beliefs that come to constitute a meaning for life may represent some of the central supporting structures of well-being and psychological integration (Storr, 1976).

Perris (1989) describes the development in health and sickness of basic cognitive schemata that are organized, interlocked ideas or thoughts and which provide the fundamental intellectual resources for labelling, classifying, interpreting, evaluating, and assigning meaning to objects and events. These schemata continuously structure our experience and are structured by it. He holds these to be broadly equivalent to belief systems, rules of life, meaning structures, basic assumptions, working models, and assumptive worlds; they also appear equivalent to the basic stories we tell, the myths we live by. As such, they tend to be self-reinforcing, stable cognitive structures, providing a foundation for identity and a touchstone for action. Psychic reorganization within psychosis, when fully developed, represents a reconfiguration of this meaning structure, resulting in a dysfunctional schemata.

It may at first seem perverse to suggest that existential benefits could accompany the elaboration of a delusional system. The proposition is that, in a psychological sense, delusional systems can become an overarching framework of meaning and secure attachment, a place to live in and return to, and that the psychological benefits associated with the possession of any organized system of belief may accompany delusional systems. This may then act to stimulate elaboration, increase resistance to refutation, and explain some of the paradoxical difficulties that follow from losing these beliefs, i.e. what some call 'recovery'.

This is a close parallel to Hughlings Jackson's (1932) formulation of symptoms arising from evolution in the context of dissolution: 'Illusions, delusions, extravagant conduct, and abnormal emotional states in an insane person signify evolution, not dissolution; they signify evolution getting on with what remains intact of the mutated higher centres . . . in what disease, effecting so much damage has spared.'

Evolutionary principles are seemingly preoccupied with adaptation for survival, this process is that of a salvaging of the self through the creation of an altered view of reality. This is similar to Scharfetter (1980) view that through elaboration of the delusions, imagined or imaginable triumph over the individual's sufferings becomes, experientially, a life reality.

An early experimental finding, which seemed to confirm this, was unexpectedly derived from testing many different clinical groups with the purpose in life test (PILT), derived from Frankl's emphasis on the basic need for meaning in life. Crumbaugh (1968) sought to validate the test by using it on a large number of subjects ($n = 1151$) in six patient and four non-patient groups, and placed each in a predicted rank order of perceived meaning and purpose in life. The results were as predicted; non-patients all scored higher than patients, the highest being successful businessmen and Dominican noviciates. The lowest were of hospitalized non-schizophrenic psychotics. However, a small group ($n = 11$) of hospitalized schizophrenics unexpectedly returned the highest patient scores and were equal to college undergraduates. He interpreted this within Frankl's framework, commenting that:

> The hidden or to the normal person, trivial meanings which typify schizophrenic thought processes do, however constitute genuinely perceived meanings from the phenomenological point of view. The schizophrenic has created his own significant world within which he resides purposefully . . . thus the schizophrenic may think that his life has meaning and purpose even though to the external eye this meaning is shallow, inadequate, distorted and unsatisfactory.
> (*Crumbaugh, 1968.*)

Following on from this, Roberts (1991) compared 17 patients with long-standing delusional belief systems with a matched group of previously deluded schizophrenic patients in remission and two non-patient groups, psychiatric rehabilitation nurses and Anglican ordinands, these being selected by virtue of also possessing sincerely held system of beliefs. All subjects completed the PILT and an abbreviated form of the Beck depression inventory.

The results were striking and paradoxical, with the chronically deluded group scoring very high on purpose in life and low on depression compared with the group in remission, in marked contrast with the impression given by their objective circumstances, and the assumptions of those treating them. A review of the PILT item which asked about suicidal intent showed there was a much greater degree of professed suicidal intent in those chronic patients who have recovered compared with those currently deluded, and a case record review found that only two out of 17 of the deluded had recorded episodes of self-harm, compared with eight out of 17 of the recovered group. The ordinands had very similar scores to the deluded group, and the rehabilitation nurses were intermediate, being on the whole more depressed and regarding their lives as less purposeful than the deluded patients they were treating. The person who scored maximum on the purpose in life test and zero depression, was a well-known vagrant who believed himself to be 'The English Leader' and that he was responsible for controlling the world from his makeshift tent, but had no contact with psychiatric services.

Comparing the quality of the delusional contents in the two patient groups showed that patients with systematized delusions possessed much more favourable beliefs than the comparison group: in particular, the possession of special knowledge and positively directed erotic beliefs. A careful review of past records demonstrated that, whereas earlier episodes of psychosis included negatively charged delusions and hallucinations, these became less prevalent over time with elaboration of the system. Thus, the longitudinal progression was to edit and re-edit the delusional story in the direction of 'detoxifying' the earlier beliefs.

Summary

A narrative approach to psychopathology emphasizes the search to understand delusional contents in the biographical past and considers delusions as arising from the healthy part of the person attributing meanings to anomalous experiences and compensating for significant losses, traumas, and destructive events. Some go on to elaborate alternative life stories built on delusional foundations. It is possible to see people using their story-telling capacities to cope with psychosis and there appear to be considerable benefits associated with attachment to some psychotic narratives that enable a transformation of the personal world and the acquisition of a sense of meaningfulness and purposefulness in living.

There is clearly a paradox here. Two models of healing are possible. The progression from psychosis to sanity, from illness to health, is accompanied by a recovery of the 'real' life story, and therapy may be directed at this process of recovery of information, organization, re-evaluation, understanding, and telling. This implies a process of leaving behind the psychotic ideas and experiences, and attempting to make sense of them, to integrate or ignore them, from a standpoint of sanity. This leads to recovering a story and a way of telling it that is intelligible and acceptable to others.

By contrast, the psychotic, in his search for self-healing, goes in the opposite direction. Through the creation or recreation of his life story within psychosis, he achieves a form of pseudo-sanity, accompanied by psychotic insight, understanding, and integration. The cost may be isolation, but, according to Cameron (1959), even that may be compensated for by experientially residing in a psychotic pseudo-community consisting of real and imagined persons, possessing motivations representing the paranoid's projections: 'This re-establishes stable object relations though on a delusional basis and thus makes integrated action possible. It organises drive directed cognitive processes and leads to meaningful interpretations in a well developed pseudo-reality structure and gives a satisfactory explanation for his strange altered world and a basis for doing something about it' (Cameron, 1959). Cameron also allows for the ambiguity of this success, by concluding that, 'this is his victory and his defeat.' And although delusion may be ameliorative, serving as 'a patch on a rent in the ego' (Freud 1924, p. 215.), psychotic constructions are none the less 'only a pseudo-solution . . . the main defensive aspect of the psychosis is the transformation of an intra-psychic danger into an external one' (Arieti, 1964).

The paradoxical notion that delusion is restitutive, a narrative means of attempting self-healing from psychotic fragmentation and disorganization can be further supported by considering some of the general principles that underlie effective psychotherapy. Frank (1986) states that 'all psychotherapies provide new concepts and information that enable the patient to make meaningful connections between symptoms and experiences that had been mysterious, thereby replacing confusion with clarity. In turn the creation of a powerful explanatory model acts as a means of reducing tension, promoting morale and restoring security.'

However, there are significant risks in finding meaning in madness and existential compensations in delusional beliefs, of romanticizing psychosis and diverting awareness away from the sufferings and deprivations that are its hallmark. It is essential that responsible clinicians are not themselves seduced by the narrative of psychotic fulfilment for 'it is important to remember that even in the sickest patient the wish to rejoin the human community is seldom completely extinguished' (Arieti, 1964).

Laing's (1964) apparently appealing assertion that, 'the cracked mind of the schizophrenic may let in light which does not enter the intact minds of many sane people who's minds are closed', should sound a warning bell.

There are complex tensions implicit in working with, and within, this paradox which may buffet and disorient the clinician; however, the benefits are in gaining greater understanding of some aspects of resistance and signalling some of the complications of recovery rather than justifying therapeutic nihilism.

Some implications of a narrative approach to rehabilitation

Psychosocial rehabilitation and the careful use of antipsychotic medication are the foundation for any treatment approach in psychosis. The implications of narrative approaches need to be interwoven with standard treatments. Institutional patterns of care and treatment have been rightly criticized for their neglect of all that is personal and much has been done to rectify that. However, the mad may initially appear unreachable, unknowable, their previous history eclipsed by their psychopathology. A narrative approach emphasizes that delusions are meaningful statements, arrived at purposefully, and that these delusional stories can often be understood to articulate the value system and dominant psychodynamic themes of the individual.

Working both to understand the life story and its relationship with delusional phenomena then becomes the means of connecting with the person within the psychosis: 'the crux of therapy becomes the task of empathising with the schizophrenic's perspective and attempting to understand its essential plausibility and validity . . . the therapist in searching for kernels of truth is better able to construct an empathic appreciation of the patient's experience than by focusing on what appears distorted and unrealistic' (Josephs and Josephs, 1986).

However, chronically deluded patients are often lost to follow-up, refuse medication, and preserve their beliefs even when treated against their will, although they often realize the wisdom of ceasing to talk about them. It follows that beyond offering or administering appropriate medication, any treatment is dependent on developing a relationship, a therapeutic attachment, that becomes the means of delivering all subsequent therapeutic benefits. It is difficult, if not impossible, to build a relationship with someone who cannot be understood.

The case his-story

Case histories are the basic text we work from and every effort needs to be made to build up a full and comprehensive clinical biography for each patient. Those suffering from chronic psychosis are often eclipsed by their disorder, they have become their diagnoses and we talk of 'schizophrenics'. They have lost their stories and, not infrequently, we have too.

One of my first jobs as a psychiatric trainee was to review the residents on an asylum backward, which was due to close, and present them to my boss. It shocked me to find that person after person had case files recording decades of psychiatric care and treatment that were relatively empty. They offered no understanding of who the person was, what they were doing in hospital, and how to understand, their predicament in life: several had been admitted during the Bristol blitz and it was as though the bombs had landed directly on the case records! Little was noted in the years that followed beyond annual health checks.

Recovering a biographical perspective reinstates an awareness of the person within the patient and fosters respect. There are parallels with reminiscence therapy for both patients and staff. Both need to remember where the patient has come from, what responsibilities and relationships they had before attending the hospital, what happened such that they were admitted, and what events and experiences have marked the years in between. The construction of this story may in turn shed light on the meaning of some of the psychotic contents, which will start to dismantle the unknowable quality of these patients and facilitate the beginning of empathy. These meaningful associations may then open up some common ground and help to orientate a therapeutic relationship. Without a biographical perspective the person ceases to exist and can only be known as a case or a diagnosis.

One of my blitz patients had been noted to have dropped out of all off-ward activities and became annoyed and irritable when encouraged to persist with occupational therapy. A review of his history and somewhat laborious interviewing eventually established that before coming to hospital he had been a butler and in the early years of his stay he had been recruited to serve in the doctors' dinning room, with increasing years and frailty he had ceased these duties but now, having turned 65, he decided that he had retired and would not go to work any longer. None of this was initially apparent and he had outlasted the staff who may have known the significance of his behaviour. It was only in recovering a biographical perspective that it became possible to understand him and accept the legitimacy of his choices rather than seek to treat his behaviour as a symptom of illness.

The pain of recovery

> Alas for the dreamer: the moment of consciousness that accompanies the awakening is the acutest of sufferings.
> (*Primo Levi, 1987.*)

The seemingly obvious project of coaxing a person captivated by psychotic experiences back to consensual reality meets with complex resistances. The struggle to return from madness, once it has become an established perspective, may involve engaging with the same transitional processes that determined the inward journey.

There is a *New Yorker* cartoon that records an affable exchange between a psychiatrist and his patient: 'Congratulations,' says the psychiatrist, 'Your cured!' 'Big deal', the patient complained. 'Before I came to you for therapy, I thought I was John F. Kennedy. Now I'm a nobody!' In reality, these realizations can be catastrophic. How must the Emperor have felt when the boy convinced the crowd that he was naked.

A person recovering from schizophrenia (Anon, 1986) wrote; 'There are days when I wonder if it might not be more humane to leave the schizophrenic patient to his world of unreality, not to make him go through the pain that it takes to become part of humanity. These are the days when the pain is so great, I think I might prefer the craziness until I remember the immobilising terror and the distance and isolation that keep the world so far away and out of focus. It is not an easily resolved dilemma.'

Phenomenologically we each see the world from our own perspective and thus live in 'perspectival worlds' (Cox and Theilgaard, 1987). Patients suffering from psychosis describe an altered perspective on reality, drawing on narrative faculties to reconfigure the psychotic break into a new gestalt, drawing on salient memories and images from religious sources and popular culture which stand for the powerful unknown. Some have gone further and in elaborating their delusional beliefs they have compensated for past hurts and disappointments and found new satisfactions. They also anticipate that loss of these beliefs, recovery, may be very painful. Resistance to recovery is most striking when there seems to be nothing of value to be gained in preserving the delusional beliefs; however, the 'gains' are in both the contents and in the process of possessing strongly held beliefs.

I once met a person who believed that he was 'polluted' in an ecological sense. So strong was his conviction, that he held out his arm for me to smell, insisting that anyone could smell the pollution all through him. This seemed the sort of complaint that anyone would have been pleased and relieved to be rid of. I asked him, 'What would it be like if one day you discovered this was not the case, that it was like a bad dream, a trick your mind has played you?' I was very surprised at his response. He thought it would be terrible, and when asked why, he said, 'Because, I know the truth!'

It would appear that the truth value attributed to delusional beliefs renders them resistant to change, or, more properly, renders the individual reluctant to change them. It is also possible that in some metaphorical or symbolic fashion the individual is telling the truth.

Jaspers (1963) warned of possible adverse consequences on recovery: 'We cannot say that the patient's whole world has changed, because to a very large extent he can conduct himself like a healthy person in thinking and behaving. But his world has changed to the extent that a changed knowledge of reality so rules and pervades it that any correction would mean a collapse of Being itself, in so far as it is for him his actual awareness of existence.' Similarly, Cox and Theilgaard (1987) noted: 'the risk of psychotic defensive processes so overprotecting a man that he runs the risk of keeping "the ground of his being" at too great a distance from the ground on which he must tread.' The prospect is allied to the image of the madman inhabiting a 'castle in the air' and recovery representing the long drop to earth.

Loss of delusional beliefs, i.e. recovery, for some is simply relief from dread and preoccupying distress, for others it contains significant losses and renewed risks, a maladaptation is still an adaptation.

Searles (1961), in summarizing his 12 years experience at Chestnut Lodge, commented that, 'facing the reality of his own life, is to face a reality overfull of tragedy and loss . . . the therapist will be aware that for the patient, the delusions represent years of arduous and subjectively constructed thought, and are therefore most deeply cherished.'

It may be that the phenomenon of post-psychotic depression and the overrepresentation of suicide during remission in schizophrenia are related to the complexities of recovery. Sims (1988) has described how, 'as the delusions fade the patient may gain insight and regard them as false beliefs "due to the illness", such a person needs help in accepting himself as a fit repository for his own self confidence once more. He may feel himself to be damaged, vulnerable and untrustworthy and suffer a massive loss of self-esteem.'

The problem is contained in the tension between the universal search for truth and meaning and T. S. Eliot's observation that 'humankind cannot bear very much reality' (1969).

Pirandello's (1985) *Henry IV* abruptly recovered after 20 years' madness to find:

> a great shock, because I realised at once that it wasn't only my hair, but everything else that had gone grey, everything had crumbled, it was all finished . . .' This proved too much to cope with and so he goes on: 'I preferred to stay mad . . . To clothe this solitude again . . . however squalid and empty it seemed when I opened my eyes again . . . To make it no longer fancy dress, but a permanent reality, the reality of true madness.'

One of the deluded patients in the PILT study unexpectedly recovered but found insight a difficult and distressing experience, which appeared to reveal something of the purpose his delusional ideas had fulfilled. He previously possessed an elaborate delusional system centring on a messianic identity. He said: 'I liked to imagine it because I felt so useless without it . . . I still feel inadequate now—it's as though I don't know anything. I always felt everything I said was worthless, but as Jesus everything I said was important—it came from God . . . I just want to hide away, I don't feel able to cope with people . . . I always feel lonely, I don't know what to say.'

An awareness of 'Awakening' (*Time*, 6 July 1992), and the associated issues of post-psychotic depression and suicide in remission, suggests the need for sustained or heightened vigilance in the early recovery period. There is a particular need to preserve contact and a supportive relationship whilst the person is struggling to adjust to a confrontation with the reality of his circumstances. This may be all the more significant in the post-Clozapine era of enhanced drug potency.

The story of Jimmy 'JC'

Jimmy came for treatment after attempting to walk across a local river on top of the water, and realizing something was wrong when he was waist deep. He had been 'ill' for some years but was something of a local tourist attraction, due to his flamboyant dress and continuous good mood. He had established a reciprocal and collusive relationship with 'the public' such that people would have their photographs taken with him and he would grant them wishes, 'I was Jimmy the Healer, JC'. Until then his only reason for visiting the psychiatry unit was to offer his services in healing patients. But he had frightened himself and accepted regular medication which cured him of grandiosity. Initially he felt completely lost but gradually he became an appreciated and integrated member of a day centre and was able to re-establish relationships with his children which had been lost for many years. He sometimes looks back on his madness with nostalgia, 'They were happy times, but I was ill, I was like a Martian, somebody nobody had seen before who had come back to Earth,' and despite living very poorly he spoke of being in charge of his own world, 'I could do what I liked . . . I used to be Jimmy the boring, then I became Jimmy the saviour. I used to be an ordinary person, them I became a super-person.'

He speaks also of the benefits of medication, which he is afraid not to take, in case he would 'cross over and go back again', and fears losing contact with his children again, 'they didn't speak to me for years, I used to embarrass them . . . the medication brings me back to the real world, I'm stable now, the kids say "dad is better".' His pattern of recovery also contains and retains something of his previous life, in that other club members affectionately refer to him as JC, following him signing himself in as Jimmy 'JC' in the club attendance register. The apostrophes that he is now able to put around JC represent the integration of his two stories and having achieved a warm acceptance within a community with both. This appears to have helped him achieve the transition into sanity without shame or humiliation concerning his previous beliefs and behaviour.

Working with the deluded within chronicity

The intractability of some delusions may be less puzzling if their explanatory power is acknowledged. As coping mechanisms they are understandably protected from challenge. It may be that engagement may be assisted by a form of therapeutic collusion, respecting these belief structures as meaningful and valuable to the person, and seeking to build trust on whatever common ground can be won rather than, 'beating the drums of logic' (Huszoneck, 1987).

Cameron (1959) described an approach developed from his concept of the delusional system as a pseudo-community: 'The primary therapeutic consideration is not the character of the delusional structure, but what makes it necessary. A reduction in anxiety is among the first objectives. Having an explanatory model that enables understanding will help the therapist to avoid becoming threatened by the patient's fear and hostility, and can then act as a living bridge between social reality and psychotic reality . . . as anxiety and the threat of disintegration subside, paranoid certainty becomes less necessary to personal survival—the patient can begin to entertain doubts and consider alternative interpretations . . . in this way the conceptual structure of the pseudo-community may be gradually replaced by something approaching the structure of social reality.'

This emphasis on 'gradual replacement' appears particularly useful, as it allows the possibility of introducing opportunities for the patient to meet his needs in non-delusional ways, whilst accepting that he may continue to assert verbally the same convictions. For Cox and Theilgaard (1987) this is when the therapist is able to embrace the patient's perspectival world, as well as respecting his perceptual autonomy, and the patient sensing this, invites the therapist in.

This almost brings us back to where we started—entering Connoly's patient's apartment, this time not as a voyeur or tourist, but as an ambassador of reality respectfully entering a foreign land, and, where there is so little common ground, working initially to find acceptance within the delusional frame of reference and the beginnings of building a trusting relationship through which basic needs can be met.

Finding your voice: telling your telling tale

This chapter began with stories of madness and will draw to its conclusion with two examples of restoration from madness. Most authors who write of psychotherapeutic effort with psychosis and long-term mental illness consider the recovery and construction of the 'real' life story as the major goal in the healing process, this is the aim towards which therapeutic endeavour is directed. Cox and Theilgaard (1987) spoke of this as, 'a complete story—intelligible, constituent and unbroken is the theoretical, created end story, . . . at the end, at the successful end—one has come into possession of one's own story.' The emphasis is of secure ownership rather than any fictional notion of truth. The examples that follow speak not only of the benefits of having a full or satisfactory story to tell, but also that the telling of it waymarks the end of madness.

Davidson and Strauss (1992) have observed that the rediscovery and reconstruction of an enduring sense of the self as an active and responsible agent; a 'me' separate from 'the illness' provides an important aspect of improvement. Establishing sufficient coherence and objectivity to tell one's story establishes the sufferer as an authority rather than victim, as author rather than character, as a person giving account of experience rather than as patient needing help and protection. It signals recovery of boundary and steps towards autonomy, a separation, holding, and transformation of what was an overwhelming experience into a story that can be told such that *I* can tell you about *it*.

Storr's (1997) patient came through recurrent and dramatic psychotic episodes and found that writing it out provided both a support to find a way through the process and by having a tellable, sharable story, a route into relationship:

> Whilst she was psychotic, she was beyond the reach of psychotherapy, but, in between episodes was co-operative and anxious for help. Most of the doctors she had seen had encouraged her to ignore the content of her psychosis, and to forget all about her periods of madness once they were over. I took the risk of encouraging her to write an account of her illness, taking the view that by this means, she might feel less at the mercy of the illness should it recur. This she did, using a pseudonym, and the book was published. Some years later during which she had been free of attacks, she wrote to me about another matter, and I enquired whether she felt that writing the book had had any effect upon her health. She has given me permission to quote her reply. 'Yes, it was very good for me to have written the book, and to have done so whilst events were still vividly in mind. Having done so I'd 'got it in the bag' so to speak, and could afford to forget all about it for some years—which was also good for me . . . if I hadn't written the book, I might have been frightened to get married. But as A. had read it, and was still prepared to take the risk of getting married to me, I reckoned it was OK to go ahead.' He then comments that he is sure that her marriage, after her series of illnesses, was more important than her writing in maintaining her stability; 'but I am also sure that one cannot afford to "forget all about" very disturbing things in one's own psyche unless one has faced them. Writing such things is one way of accomplishing this.'

My concluding account has emerged and changed over time, and perhaps will continue to do so. It is a story of prolonged difficulties but also of transformation. It illustrates many of the issues involved in a narrative approach to psychosis and the deployment of narrative processes as coping mechanisms within both psychotic disorganization and in the successive phases of recovery.

'A sharp darkness—and how to survive it'

Peter was initially only willing to come into hospital when it was framed as 'taking a holiday in a protected environment'. He brought with him a massive document which he had been working on for the previous year, describing in fine detail the conspiracy amongst his partners and rival practices against him. He had written at the top of the document 'the whole story' and felt great satisfaction in having struggled hard to get all the detail and the sequence of events accurately recorded. He also spoke of a sense of heroism in doing battle with such wicked men and he had caused alarm by revealing that he carried a knife in his briefcase against the day when he would have to take preventative action. He also expressed a grudging admiration for the subtlety of their plot as he readily conceded that to any ordinary person he would appear mad.

We could have stopped there, diagnosed some kind of paranoid psychosis and treated it accordingly, but he could also respond to the question 'What would you have to think about if you were not so taken up with the conspiracy?' and listed the collapse of his career and the frustrations of his professional ambition, the failure of his marriage, a sense of alienation from his children and his recently, and spontaneously, recovered memories of being sexually abused by his father who was also his headmaster. He was later able to speak of the emptiness, frustration, and futility of his life prior to these delusional developments.

He presented a story within a story, a painful personal account of his life and experience and a symptomatic account of threat and conspiracy, and initially could see no relationship between them. Whilst offering antipsychotic and antidepressant medication, much of our subsequent work focused on telling both these stories fully and allowing them to illuminate each other. Eighteen months later he was substantially well, he had lost his practice but taken up other work that used his skills, and regained a sense of pride and optimism. He continued to believe the conspiracy was true but in his words he had 'cocooned it' and it shifted from being all-consuming to catching little of his time or attention. At that stage it appeared that the 'cocoon' served the double function of protecting him from these beliefs and protecting the integrity of the beliefs for him.

Jung Chang's *Wild swans* headed the bestseller lists at the time and he was simultaneously fascinated by the story itself, the author's choice or perhaps need to write her life, and himself as reader drawn into a compelling narrative. He linked this with puzzling over his awareness of the narrative processes he was using to make sense of his own predicament and often wondered what drove people to turn their experience into particular stories.

Whilst recovering he began to write again of his experience, this time with the intention of offering something to fellow suffers and their carers. In doing so he gave a compelling description of the agony preceding his presentation:

> What I most remember is the pain. It was not an identifiable pain, not a wholesome pain like an agonising headache, or the excruciating pain of a burn, but an indescribable pain for which there was no explanation, no apparent cause and from which there was no relief. It came, it stayed, it sometimes remitted leaving a dull ache in the stomach, but it was a companion who walked with me for eleven years, an evil incubus on my shoulder at every turn, in every waking hour deciding in its own time when and how it was going to turn the screw, now a little, now a lot, and I could do nothing but suffer it.

The need to finish that account passed as he became more outwardly focused and socially active. He became increasingly involved in starting up a user movement and has become a very effective advocate to statutory services.

A year later he accepted an invitation to tell his story to the psychiatry department. He chose the title 'A Sharp Darkness' and spoke of becoming ill with depression and of becoming overwhelmed by confusion and fear and that 'a darkness began to force its way, very slowly, very painfully like broken glass being slowly pushed into you.' He described the paradoxical comforts within suffering: 'In the most extraordinary way this agonising darkness slowly forcing its way into my soul became a sort of friend. At least when the darkness had completely taken over, and all struggle ceased, the pain diminished.'

He spoke of the way 'Mr Rational' gets to work on fractured perceptions to make acceptable patterns, and pointed to the narrative drive to make sense out of experience and the comfort of pulling together dislocated elements into some coherent narrative: even a story of persecution is better than 'agonising emotional pain that has apparently no cause'. He eloquently described the transition from conflict, to unmanageable confusion, to reason kicking back in, and making some kind of holding narrative, however unacceptable that may be to others. He concluded that, 'the cure such as it is is to look at reality and do what you can about it.' And his process of recovery has been underpinned by telling and retelling his story to himself and others. His successive accounts documented the changing analysis of his experience and illustrated the progressive process of metabolism and integration of what began as an incomprehensible change, and ended as a story he could present in public as a foundational tale for a user's forum, in which he is an active member. Restoration of meaning has been accompanied by a transition from patient to person. The shaping of an acceptable and tellable tale and the opportunity and confidence to tell it has enabled detachment from the experience it represents, and an alchemical transformation enabling mastery and containment over what was formerly experienced as disempowering and persecutory.

Conclusion

This chapter began by acknowledging the difficulty of finding meaning in madness, and the costs of continuing to regard people suffering from psychosis as un-understandable nonsense speakers. I began with the story of a psychiatrist who was able to dance with his patients, which may seem far from our contemporary experience or expectations although our difficulty may be related to our fear of getting too close to patients we cannot understand. And yet it is in finding some means of drawing closer, building bridges, making sense, that these fears may be overcome and contact and communication made more possible.

Paul Holmes (1993), commenting on an account of the initial fear and inhibition of Shakespearean actors performing in a high security hospital, reflected on his own experience. 'Their accounts of how they moved beyond their fears of Broadmoor and the madness it contains reminded me of my terror when as a student I was invited to the patients' disco on a back ward of a psychiatric hospital in Dundee. It was only when I had been there some time that I felt the privilege of being invited to enter, for the duration of my visit, that sheltered and protected world of psychosis and madness. As my sense of privilege increased my terror abated, and I was able to dance. It is only when we confront our own fears of chaos and madness that we can allow therapeutic catharsis in those we seek to help.'

The political expedients which have now recentred public mental health services on the care and treatment of patients suffering from chronic psychosis have come at a time of rekindled therapeutic optimism based on the development of new antipsychotic drugs and the evolution of cognitive and family psychotherapies. However, most people suffering from psychosis are treated by psychiatrists in settings devoid of psychotherapeutic expertise and most psychotherapists are not involved with psychosis. There remains a need to heal Ciompi's 'disastrous split' and reintegrate psychotherapeutic and psychiatric approaches. In doing so we may replace our assumption that delusions are meaningless with an assumption of meaningfulness, and thereby promote a search for understanding and interpretation. Fundamentally this is a search for relationship and relatedness, a process of dealienation, and a means of reintegration. Rehabilitation approaches will continue to miss the mark if they fail to establish confidence and conviction that the psychotic is 'one of us' and to re-establish his full membership of society authentically.

An application of narrative invites us to deinstitutionalize ourselves from a preoccupation with taxonomies and patterns of understanding that illuminate the disorder but obfuscate the person, such that we confirm sufferers in their madness. It invites us to suspend our disbelief, our traditional stance that in delusion we are meeting the bizarre and incomprehensible, and to expand our clinical approach to listen carefully to the delusional contents alongside discerning their form and characteristics, recognizing that both offer valuable information with which to make sense of the person and his predicament. It reasserts the utility of a comprehensive case history as the basic text from which we work and not only disinters the meanings buried in symptoms but also re-evaluates delusional constructions as coping responses to psychotic disintegration, and hence, for some, the paradoxical satisfactions of madness and the pain of recovery.

A narrative perspective on psychosis recontextualizes symptoms within the lived biography of the person and thereby enhances the possibility of understanding, which in turn offers a more secure foundation for making and sustaining therapeutic relationships. This rehabilitation of rehabilitation is a progression towards rediscovering a meaningful medicine and a medicine of meaning through an integration of the story-tellers' art alongside a consolidation of the physicians' science. In part this is a rekindling and rediscovery of an approach that was available at the inception of the schizophrenia concept, but it also offers a new model for thinking about and working with psychosis which is accessible to sufferers, carers, and the multiprofessional team alike.

A note on confidentiality

The personal accounts contained within this chapter all contain a degree of disguise but are in any case recounted with the permission of those whose stories they are.

References

Anon (1986). Can we talk? The schizophrenic patient in psychotherapy. *American Journal of Psychiatry*, **143**, 68–70.

Arieti, S. (1964). *Interpretation of schizophrenia*. Crosby Lockwood Staples, London.

Arthur, A. Z. (1964). Theories and explanations of delusions: a review. *American Journal of Psychiatry*, August, 105–15.

Bennet, G. (1983). *Beyond endurance—survival at the extremes*. Secker and Warburg, London.

Bentall, R. P. and Kany, S. (1989). Content specific information processing and persecutory delusions: an investigation using the emotional Stroop test. *British Journal of Medical Psychology*, **62**, 355–64.

Berner, P., Gabriel, E., Kieffer, Schanda (1986). Paranoid psychosis: new aspects of classification and prognosis coming from the Vienna research group. *Psychopathology*, **19**, 16–29.

Bleuler. E. (1951). Autistic thinking. In *Organisation and pathology of thought*, (ed. D. Rapaport).
Colombia University Press, New York.

Bleuler, M. and Bleuler, R. (1986). Books reconsidered: Dementia Praecox die Gruppe der
Schizophreien: Eugen Bleuler. *British Journal of Psychiatry*, **149**, 661–64.

Cameron, N. (1959). The paranoid pseudo-community re-visited. *American Journal of Sociology*, **65**, 52–8.

Ciompi, L. (1989). The dynamics of complex biological-Psychosocial systems. British Journal
of Psychiatry, 155 (Suppl. 5), 15–21.

Connoly, J. (1830). *The indications of insanity*, (reprinted 1964 with introduction by R. Hunter
and I. Macalpine). Dawsons of Pall Mall, London.

Cox, M. and Theilgaard, A. (1987). *Mutative metaphors in psychotherapy*. Tavistock Publications, London.

Crumbaugh, J. C. (1968). Cross-validation of Purpose-in-life test based on Frankl's concepts.
Journal of Individual Psychology, **24**, 74–81.

Cutting, J. (1989). Gestalt theory and psychiatry: a discussion paper. *Journal of the Royal
Society of Medicine*, **82**, 429–31.

Davidson, L. (1993). Story telling and schizophrenia: using narrative structure in phenomenological research. *Humanistic Psychologist*, **21**, 200–20.

Davidson, L. and Strauss, J. S. (1992). Sense of self in recovery from severe mental illness.
British Journal of Medical Psychology, **65**, 131–45.

Davidson, L. and Strauss, J. S. (1995). Beyond the biopsychosocial model: integrating disorder,
health and recovery. *Psychiatry*, **58**, 44–55.

Donne, J (1624). *Devotions, chapter XVII*. In Donne (1972). *Complete verse and selected prose*,
(ed. J. Hayward). Nonsuch, London.

Eliot, T. S. (1969). *Burnt Norton, The Four Quartets*. In *The Complete Poems and Plays of
T. S. Eliot*. Faber, London.

Estroff, S. E. (1981). *Making it crazy: an ethnography of psychiatric patients in an american community*. University of California Press, Berkeley.

Forgus, R. H. and DeWolfe, A. S. (1974). Coding of cognative input in delusional patients.
Journal of Abnormal Psychology, 83, 3, 278–84.

Frank, J. D. (1986). Psychotherapy—the transformation of meanings: a discussion paper.
Journal of the Royal Society of Medicine, **79**, 341–46.

Freud, S. (1924). Neurosis and Psychosis, *Standard Edition*, **19**, 203–27.

Freud, S. (1939). Constructions in analysis. *Standard Edition*, **23**, 267.

Fuller Torey, E. (1995). *Surviving schizophrenia*. HarperCollins, New York.

Gamboni, D. (1997). *The destruction of art*. Reaktion Books, London.

Garety, P. A. and Hemsley, D. R. (1994). *Delusions—investigations into the psychology of delusional reasoning*. Oxford University Press, Oxford.

Hardy, T. (1918). The white washed wall. In *The Complete Poems of Thomas Hardy* (1981).
MacMillan, London, p. 685.

Holloway, F. (1988). Day care and community support. In *Community care in practice*, (ed.
A. Lavender and F. Holloway). John Wiley and Sons, Chichester.

Holmes, P. (1993). If drama be the food of life, act on. *British Journal of Psychiatry Review of Books*, **5**, 20.

Hughlings Jackson, J (1932) Factors of insanities. In *Selected writings of John Hughlings Jackson*, (ed. J Taylor), pp. 415–16. Hodder and Soughton Ltd., London.

Hunter, K. M. (1991). *Doctors stories: the narrative structure of medical knowledge*. Princeton University Press, New Jersey.

Huszoneck, J. J. (1987). Establishing therapeutic contact with schizophrenics: a supervisory approach. *American Journal of Psychotherapy*, **XLI**, 185–93.

Jaspers, K. (1963). *General psychopathology*, (trans. J. Hoenig and M. Hamilton). Manchester University Press, Manchester.

Jenner, F. A., Monteriro, A. C., and Vlissides, D. (1986). The negative effect on psychiatry of Karl Jaspers development of Verstehen. *Journal of the British Society for Phenomenology*, **17**, 52–71.

Johnson, W. G., Ross, J. M., and Mastra, M. A. (1977). Delusional behaviour: an attribution analysis of development and modification. *Journal of Abnormal Psychology*, **86**, 421–6.

Josephs, L. (1988). Witness to tragedy—a self psychological approach to the treatment of schizophrenia. *Bulletin of the Menninger Clinic*, **52**, 1252–60.

Josephs, L. and Josephs, L. (1986). Pursuing the kernel of truth in the psychotherapy of schizophrenia. *Psychoanalytic Psychology*, **3**, 105–19.

Kaffman, M. (1984). Paranoid disorders: the core of truth behind the delusional system. *International Journal of Family Therapy*, **6**, 220–32.

Klienman, A. (1988). *The illness narratives: suffering, healing and the human condition*. Basic Books, New York.

Laing, R. (1964). *The divided self*. Pelican, London.

Lansky, M. R. (1977). Schizophrenic delusional phenomena. *Comprehensive Psychiatry*, **18**, 157–68.

Levi, P. (1987). *If this is a man: the truce*. Sphere Books, London.

Maher, B. A. (1974). Delusional thinking and perceptual disorder. *Journal of Individual Psychology*, **30**, 98–113.

Maher, B. and Ross, J., S. (1984). Delusions. In *Comprehensive handbook of psychopathology*, (ed. H. Adams and P. Sutker). Plenum Press, New York.

Murphy, H. B. M. (1983). Sociocultural variations in symptomatology, incidence and course of illness. In *Handbook of psychiatry*, (ed. M. Shepherd and O. Zangwill), Vol. 1, Ch. 5. Cambridge University Press, Cambridge.

Murray, M. (1997). A narrative approach to health psychology. *Journal of Health Psychology*, Vol. 2, **1**, 9–20.

Norman, C. (1899). Systematised delusional insanity (paranoia). In *System of medicine*, (ed. T. C. Allbutt). Macmillan, London.

Penrose, L. S. (1931). A case of schizophrenia of long duration. *Medicine and Psychiatry*, **11**, 1–31.

Perris, C. (1989). *Cognitive therapy with schizophrenic patients*. Cassell: The Guilford Press,

Pirandello, L. (1985). Henry IV. In *Three plays* (trans. J. Linstrum). Methuen, London.

Porter, R. (1995). Parkinson's Disease (Paralysis Agitans). In, *A History of Clinical Psychiatry* (eds. G. Berrios and R. Porter), pp. 113–22. Athlone, London.

Roberts, G. A. (1991). Delusional systems and meaning in life—a preferred reality? *British Journal of Psychiatry*, 159, (Suppl. 14), 20–9.

Roberts, G. A. (1992). The origins of delusion. *British Journal of Psychiatry*, **161**, 298–308.

Rogers, A., Pilgrim, D., and Lacey, R. (1993). *Experiencing psychiatry: users' views of services*. MIND and Macmillan, London.

Roth, S. (1970). The seemingly ubiquitous depression following acute schizophrenic episodes: a neglected area of clinical discussion. *American Journal of Psychiatry*, **127**, 91–8.

Sayers, P. (1989). *The comforts of madness*. Sceptre, London.

Scharfetter, C. (1980). *General psychopathology*, (trans. H. Marshall). Cambridge University Press, Cambridge.

Schilder, P. (1951). On the development of thoughts. In *Organisation and pathology of thought*, (ed. D. Rapaport). Colombia University Press, New York.

Searles, H. F. (1961). Phases of patient-therapist interaction in the psychotherapy of chronic schizophrenia. *British Journal of Medical Psychology*, **34**, 169–93.

Sims, A. (1988). *Symptoms in the mind—an introduction to descriptive psychopathology*. Balliere, London.

Stafford- Clark, D. (1970). *Five questions in search of an answer: religion and life some inescapable contradictions*. Collins, London.

Storr, A. (1976). *The dynamics of creation*. Penguin, London.

Storr, A. (1997). *The art of psychotherapy*. Butterworth-Heinemann, Oxford.

Strauss, J. S. (1989). Mediating processes in schizophrenia—towards a new dynamic psychiatry. *British Journal of Psychiatry*, **155** (Suppl. 5), 22–8.

Strauss, J. S. (1994). The person with schizophrenia as a person. *British Journal of Psychiatry*, **164** (Suppl. 23), 103–7.

Tsuang, M. T., Faraone, S. V., and Day, M. (1988). Schizophrenic disorders. In *The new Harvard guide to psychiatry*, (ed. A. Nicholi, Jr). Belknap Press, Cambridge.

Wallace, E. R. (1988). What is truth? Some philosophical contributions to psychiatric issues. *American Journal of Psychiatry*, **147**, 137–47.

Weinstein, E. A. (1962). *Cultural aspects of delusions: a psychiatric study of the Virgin Islands*. The Free Press of Glencoe Inc., New York.

Wing, J. K. and Brown, G. W. (1970). *Institutionalism and schizophrenia*. Cambridge University Press, London.

Woodley, H. G. (1947). *Certified*. Gollancz, London.

Yalom, I. D. (1980). *Existential psychotherapy*. Basic Books, New York.

York, C. (1988). A defect in training. *British Journal of Psychiatry*, **152**, 159–63.

9 Holding on to the story: older people, narrative, and dementia

Errollyn Bruce

In this chapter I put forward some attempts to weave together ideas about attachment throughout the life course, and narratives in dementia. However, for the vast majority of people, the backdrop to dementia is ageing, and to set dementia in context I begin with a discussion of the place of older people's narratives, in particular their reminiscence stories.

The place of older people's stories in a changing world

Older people have a place in fairy stories as tellers of wonderful tales. Other parts of children's literature offer a multiplicity of images for older people, from the evil killjoys of Dahl, through the wildly eccentric, good-fun grannies, to the supportive older person who, often unexpectedly, comes up trumps when all other adults seem to be against the young. Over a period of time, social change and the communication revolution have eroded the traditional role of elders as repositories of culture, passing on customs and tribal wisdom to younger generations. Increasingly, younger people have been able to turn to other sources to access the accumulated knowledge of humankind, and old customs have been challenged as irrelevant to a fast-changing world. There must be few places left in the world where young people are not bombarded with images of dominant cultures which tempt them to bypass the wisdom of local elders as their framework for living.

The transmission of culture by elders was not always the benign and nurturant process people looking back to a world we have lost might like to suppose. In this volume Jeremy Holmes argues that narrative forms one half of a duality that lies at the heart of psychotherapy: a duality that is relevant to human relations beyond psychotherapy. Elders' narratives can constrict and control as well as support and nurture. The traditions they uphold may be life-enhancing and socially cohesive but they can also have confining and life-destroying elements affecting large numbers of people for generation after generation. Alice Walker's (1992) fictional account of elders justifying genital mutilation is a powerful reminder of narratives that help to perpetuate practices that cause untold suffering.

As a small child, the narrator (in the novel) brings a tray of food and water to the elders of her village who 'sit beside a baobab tree and gaze wisely out over the plain'. Because she is small they do not completely stop their talk:

ALL: Woman is queen.

NUMBER ONE: She is queen.

NUMBER TWO: God has given her to us.

NUMBER THREE: We are thankful to God for all His gifts.

NUMBER FOUR: Since God has given her to us, we must treat her well.

NUMBER ONE: We must feed her so that she will stay plump.

NUMBER TWO: Even her excrement will be plump.
(*They laugh*)

NUMBER THREE: If left to herself the Queen would fly.

NUMBER TWO: True.

NUMBER THREE: And then where would we be?

NUMBER FOUR: But God is merciful.

NUMBER ONE: He clips her wings.

NUMBER THREE: God struck the blow that made her Queen!

NUMBER FOUR: Beautiful enough for him to fuck.

NUMBER ONE: God liked it fighting!
(*laughter*)

NUMBER TWO: God liked it tight!

NUMBER FOUR: God is wise. That is why He created the *tsunga*.[*]

ALL: With her sharpened stone and bag of thorns!

NUMBER ONE: With her needle and thread.

NUMBER TWO: Because He liked it tight!

NUMBER THREE: God likes to feel big.

NUMBER FOUR: What man does not?
(*laughter*)

Reminiscence: a bad thing or a good thing?

Older people's narratives have played a part in the transmission of culture, both good and bad, and it is perhaps no surprise that it was at the same time that youth culture was emerging, and the label 'teenager' appeared, that there was a particularly negative attitude to the story-telling of older people in this country. At end of the 1950s many professionals took the view that older people should be told to avoid reminiscence. 'Living in the past' was seen as pathological, an un-healthy denial of present reality. Talking about the past might cause or worsen depression, and contribute to unhealthy disengagement. The task of care workers was to distract the old from their preoccupation with the past with activities like bingo and basket-making. The 'defect' of turning back to the days when life was more rewarding was particularly acute among the senile—even claimed as the most characteristic feature of senility. Once identified as a symptom of men-tal decline, it was by association a suspicious sign in the old but mentally intact (Coleman, 1989).

As the young demanded more power and control over their lives, perhaps there was a need to discredit the traditional role of elders, with its dual purpose of keeping certain sections of society under control—the young, as well as women—and giving them the knowledge and experience that would help them to thrive. In fact, the latter function had already been long superseded as the rate of change overtook the knowledge of the elders, and written communication replaced

---

[*] *tsunga*: woman who performs genital mutilation operations on young girls

oral as the dominant mode of passing on accumulated human experience from generation to generation. In the complex urbanized society of the 20th century the vast majority of older people had little power as agents of social control either. Real power lay elsewhere, and the reality of old people's lives was that it was a struggle to maintain well-being in the face of the losses and deprivations of old age, something made worse in a climate of denigration by younger generations, and a context of rapid social change. But social psychology's attempt to deprive older people of their stories was short-lived, and, as Peter Coleman (1989) tells us, the reversal of attitudes is:

> most graphically illustrated in the career of Robert Havighurst. . . . At the end of the 1950s he was advising older people to avoid reminiscence. A little over ten years later he was researching the benefits of reminiscence.

Just how much the negative view of reminiscence in psychology filtered down through society is hard to judge. In any case, nursing care practice, with its emphasis on physical care, hygiene, and efficiency, left little time for listening to stories. Nurses were certainly discouraged from wasting time talking, or listening, to patients, and the same attitude to 'emotional labour' was, and still is, found among care staff in homes.

Most older people live out their lives outside institutions and many may never have received professional advice on reminiscence. Certainly, the three elderly ladies with whom I grew up in the late 1950s felt as free to amuse me with their stories of the past as their comments on the present. But then reminiscence may be more of a problem for their listeners than for the old themselves. It is not uncommon to hear negative comments about the tedious and repetitive nature of old people's stories. Busy nurses and social workers are expected to fill in forms, make assessments, and deal with the problems of the moment at full tilt; not surprisingly they find the desire of their clients to tell them stories from the long past interferes with management goals of efficiency and throughput. That the negative view of reminiscence was taken up by the authors of nursing and social work textbooks, may well have reflected a reluctance on the part of the guardians of professional practice to see listening to stories as a legitimate part of the worker's professional role. Older people's stories can be a nuisance, as they demand the listener's time, and apparently contribute little to the listener's primary task of organizing present practicalities.

However, for many practitioners, older people's stories were not always a nuisance and their own experience was at odds with the negative view of reminiscence. Erikson's (1950) life stage theory was anyway well-known throughout the period in which reminiscence was unpopular. His ideal of integrity for people in their last phase of life includes goals such as accepting one's past life, and reconciling past and present. How this could possibly be achieved without an opportunity to reflect on the past is hard to imagine. That the negative view of reminiscence was so readily overturned suggests that many people were unconvinced and were only too glad to embrace listening to stories as a legitimate part of their professional role once rehabilitated and reframed, whether as activity, psychological support, or therapy. When Butler's (1963) much-quoted article on life review appeared, his view of reminiscence as a normal and healthy activity in old age was well received. Whatever the official position on reminiscence, ambivalence about reminiscence is likely to remain. Although the subject of reminiscence is the past, it is actually a here and now activity, which requires a listener, and has to compete with other demands on the listener's time.

New roles for elders' stories

Once life review had been identified as a goal of later life, it followed that professional expertise might be valuable to help older people process their memories into a coherent form. Coleman (1989) suggests that the enduring popularity of Erikson's 'few pages' on integrity may reflect a hunger for a meaningful view of later life among younger people whose own old age is yet to come. Those who work with the elderly are only too aware of the pitfalls of depression, isolation, and rejection, and of the social factors that work against reconciliation and acceptance in old age. The same changes that stole from older people their traditional role as transmitters of knowledge and cultural wisdom left them with the problem of adjusting not only to the inevitable losses of ageing, but also to a present that outpaces them, and which is characterized more by discontinuities than resonances with the past. For those who are witnessing the difficulties of the elderly and who before long will be old themselves, there is a need for hope.

Society as a whole may no longer see elderly people's stories as a necessary channel through which to transmit traditions and affirm culture, but among professionals working with older people there are many who now recognize that elderly people need their narrative heirlooms to be polished and treasured and handed on to the next generation. The process of creating a coherent story, and sharing it with a respectful listener has a new value as a route by which people in later life may adjust to inevitable losses and come to face death with equanimity. A wide variety of professional inputs have sprung up in which the cherishing of older people's stories play a part.

People may be rather less likely than in the past to turn to their elders to ask advice on how to handle the challenges of life. Whereas people in simpler societies faced with an unusual water shortage might have sought out older people to ask if this had ever happened before, we now turn to written records and statistical methods to help us to understand the significance of water shortages. However, there is a view that we still need the stories of elders to help us to face the challenges that we may prefer not to think about. It is their ability to find a way to survive the losses of old age and express their unique personhood despite the rapidly changing world, that can give us the hope that Coleman suggests that we need to face up to the prospect of our own ageing.

Do story tellers need listeners?

Coleman's study (which was done at the time that professional views of reminiscence were shifting from negative to positive) found a substantial group of elderly people who expressed negative views of reminiscence and yet were coping well with later life. This group included people who gave details of their past lives by way of introduction, but did not otherwise bring the past into their conversation. Coleman's view is that reminiscence is not a *necessary* feature of successful adjustment to later life: though there were also many people in his study who had a positive attitude to their memories and seemed to be using reminiscence and life review processes to withstand the present. However, it may be helpful to distinguish between reminiscence as an essentially social activity, and private introspective reminiscence. There is a considerable body of evidence suggesting that social support is beneficial to health and well-being (e.g. Cohen and Syme, 1985). Talking about the past to a listener can be seen as a form of social support and to have all the potential benefits of satisfying social contact. Private introspective reminiscence can be anything from a lonely brooding on an unhappy past, to a satisfying telling of the story to an imaginary listener—perhaps a niece who will visit next month, a husband who would listen if he were still alive, or God

At least some of those older people who have a negative view of reminiscence—those who see no point in it—may have formed their view as a result of a social context more welcoming to here-and-now conversation than reminiscing. The move to sheltered housing had removed most of the participants in Coleman's study from what remained of the communities in which they had been living. There was little opportunity for the joint remembering of events with others who were there at the time. Nor were they living alongside family members and playing an active part in supporting their lives. Given a social context that was more welcoming to reminiscence, at least some of these people might have found some point in it. However, for whatever reason, they chose not to talk about the past, and had found other strategies for coping with later life.

Social reminiscence requires a willing listener. If the listener refuses to co-operate, reminiscence will come to a halt. The listener may be unwilling to listen at all, or be prepared to listen to some things and not to others. A neighbour may interrupt a story by saying, 'Sorry, I must dash, I've left something on the cooker,' while a social worker attempting to arrange home help might say, 'We're not talking about that now', and steer the conversation back to the need for present help. Thus the listener plays an active part both in influencing whether reminiscence takes place at all and in determining the value of the social interaction. Human contact is not always supportive, and some of the research on social support is concerned with what constitutes a supportive intervention. Ann Oakley is a leading figure in research on social support, and looking at her instructions to the research midwives who were providing social support to pregnant mothers reveals what features of the intervention she judged to be supportive and unsupportive. Her research midwives were asked to 'unlearn' some of their normal professional responses, as they were instructed, for instance, not to proffer advice or information on any topic unless it was asked for. They were asked to be attentive, non-judgmental, respectful, to encourage the mothers to talk, but not to stick rigidly to their questions if other topics came up. Oakley was trying to make their interventions as supportive as possible, and her model included: allowing people to control the agenda, support for the supporters, phone contact made easy, and professionals required to approach the relationship with their clients from a standpoint that sounds very similar to that of counselling. The model was influenced by her observation of the supportive potential of the semi-structured research interview, of which a key feature is that interviewers genuinely need to know, and want to hear, what their informants have to say (Oakley, 1992).

Where reminiscence is social, part of the value of reminiscence is the value of social support, and the intrinsic worth of having a listener who genuinely wants to hear what a person has to say. This need not necessarily be on a one-to-one basis: a group with a culture of listening can be just as affirming.

It is a tribute to human adaptability that where a listener is missing, some people can create a fantasy listener, or indeed become the listener for themselves. Through internal dialogues with God, writing a diary, imaginary conversations with someone long dead, or an invented confidante, private introspective reminiscence effectively becomes social reminiscence. One of Coleman's informants was a very solitary person for whom reminiscence was a private activity, apart from her conversations and correspondence in the course of the research. Asked during the first interview if she often thought about the past she replied that is was the main thing she did, thinking further and further back, and about all the things that had happened. Later she talked of her memories as 'like a pattern, all rolled out behind' (Coleman, 1989, p.129). It is of course hard to tell how much her private reminiscence was enhanced by participating in a research study. Coleman presents her as an example of someone for whom reminiscing was a path towards integrity, and it is interesting that Beirut hostages used internal reminiscence as a way to deal with solitary confinement. However, it seems that for many people private reminiscence is not a route to peace and resolution. For them, validation from real-life listeners may be needed to make reminiscence worthwhile.

The value of reminiscence

The recasting of reminiscence as broadly a 'good thing' rather than a 'bad thing' does not automatically bring with it a social context for older people's stories. Most people do not feel an urgent need for their elders' stories to help them maintain a sense of stability in an unpredictable natural world. Science and technology are widely seen as the answer to unpredictable natural events but they come at a price, because they bring with them an unprecedented pace of social and technological change. How can older people be any help, when even younger generations grumble? Their contribution may be as people with long experience of living with change. The upsurge of interest in oral history offers a new role for elderly people's stories as a model for finding continuity and meaning in a context of change. The problem now, as presumably in the traditional societies of the past, is that not every older person's story is genuinely needed by someone else, and there tends to be a shortage of willing listeners.

Renewed interest in reminiscence in the late 1960s inspired research and debate. For instance, it has been questioned whether reminiscence is a route to resolving the problems of the past and achieving serenity in the face of death, or whether it is mainly acting as a defence against the losses and difficulties of the present. Research evidence is inconclusive with respect to studies attempting to show 'reminiscers' to be better adjusted than 'non-reminiscers'. It seems that the simple dichotomy is not able to capture the complexities of people's lives. As I have already suggested there may a difference between social and introspective reminiscence, though the two seem to overlap where introspective reminiscence involves a satisfying imaginary listener. Reminiscence appears to be doing different things for different people, and also too for the same person at different times. Life review does not always have a successful outcome; integrity in Erikson's sense is hard to achieve. If reminiscence is a preoccupation with distressing memories, it can contribute to a depressed view of life as unremittingly unfair from start to finish. Alternatively, if the present compares unfavourably with past memories of happiness, it can underline the poverty of the present. In either case, reminiscence can serve to perpetuate, rather than alleviate, present misery.

On the positive side, reminiscence can be doing a number of different things.

1. There are certainly signs in older people's reminiscence narratives of reworking the past to create a good story. The person becomes the hero in a drama worth telling. The story becomes a myth or an image which enables the older person to hold on to self-esteem in the face of decline. This kind of story may be particularly valuable in holding on to identity when a person moves into a strange environment such as hospital or institutional care.

2. Undoubtedly, some people do return to unresolved conflicts when reflecting on the past, and this may or may not lead to resolution. One strategy is to reconstruct the story, cutting out the painful material. While this may result in the person feeling at peace with the past, it looks more like defence and denial than integrity in Erikson's sense.

3. Reminiscence is also a way to find continuities between past and present. The role of metaphor in the narrative may be very important here, particularly among people with failing mental powers. Stories from the past may be a way of talking about the present, and even making more palatable a scale of loss that is too terrible to talk of directly. The following is an example taken from one of John Killick's poems, which are constructed entirely from the words of people with dementia

Have you seen my barrow
I joined the group
and now it belongs to all of us.
But I don't know where it's gone

Killick interprets the barrow as representing the disempowerment that follows loss of employment and loss of role, but suggests that it may also stand for lost coherence and autonomy

Altogether you won't find
much toing and froing
and doing or being
with me. I never carry
as full as you do.
(*John Killick, 1997*)

4. Loss is inevitable in later life, and reminiscence can be important in coping with grief. And, as Coleman suggests, both the 'flight from happy memories' and a preoccupation with distressing ones can be indicators of unresolved grief and the need for intervention.

5. Finally, story-telling is an activity, and a competence. People do it because they can do it— and there may be many things that they now cannot do—and because it is something to do. Where it successfully entertains the listener(s) as well as the teller, it is particularly powerful. Audience reaction to reminiscence is very important. Respect for the person is embodied in attentive listening, rejection in inattentive body language, and derogatory remarks like 'yes, you've told me about that before' or 'no, you've got it all wrong—you were never in Italy during the war'. Given a good listener, reminiscence is a pleasure—particularly valuable when many other sources of pleasure have been lost.

Keeping reminiscence

Reminiscence is now on the agenda of professionals working with the elderly, but will it remain? And what is its status with non-professionals? Ageism is a significant dimension of oppression (Byethway, 1995), fuelled by concerns about demographic change. The changing age structure of society has been characterized as a 'demographic time bomb', in which older people are seen as an intolerable burden on the working population. At its worst, demographic panic leads to a view of older people as an expensive nuisance, taking an unfair share of the resources generated by the labours of younger people. The old are seen as a race apart, barely human: this perspective leaves little chance of respect or gracious acceptance of the narrative heirlooms of the old. A positive view of reminiscence may need to be defended in the face of this view of the elderly. The critique of demographic panic is powerful (e.g. Arber and Ginn, 1991). Among other things, the role of the elderly in caring for people—both the young and those older or more frail than themselves—has been identified as one of the economically valuable contributions that they make to society.

However, ageism is not readily overturned, and we cannot assume that the recognition of reminiscence as a good thing, and the upsurge of interest in oral history, means that older people will naturally find respectful listeners for their stories. Ideally, older people have listeners because their experiences are needed, but inevitably some people's experiences are needed more than others. To give older people ample opportunities to have a hearing it is necessary to have professional input, encouraging reminiscence for those who like it wherever older people are receiving care.

In this volume James Phillips suggests that we live in and through the stories we tell or imagine about ourselves. When a patient comes for therapy, in general the story is not going well. For many older people a reason for the story not going well is the lack of listeners, and imaginary listeners are not enough. The answer may lie not in a vast influx of elderly people into psychotherapy, but in giving more weight to emotional support (rather than physical support) in basic care, whether institutional or in the community.

The degree to which care staff can succeed in giving emotional work the same priority as physical work remains to be seen. It may be that to keep reminiscence work going it needs to be framed as some kind of essential but specialist activity or therapy. Perhaps we need to see listeners to older people's stories as being as essential for their basic health care as chiropodists are for their feet. Professional listening has a role, not only for the individual in compensating for the deficiencies in the social world, but also as a cultural function in valuing history and continuity. However, there will be many people for whom the story is not going well for deeper reasons than the lack of a listener, and that their contribution to history has been bypassed. One group of people for whom this is true are people who suffer from dementia and those who care for them.

Narratives and dementia

My particular interest in older people's narratives arose in the context of people with dementia and their (unpaid) carers. It was from listening to carers' accounts that I began to consider what is happening to the narratives of both those who have failing mental powers and the people with whom they have shared their lives and who are witness to their decline.

Faith Gibson (1997) has described people with dementia as living in a contracting world. They become increasingly unable to do things, and those around them take over and gain power over them. Social life tends to fall away, and many people will ignore the person with dementia, addressing conversation to the carer instead. Gibson sees reminiscence work with people with dementia as a way of 'holding at bay, at least for a time, this shrinking world.'

> It is a means of conveying respect, of holding people in relationship, of affirming them as social beings and confirming their personhood. It is a means of reassuring them that come what may, they shall be cared for and not abandoned to the terrifying loneliness of aloneness.
> (*Gibson, 1997.*)

Holding people with dementia in the social world is a major challenge to both paid and unpaid carers, given the disabilities brought about by cognitive decline. Dementia damages memory and communication, but it is usually the case that at least some past memories are retained. These fragments from long ago are often more vivid and enduring than the memories of recent events. Like everyone else, people with dementia find recognition easier than recall, and may need others to hold their memories, and tell them their own life stories.

Recognition may then trigger recall. In remembering the past, people often find the feelings of the past, are able to hold on to a former sense of self-worth and social confidence that is severely challenged by the experience of dementia.

Reminiscence has the power to combine the here-and-now with the then-and-there. The person is held in relationship with the person or group that is focused on their experiences. The affirmation of their past is a pleasure in the present, while the feel of the past may help to dispel the unsatisfactory feel of the present.

For many people with dementia it seems that the present has a strange and unreal quality about it and their narratives are shaped by changes in their ability to remember, think, and reason. Past memories may feel more solid and reliable and work better for people as a metaphor for present experience than the narrative, restricted by cognitive impairment, that they able to construct about the present.

Stories of changing relationships

I began to listen to carers as a researcher investigating gender differences in the experiences of elderly people caring for their spouses. The stories of caring were told with constant reference to the past, perhaps because it was in the past that the impetus to care lay. Few people choose to restrict their own lives and freedoms in order to meet the needs of another person, unless there is a joint past to give meaning to the endurance test inherent in caring. In my own research the number of older people caring for neighbours—rather than people with whom they had a significant long-running relationship—was negligible, and the level of care provided, valuable though it was, a mere fraction of the time and effort put in by carers who had significant attachments to the people they cared for.

The story of older people as carers is mainly one of spouse care, and some of the most demanding situations are those where the person cared for is a spouse who is losing his or her mental powers. Following the research, I became 'community support worker' with family carers of people with dementia. Repeated contacts with carers over a period of time added to the single, snapshot view of the research interview.

Caring for a partner with failing mental powers is the story of a changing relationship. Caring is undertaken because of the relationship, a significant attachment, but as a result of the need for care, and through the caring process, the nature of the attachment is transformed. Caring comes at considerable personal cost to the carer who faces task overload, restricted freedom, social isolation, and an unremitting feeling of responsibility. Giving care demands a great deal, both physically and emotionally. And yet the object of care is someone to whom the carer has until now turned for support in times of difficulty. Spousal relationships have implicit agreements about how each partner should look after the other, but when one develops dementia she inevitably reneges on the old agreements to a considerable degree. Carers often describe the attachment shift as a role reversal, 'I am his mother more than his wife', or a quicksand of role changes, as in these lines from a poem by an unknown carer:

> Sometimes he sits in his corner like a tired old man.
> Sometimes he trots and pesters like a little boy.
> Mostly he nods and smiles, and proffers his few phrases almost like a functional human being.
> My companion, friend and lover is now my child, or my aged father
> Or at times I'm with a stranger, living in my space, but not in my reality

From the perspective of the person who is cared for, there are also ways in which the old agreements are not being upheld.

Elsie Bailey described her second marriage to Ronald Bailey as on the whole a good marriage, where they had both worked, shared the domestic tasks, and enjoyed an easy companionship. They both had friends at work, Elsie had children from her previous marriage, and they didn't feel the need for a lot of friends because they had each other. When Ronald developed Alzheimer's Disease, everything changed, and the following extracts from her interview illustrate the 'broken agreement' and how much she minded about it.

> Where one went the other went, we always went together, we went out together, and when we retired at first what he used to do, he used to say, we used to share the work and we used to share it and then we used to go out for lunches and go out to bingo at night you know, and bus rides, we used to go coach rides, you know day trips, well everything's stopped.
>
> To be honest with you I leaned on him, I didn't have to do anything, nothing you know. I leaned on him too much, I mean when I was poorly with arthritis when I was 60 I couldn't bath myself, I couldn't dress myself, and he was marvellous, he did everything, and it's turned the tail, I couldn't do nothing.
>
> You see his nature's changed considerably, he's not the same . . . . I mean he was kind and helpful, I mean I can say to him oh I don't feel well today, ... and he won't say anything, he couldn't care less, it doesn't seem to sink in.
>
> He's got no affection, no kiss, no thank you, nothing, and you know I feel as if all my work's done and it's not appreciated, do you know what I mean. . . . .It isn't, I mean I'm not saying he, perhaps in himself he appreciates it, but he doesn't show it at all.
>
> Another thing 8 o'clock he'll switch the telly off and he expects. .well I do, I come to bed with him at half past 8. He wants me you see to come to bed with him, he seems as if, he's like a baby somehow. So what I do, I have my books and a little radio you know to plug in and that's what I do in bed and then I'm up at quarter to 6 because I'm ready to get up, in fact I could get up before that really because I'm not asleep.

The person with dementia does and says things that are 'out of character'. The caring spouse has to respond to actions and utterances that would not have occurred in the pre-dementia relationship. Or if they did occur, these actions have different meanings given that the person now has dementia. From carers' accounts, it seems that it is often hard to take on the change of meaning and the common sense responses of the previous relationship often prevail. The results are uncomfortable for everyone. Here are some examples from Elsie Bailey's interview, with speculations as to how her behaviour might feel to Ronald Bailey:

> I've said to him many a time 'what's the matter, you're not talking to me?' . . . he doesn't talk, sometimes my mouth is dry, my lips are dry with not talking to anybody, I have to talk to the cats you know.

Ronald Bailey feels got at. He can't work out what Elsie wants him to say.

> I'm frightened of leaving him because he smokes, he'll have a cigarette while I'm there and it drops off the tray, in fact only last week the tray turned upside down and I smacked him on his leg and he didn't half hit me and that's a thing he would never have done because he was so placid

Ronald has no memory of knocking the ashtray on to the floor, so he's sure he did not do it. He's sick and tired of Elsie blaming him for things, and treating him like a naughty child. She's getting altogether too bossy these days, he can't imagine what's got into her. She never used to be like that.

> But you know it's hard work and it's tiring, some days I just feel as if I could just scream and burst and leave him. I mean I shout at him and I've seen him shudder when I've shouted, and then I'm sorry after, I cry after, I'm sorry that I've shouted at him, but I don't know, I think it must be an outlet.

Ronald relies on Elsie. She's his security, he feels anxious when she leaves the room. It's such a relief when she returns, it makes him feel cross with her for going. It's terrible when she shouts. It makes him think that she might walk out and never return.

Ronald Bailey was not able to give us his view of how the relationship has changed, so the speculations above are guesses, but other people with dementia have been able to talk about their experiences, especially early on. The following extracts are from a remarkable account of 'Maureen's' experiences of early dementia recorded by Richard Corney (1994). They show how dementia changes relationships for sufferers as well as carers:

> I feel afraid, perpetually afraid of something, but I don't know what; even if I don't feel I've done something wrong, it's in the back of my mind that I've forgotten to do something, so I'm just so afraid all the time.
>
> I wake in the morning and nothing is familiar to me, I have to sit on the side of the bed and keep saying to myself, 'I know where I am, but it all looks wrong'; then you get used to it looking wrong and think 'Well, that's all right, that must be the way it is. . . . .
>
> My husband wants to go on holiday, but I don't want to leave this house. . . .
>
> I think I must be driving my husband mad. I can't deal with ordinary household things any-more, like paying bills; my husband has to do all that now or they wouldn't get paid . . . or get paid twice. It's not so bad for me, but it must be hell for him, you see he has a memory like an elephant, never forgets anything. He's in hospital now, and I feel so guilty that the stress I put him under has put him there . . . I really worry about that, and what I could do or should do, but what can I do? Nothing. I wish there was something. . . .
>
> The stupid thing is that I can remember childhood things. I can remember my mother plainly, like yesterday, and the big hats she used to love to wear; but I can't remember where I put the packet of Bisto, or what my husband has just said he will have for dinner. He says it's because I don't listen, but I do. . . .
>
> It must have come slowly, this thing, I didn't realise anything was happening, I just knew my husband was losing patience with me. . . .
>
> I used to be a happy little thing, but now I'm a mass of doubt and insecurity. I feel guilty but I don't know why, I just know it's all my fault . . . it's my 'headbox' that's acting up, I'm causing dis-tress to others; my husband has visibly aged 20 years in the last four years. But they don't under-stand it's out of my control; I'm not doing it on purpose. They get cross with me at times and lose their patience. If I was a four-year-old child, they wouldn't. But because I'm not they do.
>
> Are there really others like me out there, or am I alone in this?

Careful observation of body language, and listening for meaning in what people say suggests that at later stages too, people with dementia are often aware of their changed roles and relation-ships, and mind about the changes. Tom Kitwood has described the changing social world of people with dementia in terms of 'malignant social psychology', and has identified 17 different types of carer behaviour—ignoring, labelling, outpacing, invalidation, etc.—which disempower and depersonalize people, particularly if this is happening in the already alien setting of institutional care (Kitwood, 1997).

A dementing illness inevitably means that there is 'something wrong with the story'. For carers it brings a complex and variable mix of losses and changes. For people with dementia, a key element is that something is going wrong with their relationships, and in particular with their relationship to the person who is closest to them. I will return later to the question of restrictive and supportive narratives of dementia, and how they can act to undermine or bolster a person with dementia's identity. At this point I want to look at the impact of dementia on a person's relationships and their narrative identity, focusing on the attachment system.

Attachment and dementia

Few carers, whether paid or unpaid, deliberately set out to disempower and depersonalize those in their care. These things generally come about because carers fail to understand the world of people with dementia and lack the personal resources and skill to respond to their needs. Family carers have a lot to contend with. They face the major challenge of dementia care without the benefit of support or training, while concurrently losing the practical help and emotional support that the person they care for used to give to them as parent or spouse. In listening to carers I hear many accounts of baffling and irritating changes in behaviour that have to be endured. One set of irritating behaviours must be all too familiar to anyone who has had the experience of parenting. Many people with dementia seem to be doing things which look remarkably like the attachment behaviour of small children, as identified by Bowlby and Ainsworth. The meaning of these things, if they were to occur in a pre-dementia, adult-to-adult relationship, would be quite different from the same behaviour occurring in a parent–child context, and from carers' accounts it is clear that many people are responding as they might have done in the pre-dementia context, rather than in the manner of an attuned parent. Two possible reasons for this are that carers do not 'read' the attachment message in their person's actions, i.e. they don't recognize their need to stay close to feel secure, or, alternatively, they understand the message, but do not respond helpfully, often because they feel that their person should not have this need.

> I am his security. I know that, but it doesn't stop me making sharp comments. He exasperates me to the point of screaming.
>
> I think with this loss of memory. . . you tend to cling onto little bits that you know, like myself, and thinking that her mother's round the corner
>
> He even tries to follow me into the toilet. I just can't do with that.
>
> I spent all Saturday with her doing what she wanted, but the minute I went into the kitchen to do the tea she was calling after me. It's not on, this constant attention-seeking.

People with dementia commonly do the following things:

(1) gaze at the carer;

(2) follow the carer's movement with his or her eyes;

(3) call, or shout, when the carer is out of sight;

(4) follow the carer;

(5) hold or cling on to the carer;

(6) become angry or unco-operative with the carer following a separation;

(7) refuse to look at or talk to the carer following separation;

(8) become angry or violent with the carer when she say she is going out.

Bere Miesen (1992) has observed similar behaviours in the context of family visits to people with dementia in a hospital setting, and has suggested that they can be understood as attachment behaviour. He puts forward the view that dementia transforms everyday reality into a strange situation, and, as in young children, this triggers the need to stay close to a trusted person in order to feel safe. In addition, Miesen identified another cluster of behaviours typical of people with moderate to severe dementia, which he interprets as attachment behaviours. Examples of these are:

(1) trying to find parents;

(2) imagining themselves back in the parental family;

(3) expressions of concern about parents, expectation that parents will arrive, fears of parental disapproval etc.;

(4) saying that they have just seen parents (who are actually long dead);

(5) wanting to go home;

(6) preoccupation with other significant people, animals, or places—spouses, siblings, old friends, or pets, the town or country where someone grew up.

Miesen calls these behaviours parent fixation. He found parent fixation to be most common among people with severe dementia, but also among those less disabled by their failing mental powers who he judged were not satisfied by their 'here and now' attachments.

Neurological impairment and the attachment system

Given that people with dementia are adults, what is causing them to act in ways that are reminiscent of infant behavioural patterns? Meisen suggests that the dementia-induced strange situation is a trigger; however, this may not be the whole story. It seems likely that dementia also interferes with adult strategies for coping with strange situations. Between infancy and adulthood lies a process of development whereby the adult no longer needs constant physical proximity to an attachment figure to feel safe. Experience enables a person to understand what is happening, to contain emotional reactions and to work out what needs to be done (Holmes, chapter 3, this volume) The need for physical closeness does not disappear altogether in adult life. It remains for most people as a regular part of intimate relationships, and faced with stress, many adults take comfort from physical proximity to a trusted person. However, this need for closeness does not have the urgency of infancy. Adults can wait, whereas in infants, all exploration and play is halted until proximity is achieved.

People with dementia seem to regain this urgent need for closeness. Forgetfulness and confusion mean that they may be unable to understand what is happening, lose the ability to contain their feelings, and don't always know what to do about things. In the context of therapy, the idea of containment suggests that the therapist is temporarily taking on some of the client's psychological functions until she becomes able to regain them for herself. For people with dementia, containment may need to become part of care, just as the attuned mother names her baby's feelings for him and, in accepting them, conveys that his rage is not all-encompassing and destructive. However, dementia cannot be seen as a tidy return to infancy. Adult mechanisms for maintaining a sense of security without the need to stay close to an attachment figure may work at some times and not at others. Unlike babies who are on a somewhat predictable pathway from dependency to independence, people with dementia are experiencing a variable and unpredictable cognitive decline, which has a complicated relationship with their sense of self and security.

Attachment theory suggests that in adult life a sense of security is maintained by internal working models. The constituents of working models proposed by Collins and Read (1994) include cognitive functions such as memory, judgement, and planning, and it seems certain that dementia will interfere with the structure and function of working models. Meisen (1996) has argued that dementia seems to make many ordinary situations become strange. This may be because cognitive decline prevents people from using past experience to help them interpret what is going on and to work out what to do. Disinhibition among people with dementia means that they reveal feelings that other adults would control. Whether the outpouring of feelings is a direct effect of neurological decline, or a result of life becoming more alarming is an open question. However, it does seem that for many people with dementia, the ability to calm themselves when distressed is reduced. Coherent internal narratives are a key feature of adult security, and dementia typically disrupts narrative coherence. Internal consistency and plausibility are the two main components of Main's concept of coherence. One or both of these features are often missing from the spoken stories of people with dementia, and almost certainly from their internal narratives as well. If this is happening is it possible that the incoherence resulting from neurological impairment gives a person the same feeling of insecurity as incoherence arising from unsatisfactory childhood experiences?

John Byng-Hall (Chapter 7, this volume) refers to two further mechanisms—metacognitive monitoring and reflexive self-function—that are associated with secure attachment. There is reason to think that both of these processes are disturbed by dementia. Bowlby observed children who retained incompatible models, and Main suggested that certain parental defensive strategies inhibit metacognitive monitoring, leaving children with disorganized internal narratives. Sometimes, people with dementia appear to think of the person that looks after them as not a single person, but two or more different people. This phenomenon suggests that metacognitive monitoring is not working properly, and perhaps also that they are holding on to incompatible models.

Carers often complain that people with dementia do not seem to be able to understand their difficulties, e.g. they won't make allowances when the carer is ill, and become cross if their needs aren't met in the usual way. Also, people with dementia often insist that there is nothing wrong with them; 'I'll be fine here on my own' when the evidence is that they fly into a panic the minute the carer leaves the house. Observations like these suggest impaired reflexive self-function. This may be not only because of the person's declining ability to make judgements, but also because the scale of a person's losses is so enormous that denial becomes an important defence. Dementia seems to give good reason for defensive exclusion, which Bowlby suggested would lead to internal working models that did not fit well with external reality (Bretherton, 1995).

Attachment theory suggests a number of internal mechanisms that replace physical proximity as a source of security. As cognition and recall play a part in the operation of these mechanisms there is every reason to believe that the dementing process is likely to wreak havoc with them. Dementia has the tendency to make ordinary situations feel strange and a strange situation is a classic trigger for the attachment system. But if dementia also disrupts internal working models, makes internal narratives incoherent, and interferes with metacognitive monitoring and reflexive self-function, this would suggest that adult self-calming mechanisms will not work reliably and it is perhaps not surprising that people with dementia seek security through physical proximity.

Parent fixation, interpreted by Miesen as a kind of attachment behaviour, is typically seen later on in dementia than proximity seeking. Can we see this as the development of a new form of internalized self-calming process, based on the most reliably retrievable memories? A common feature among people who are well into dementia is that they appear to find the past more real than the present. They may be overheard conversing with people from the distant past, and talk to current carers about them as though they were part of everyday life. They often appear more absorbed and alive in their internal worlds than in the here and now. Perhaps the fragments from the past are well preserved from repeated rehearsal, whereas more recent material is shadowy and faint. This would allow a new internal working model to be constructed from old memories, which brings a feeling of security based on the belief that mother (or whoever) is close at hand without interference from the contradictory evidence of recent experience. Perhaps the return to an internally generated sense of security is most likely to work well for a person who has a rich internal world of relatively intact memories, and is able to be unperturbed by inconsistencies between their fantasy world and the parallel world of their present. There may also be defensive exclusion, but cognitive decline may be such that inconsistencies between internal and external realities are no longer as disturbing as in people whose mental powers are intact.

We may need to reframe 'living in a world of her own', which tends to be seen as a sign that someone is 'really far gone'. It can be seen more positively as the person with dementia adapting to the disruption of mental processes caused by dementia, and finding new ways to cope with strange situations that do not rely on staying close to another person. Here we may have an example of a person with dementia finding a way to successfully 're-story' her life. If this is so, then it is important that carers do not invalidate her story by reminding her that mother has been dead for years. This is not as easy as it sounds, especially for those who are characters in each other's stories. It can be very difficult for a carer to live closely alongside a person who is living in her space, but not in her reality, to condone the eccentric reality of the person she cares for without feeling that her own is compromised. The person cared for has reconstructed his/her story in order to make living with dementia tolerable, but the new story is a challenge to the validity of the carer's own narrative, and to the significance of their shared past.

Attachment and caring

Two of the assumptions underlying person-centred approaches to dementia care are that:

(1) however odd it may look, there is some sense in what a person with dementia is saying and doing, and

(2) challenging, baffling, or difficult behaviour is best seen as an attempt to communicate—a way to express a need, an anxiety, a protest, or an interest, or, in the widest sense, to tell a story.

The challenge for carers is to crack the code, or read between the lines, to find the message. Often there is emotional truth in a statement that is factually incorrect. When people with dementia say 'You've stolen my money', more often than not they are falsely accusing someone who, far from stealing their money, is caring for them at great personal cost. Translated into a statement about feelings: 'I feel robbed of the things I valued most highly in my life and you are disempowering me because you keep telling me what to do', what they are saying makes sense. Once the code is cracked, the challenge is to find an appropriate response to such difficult feelings. While the ability to do this may be second nature to people with a training in psychotherapy or counselling, it is does not come easily to many carers.

The attachment framework can be useful, because so many people have experienced parenting. Recognizing that gazing, following, and calling out are signs of the need for proximity may trigger appropriate responses in carers, based on their parenting skills. However, there are pitfalls. Not all parenting is attuned parenting, and responses to the need for proximity are not always welcoming. Parents encourage their dependent infants to become independent, and carers all too easily fall into attempts to 'teach' their person with dementia—in whom a childlike need for physical closeness seems age-inappropriate—to regain a sense of independence. Finally, people with dementia are not children and generally remember how they should be treated as adults; unmodified responses from a carers' childcare repertoire, especially of the condescending kind, are likely to be met with anger.

A diagnosis of dementia is made when a person's performance has declined, and she is unable to remember, think, and reason as well as before. Cognitive tests may indicate a decline in orientation, spatial awareness, deduction, problem solving, making judgements, and so on, as well as memory. Testing emphasizes lost abilities, and what people cannot do. Caring is often made most difficult by what people can do, and do do, as they attempt to make sense of what is happening, and control the chaos and confusion around them.

As outlined earlier, when a person with dementia makes a bid for closeness, the carer does not always understand, or if she does understand, does not always manage to respond supportively. Following Bowlby, there has been an enormous amount of work done on the consequences of different kinds of parental response to the attachment needs of infants. Ainsworth argued that infants with sensitive, responsive, accessible, and co-operative attachment figures feel more secure, and this forms the basis of feelings of confidence and self-worth. Her research relates insecure attachment to unresponsiveness and insensitivity on the part of mothers. Marked 'punishment' responses that occur after a separation are typical of insecure attachment, e.g. unassuaged anger on reunion, resisting comfort, turning away, not looking at the attachment figure, or appearing dazed or fearful.

Attachment creates the first chapter of a person's narrative identity. Parental responses lead to underlying assumptions about what can be expected from others, the child's worth, and capacity as agent. As life unfolds, an account of what is happening is constructed in the light of these underlying assumptions. Many different patterns emerge as significant life events are met and become part of the narrative, but behind the richness and diversity of people's stories, the underlying structure of early attachment status is still visible (Holmes, Chapter 3, this volume). We see narrative identity as having two components: *the story of the person's life so far (diachronic component) and the account of their present life constructed from social feedback, and judgements of herself based on direct attribution and social comparison (synchronic component)*(Tom

Kitwood, personal communication). Attachment is involved in both: it is a scaffold that deter-mines the shape of the diachronic component, and it is a determinant of relationships, reflected back in the way that others are responding. The experience of dementia upsets the coherence of the diachronic component, as forgetfulness leaves holes in the narrative, and only much-re-hearsed fragments remain. And the synchronic component is upset when the person cannot make accurate judgements, or hold on to a consistent narrative of the present. Glaring discrep-ancies between remembered fragments of her earlier identity and the reflection of herself that she sees in the way that others are treating her make it hard to work out what is real.

Kitwood's (1997) person-centred approach to dementia care requires of carers responses to people with dementia that are similar to Ainsworth's requirements for attachment figures at-tuned to children. His 'malignant social psychology' which emerged from his observations care practice describes elements of caring which he argues add to distress, fuel difficult behaviour, and ultimately hasten disengagement and vegetation. Perhaps the power of the person-centred approach is to recreate constantly the conditions that lead to secure attachment. If dementia is breaking down internal working models and narratives, and interfering with processes like metacognitive monitoring and reflexive self-function, which are essential to the construction of coherent narratives, a person may need help in maintaining and reconstructing their view of the world.

Part of the carer's role is to care for malfunctioning psychological processes. Person-centred care is a drip-feed mechanism helping people experiencing mental decline to create and main-tain a positive reflection of themselves. Doing this may involve similar approaches to good mothering, suitably modified to reflect the fact that the people in question are adults, and not babies. Mirroring a person's feelings becomes especially important when a person has lost words to express feelings, and feels frustrated and misunderstood.

Whereas it may be possible to maintain some fragments of coherent narrative about the past, because of the relative enduring nature of past memories, coherent narratives of the present become ever more elusive as the dementia progresses. Kitwood's view is that there is a need to bypass cognition, and to maintain a coherent world of feelings (Kitwood, 1997). Increasingly the cognitive processes that hold affirming experiences beyond the present moment are no longer working, and we can hypothesize that this reduces the possibility of good moments hav-ing a lasting effect. It is in this context that an emotionally supportive physical and social envi-ronment becomes so essential, and that care needs to become psychotherapeutic as well as attending to physical need.

Restrictive and supportive narratives of dementia

So-called 'old culture' responses to people with dementia reflect to them a constricting (and negative) story of who they now are. Seen as irreparably damaged by incurable illness, their utterances the meaningless outpourings of a damaged brain, their personalities lost, they be-come bodies, socially dead, with no real person inside. 'An empty shell', 'a husk', 'not the man I married' are all indicators of a restricted illness narrative. This story is relatively safe and secure for carers, but destructive for people with dementia, and unlikely to fit their experiences. When a person explodes with frustration because no-one will take him home, and is told, 'You are con-fused because you've got this illness, this is your home now, we'll give you something to calm you down,' this fails to mirror his feelings. Careful observation suggests that although dementia means that people's brains are not working as they once did, they are still working. The things people with dementia say and do are not entirely chaotic and 'demented'; a more positive interpretation sees them as attempts to create order from flawed information. Distortions of perception, gaps in information, disruption of mental models, all interfere with the construction of a coherent narrative, but stories are still produced and attempts to reach out to other people are still made, at least before the disabilities are so severe that it is hard to guess at people's experiences. The telling signs of affective responsiveness to good guesses can also be observed (Holmes, Chapter 3, this volume).

The illness narrative has its uses (Holmes, Chapter 3), but one of the problems for people with dementia is that they are often not told of their diagnosis at a stage where they have sufficient mental powers to comprehend it. It's often a secret story, known to professionals and family carers, but hidden from the person themselves. Other stories such as 'You're getting old', 'You're under the weather' collude with a person's reluctance to face what is happening. How much a person's 'lack of insight' is an intrinsic part of their dementia, and how much it arises from denial or from other people's avoidance of painful scenes may be hard to judge. Some people with dementia do find a way of talking about what is happening to them: 'My brain is stiff, it's got arthritis like my knees', 'I can't make the tea any more, I've got something wrong, I think they call it confusion', 'Oh dear, it's my Alzheimer's playing tricks again.' It must be easier to do this when other people help to find the words.

People with dementia experience problems familiar to most of us to a more than ordinary degree. They need a narrative that makes allowances for, rather than blames them, for their difficulties. The illness narrative can be useful for this. Many carers describe a twilight period, before diagnosis, where they had no idea what was going on or how to respond to it.

The story of Edward and Valerie Lloyd

Edward and Valerie had been married over 40 years and always enjoyed a busy social life. They had many friends at their 'local'. When Valerie was in her late sixties things began to go wrong. She seemed to be fine in company, but would barely speak to Edward at home. When members of her family came to visit, she would brighten up and chat to them, when they left she would not even look at Edward, let alone speak. Eventually he made plans to separate and Valerie seemed to agree that the marriage was over. Just before the house was sold, Valerie's mum came to see Edward. She persuaded him that Valerie 'wasn't right' and that she still needed him. Edward was persuaded. He cancelled the sale, and stopped divorce proceedings. Six months later Valerie had a diagnosis of Alzheimer's Disease.

Seeing no reason for Valerie's changed behaviour Edward assumed that she no longer loved him. He was hurt and angry at her treatment of him. There were signs that this was something more than ordinary marital breakdown, but there was nothing to signal illness clearly rather than breakdown of relationship. However, he did have some doubts which were sufficient to make him responsive to his mother-in-law's intervention. The diagnosis of Alzheimer's brought a reason for Valerie's hostile behaviour, and Edward settled down to care for her as best he could.

Here illness narrative helped, but the dangers of the illness narrative are that it takes over, and we lose sight of the person. This is particularly problematic in dementia, where the symptoms of the illness are the things that people do and say, and neurological decline is not the sole factor responsible for their actions. In the case of Edward and Valerie, the diagnosis of dementia gave him a reason to stay with her and look after her, but it also gave him a way to discount her protests at the way he took over her life. Edward was a very controlling carer, liking to do things his own way and excluding Valerie from the kitchen in case she made a mess of things. When she swore at him and insulted him he dismissed it as part of the illness saying: 'They do that, you know. They turn against the one that is caring for them.'

A person-centred disability narrative allows us to keep the person in view as well as the illness. Whatever the story, the person will decline, but a disability narrative allows the person to be supported and enabled as they decline.

The immediate goal of person-centred dementia care is to foster well-being as far as is possible, given the disabilities brought by declining mental powers. It does not seek to remove symptoms, in the sense of curing neurological decline. Good care may mean that some symptoms of distress disappear, but it is equally possible that they may continue to recur, because of the person's enduring difficulties with the strangeness of dementia. The person-centred carer's goal is to attend to the distress on each occasion, and to ensure that the person's feelings are looked after. The caring role is both to alleviate and compensate for the distressing experiences that occur as a result of mental decline. Most people with dementia cannot find strategies to deal with these strange experiences without help. The therapeutic relationship needs to be integrated into their on-going care. In psychotherapy we can view the therapist as the attachment figure, who creates a relationship with clients similar to the relationship between attuned mother and infant. One relevant difference is that the relationship is rationed rather than continuous. Therapeutic dementia care needs carers who are willing to act as attachment figures, and to compensate for the disabilities dementia brings; the relationship needs to be constantly available.

Family care, attachment, and narratives

Attachment research explores caregiving in the context of parent and child. While there are clearly relevant differences in caring for a person with dementia who is an adult, and has experienced independence, attachment theory suggests that our experiences of parenting shape the ways in which we negotiate caregiving and carereceiving in relationships throughout life. In addition, the underlying structure in the two kinds of caregiving is the same, involving a more autonomous person performing a number of tasks for a person who is less autonomous. The caregiver, whether parent or carer, is more powerful than the person receiving care in a number of important respects. For these reasons studies of parenting may throw up ideas which that have relevance in other caregiving contexts.

Caring for a relative disrupts long-standing habits of care-giving and care-receiving in the relationship and this gives reason to assume that a carer's resources for care-giving may be depleted, because many of the things that the person with dementia could be relied upon to provide in the past they are no longer capable of delivering. I shall argue that attachment issues shape the narratives that carers construct, and that these narratives influence their responses to those for whom they care.

Carers also experience overload of various kinds and often they share the person with dementia's shrinking social world. These factors are often cited as reasons for the high levels of depression and low morale among carers. However they may also affect the nature of carers' narratives.

Attachment research has studied the quality of interaction between mother and child. Recent research, while generally upholding the view that infant security rests upon timely and empathic responses to the child that affirm their experiences, suggests a number of factors that influence a mother's ability to be attuned to her infant. Whereas there are only weak associations between security and individual risk factors, strong relationships are found where a number of risk factors occur in combination. For example, where poor marital quality, difficult infant temperament, and unfavourable maternal personality occur together the likelihood of secure attachment (mediated by attuned parenting) is vastly reduced. Maternal depression and social support also play a role in the interactions between stresses and supports, which influence infant attachment status (Belsky 1995).

Three factors emphasized in attachment research could well have relevance to the quality of interactions between carers and people with dementia. It seems quite probable that a perceived worsening of the marital relationship is a risk factor for carers of people with dementia; the illness both precipitates the need for care and changes the marital relationship. However it cannot be assumed that all carers experience this as a change for the worse. In one study a small number of husbands reported improved relationships with their wives since the onset of dementia (Fitting, 1986). Clearly too, the story of the relationship is important. However although a good story of the past relationship may fuel a spouse's commitment to caring, it does not necessarily lead to high quality care. Where a partner's mental decline reduces the level of support previously given to the spouse, and pressing attachment needs are left unmet. I would suggest that this is a risk factor for lack of attuned care, which is most likely to result if there are other adverse factors in the situation.

Just as some infants are 'cranky' there is no doubt that some people with dementia are more difficult to look after than others. Where a person reacts to the condition with aggressive outbursts, for example, or night restlessness, this puts considerable strain on carers. Of course some people have been 'difficult' throughout life and may retain this quality on developing dementia. The example given below illustrates how a daughter's lifelong experience of her mother as difficult appeared to shape her narrative of her mother in old age, and to interpret her mother's actions as being typically difficult rather than signs of her mother's struggle to retain control of her life, in the face of mental decline.

There may be a number of carer characteristics which affect a person's ability to give good care. Depression and low morale, known to be prevalent among carers (Morris, 1987) may be particularly significant. Depressive narratives focus unhelpfully on the grim realities of people's lives. Good quality dementia care requires an emphasis on the positive, and on small achievable pleasures in the here-and-now rather than comparing the present unfavourably with what might have been.

There is another strand of attachment research which may prove to be highly relevant to other kinds of caregiving than parenting. This is the growing body of work exploring adult attachment status and its impact on parenting. There are strong associations between mothers' and infants' attachment status (Zeanah and Zeanah, 1989) and on mothers' attachment status and their interactional behaviour with their infants (Vondra and Shaw, 1995). Here again it seems highly likely that a carer's attachment status will affect the way in which they care for a relative with dementia, especially if that person has played a key role in their security as either parent or spouse.

Listening to carers leaves no doubt that some find the attachment needs of their partner/parent harder to understand and respond to sympathetically than those or others. And certain carers are memorable for their inability to settle on a 'good story' of the situation, despite high levels of support and service intervention.

Carol Smith

Carol Smith's mother lived alone, not far from Carol. As community care goes, she had a generous package of care with home care, day care, and respite stays every four weeks. Despite a disastrous marriage in the past, Carol was now well-supported by her daughter, her sister, and several friends from her church. During a chance encounter with a worker from an EMI unit Carol burst into tears and said how awful she felt about her mother. She also said that she didn't believe that she had dementia. I was asked to talk to her. From Carol's account of her mother there was no reason to doubt the diagnosis. But Carol said that her mother had always made her life difficult and this was just more of the same. Guessing that there might be an attachment problem I encouraged Carol to talk about her childhood and to speculate about her mother's childhood. I sent her a letter summarizing the things she had told me. A month later we met again. She seemed to have revised the story of her mother. At our initial meeting she told me that her mother was always difficult, selfish, and rejecting, and could see no reason why she should be so uncaring. By our second meeting she had thought more about what life might have been like for her mother as eldest girl in a family of nine, with a rather cold and controlling mother. Carol had been in her grandmother's care during the war, and this experience helped her to see some reason for her mother's selfish nature. She told me that she now agreed that her mother had dementia, but was a really difficult character none the less. This agreed, we were able to discuss strategies for handling her mother. I saw Carol again after her mother died some months later. She told me that things had been easier for her once she had accepted that it really was dementia, and she had been discussing forgiveness with her church friends. She said she thought she could forgive her mother for failing her is so many ways, and she had had feelings of compassion for her before she died.

I felt that Carol needed to change her story of what was happening to be better able to tolerate the situation. Feeling that her mother was doing things on purpose to annoy her was far worse than seeing her mother's demands as arising from her insecurity faced with mental decline. It was surprising how easy it was for Carol to change her story; it was much harder, she told me, to treat her mother differently and to quash her feelings of irritation at her mother's demands and acerbic remarks. Where old narratives are 'inscribed' in behaviour patterns that are hard to change, action may lag behind insight. None the less, there did seem to be progress, especially as she was able to feel compassion.

Ingbretsen and Solem (1995) have published an account of their work with carers of people with dementia and identified some of the particular difficulties experienced by carers classified using Bowlby's three categories of insecure attachment: anxious attachment, compulsive caregiving, and strenuous attempts to claim emotional self-sufficiency. In their experience, securely attached carers experience all the pain and distress of a changing relationship, and the uncertainty about how best to care for their person, but are more open and receptive to information about dementia and better able to adapt to the changes as they come. As they put it: 'Secure attachment seems to facilitate flexible coping while insecure attachment may cause reluctance to accept changes being in conflict with the caregiver's basic needs of stability and security.' These may be the people that can most easily adopt enabling rather than restrictive narratives of dementia, and who can adjust their own stories to accommodate changes. Not that change is impossible for those with insecure attachment status, but they may need to gain insight into their own needs for security before they can adapt to changing circumstances.

Anxious attachment

Ingebretsen and Solem (1995) give an example of a carer showing anxious attachment who struggled to keep her husband going, and tried to cajole—and at times berate—him into performing as he used to. Her need to hold on to him as a secure and solid husband was preventing her from responding to his need for support and security as he was faced with a (literally) unnerving illness! Her approach lead to much conflict. This carer's loss of her father in childhood had left a gap which had been filled by her strong and dependable husband, and his mental decline was arousing intense anxiety about the possibility of a new loss. Something was going wrong with her story, and her initial reaction was to try to restore the familiar script. Her attempts to do this just made matters worse, as they brought unfamiliar levels of conflict into the relationship. Counselling enabled her to find a new script, and with it a less restrictive narrative of her husband's illness. Once she had recognized how her own anxiety and fear of loss had been aroused by her husband's illness, she learnt to try simply being close to her husband rather than constantly coaxing him to perform, and he responded better to this than to her criticism and commands.

Compulsive caregiving

Compulsive caregiving is a strategy that attempts to solve the pain of past rejection by caring for another person with all the dedication and sensitivity that was missing from the carer's own painful past. The carer's needs merge with those of the person cared for. In the case of Mrs O, described by Ingebretsen and Solem (1995), this lead to sensitive care for the person with dementia, but was extremely taxing for his wife who felt rejected by her husband's desire to go home to his mother, and perhaps too by his failure to get better. A narrative which eclipses the carer's own needs, and fails to acknowledge the inevitable conflicts of interest between carer and cared for may sustain good quality care for a time, but contains the risk of sudden carer collapse.

Independence and self-sufficiency

This pattern of attachment is better known by Ainsworth's? term anxious/avoidant attachment. Ingebretsen and Solem (1995) describe Mr T, a man caring for his wife, who discounted the possibility of any meaningful contact with her while she was suffering from the disease, and seemed to be hoping for a recovery. This hope made it hard for him to adjust to her changing needs. In the past he had relied on her presence and efficient management of the household to provide a stable structure in his life, but had avoided emotional closeness. He continued to care for her, perhaps in an attempt to hang on to the remains of the stable structure that had underpinned his life and activities, but was not satisfied with this own performance, and found it difficult to concentrate on his own activities. Mr T never adopted a narrative of his wife's dementia which accepted her as fully human, describing her as 'spiritually dead' and a 'non-person'. It is generally assumed that dehumanizing narratives of dementia are associated with insensitive care; it may also be the case that they reduce the chances of a carer finding a satisfactory meaning in caring. Mr T's reluctance to talk about the past prevented him from gaining insight into his own needs, and it seemed that the intensity of his needs impeded his ability to adopt better ways of helping his wife, although his involvement in a support group which brought social support and an opportunity to complain did seem to mean something to him.

Common sense might predict that an adult who had experienced an insecure attachment to their mother in childhood would never take on a caring role for their mother in later life; or that a spouse with an insecure attachment status would institutionalize the dementing partner at the first opportunity. Both attachment theory and experience suggest that this view is wrong. The work on children suggests that attachments are no less strong for being classified as insecure. Many daughters with insecure attachments to their mothers in childhood do take on a caring role, and are as committed to it as any other carer. I have argued that it is highly likely that attachment status affects both narratives and caring responses, but this is a hypothesis that needs to be investigated by research. If there are significant associations, these would have implications for intervention.

Our own experience in supporting carers suggest that all carers, whatever their attachment status, face difficulties in adjusting to the changed relationship that is brought about by a dementing illness. Thinking about attachment issues and narrative perspectives in relation to caring brought up a number of questions.

1. To what extent do attachment issues shape the narratives that carers construct?

2. How closely are people's narratives related to their responses?

3. How stable is adult attachment status? Faced with far-reaching changes to established patterns of caregiving and carereceiving, is it possible that a previously secure adult may become insecure, particularly where a dependable marital relationship has enabled someone who would have been classified as insecurely attached in childhood to achieve secure status as an adult?

4. Do we expect insecurely attached carers to express higher levels of distress?

5. Are insecurely attached carers less likely to adopt supportive narratives and to learn how to give the kind of care that helps life run more smoothly?

6. Do we need to acknowledge the attachment needs of carers before they can learn to respond to the attachment need of those that they care for?

7. Do attachment issues affect relationships with service providers?

Conclusions

For family carers of people with dementia, something goes very badly wrong with the story. All chances of a happy ending seem to be lost, and dementia has a way of intruding into every corner of their lives. Supporting carers, whether through formal therapy or support groups and education, has a narrative dimension. The construction of a story that emphasizes agency rather than illness is crucial not only to carers' morale, but almost certainly as an influence on the quality of care they are able to give to those they look after. The working models of insecure attachment are assumed to be more inflexible and difficult to change than those of secure attachment (Bretherton, 1995). The enormous changes in behaviour that dementia brings require a reworking of internal models, entailing a thorough revision of the story of the relationship to enable the carer to interpret and respond to the behaviour of the person with dementia. Because caregiving and carereceiving is a central dimension in the type of relationship in which informal care takes place, issues of attachment are inevitably interwoven with narratives of dementia, both for the person with the illness, and for those who give care. I have put forward some tentative suggestions: my hope is that others will find ways to take them forward to explore further the connections and to look at implications for intervention.

References

Arber, S. and Ginn, J. (1991). *Gender and later life: a sociological analysis of resources and constraints*. Sage, London.

Belsky. J. (1995). The origins of attachment security: classical and contextual determinants. *Attachment theory: social, developmental and clinical perspectives*, (ed. S. Goldberg,? Muir, and? Kerr). The Analytic Press, London.

Bretherton, I. (1995). The origins of attachment theory. *Attachment theory: social, developmental and clinical perspectives*, (ed. S. Goldberg,? Muir, and? Kerr). The Analytic Press, London.

Butler, R. (1963). The life review: an interpretation of reminiscence in the aged. *Psychiatry*, **26**, 65–76.

Bytheway. B. (1995). *Ageism*, Open University Press, Buckingham.

Cohen, S. and Syme, L. (eds.). (1985). *Social support and health*. Academic Press, London.

Cohen, S. and Syme, L. (ed.). *Social support and health*. Academic Press, New York.

Coleman, P. (1989). *Ageing and reminiscence processes*. John Wiley, Chichester.

Collins, N. and Read, S. (1994). Cognitive representations of attachment: the structure and function of working models. *Attachment processes in adulthood: advances in personal relationships*, (ed. K. Bartholomew and D. Perlman). Jessica Kingsley, New York.

Corney, R. (1994). *The carers' companion*. Winslow Press, Bicester.

Erikson, E. (1950). *Childhood and society*. Norton, New York.

Fitting, M., Rabins, P., Lucas, M. J. and Eastham, J. (1986). Caregivers for dementia patients: a comparison of husbands and wives *The Gerontologist*. **26**, 248–52

Gibson, F. (1997). Reaching people with dementia through reminiscence work. In *Conference papers: widening horizons in dementia care*. Age Exchange, London.

Ingebretsen. R. and Solem, E. (1995). Attachment, loss and coping in caring for a dementing spouse. *Care-giving in dementia, Vol. 2*, (ed. B. Miesen and G. Jones). Routledge, London.

Killick, J. (1997). *You are words*. Hawker Publications, London.

Kitwood, T. (1997). *Dementia reconsidered: the person comes first*. Open University Press, Buckingham.

Miesen, B. (1992). Attachment theory and dementia. *Care-giving in Dementia*, (ed. B. Miesen and G. Jones). Routledge, London.

Morris, R. G., Morris, L. W. and Britton, P. G. (1988). Factors affecting the emotional well being of caregivers of dementia sufferers: a review *British Journal of Psychiatry*.

Oakley, A. (1992). *Social support and motherhood: the natural history of a research project*. Basil Blackwell, Oxford.

Vondra, J. and Shaw, D. (1995). Predicting infant attachment classification from multiple contemporaneous measures of maternal care. *Infant Behaviour and Development*, **18**, 415–25.

Walker, A. (1992). *Possessing the secret of joy*. Jonathan Cape, London.

Zeanah, C. and Zeanah, P. (1989). Intergenerational transmission of maltreatment: insights from attachment theory and research *Psychiatry*, **52**, 177–96.

IV Postscript

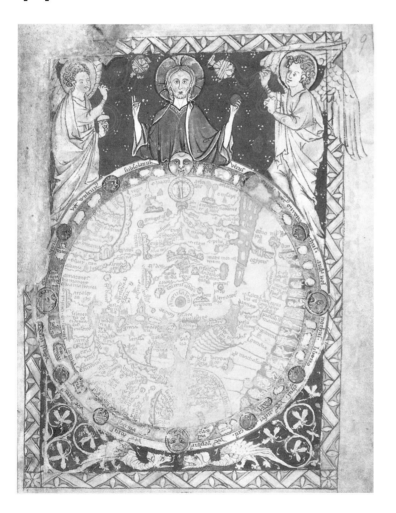

10 Narratives in history, social science, and therapy

Paul Thompson

We all work with narratives: but how similar are the issues which concern historians and social scientists to those with which therapists wrestle?

It seems appropriate, in the context of this book, to situate myself, and give a few hints at my own story. I have been working with auto/biographical stories in one form or another for over 30 years. I began as an historian working primarily from paper documents, which I unearthed not only from archives but also from parish chests or family attics, sometimes from garden sheds, once from a sooty lightless cellar in Birmingham: and at least in order to get hold of them, you had to talk to people a bit. In this way I wrote a thesis on the labour movement in London and two biographies – one about the architect William Butterfield, the other about my life-long hero William Morris.[1]

Each of these biographies involved constructing my own narrative as the historian-biographer, but at the time I did not think about it like that: I saw myself rather as simply seeking to test out the evidence of each man's life against various rival interpretations of it. Thus I defended Butterfield against accusations that he deliberately sought to inflict visual pain through his architecture, and I argued against the view that William Morris was primarily interesting as a 'pioneer of modern design', suggesting that he was also an outstanding artist in terms of the aesthetics of his own time. It was only gradually that I came to see that the historian's professional role involved not only attacking false myths, but also creating new stories about the past, stories often also involving the creation of new heroes or heroines: and stories which worked because they could convince an audience.

There have been various moments of truth along this path. One was quite recently when Roberta Pallotta, a young woman postgraduate anthropologist, appeared from Rome to present me with her dissertation, which is an intellectual biography of myself, based on my own writing and interviews with me. I read it with increasing amazement and excitement, for I had never imagined that my own development could be seen so logically. It suggested to me that the drive to create retrospective logic from the apparent disorder of much personal experience can be as powerful in the professional as in the biographical subject.

More fundamentally, however, the experience of trying out various different methods of presenting history – through writing, and radio, and television – has brought home how much it all depends not just on overall artistic skill, but on specialized arts of narrating which are particular to each medium. For one television series, *The Nineties*, based on interviews with men and women all aged over 90, I co-authored the book of the series as well as working on the programmes with the outstanding producer, Ann Paul. This double involvement taught me how a story which works on paper – and indeed might have its place in the printed book – can prove artistically intolerable on the screen. This means that the demands of the art form in itself help to shape the message you can convey and the people you can choose to present. We had a fascinating interview, for example, with a highly articulate pioneer psychiatric social worker, but her lecturing manner jarred in the programme, and we were only able to use the interview in the book. At the opposite end of the spectrum was an untrained former midwife and layer-out from Ulster, whose words on paper seemed slight, but when you saw her on the screen talking about dead bodies in a matter-of-fact way and then, after a split second, smiling, the effect was hypnotic: she was an oral storyteller whose art compelled you to listen to her.[2]

Thus, even though I still cling to the pre-postmodern hope that research can lead us closer to a truer understanding of past and present, I have gradually become much more conscious that my own role as a professional historian does involve, in its presentation, the artistic *creation* of historical stories. And I entirely concur with Jeremy Holmes when he argues that we are all looking, in one way or another, despite our different professional aims, for narratives that 'fit' – fit with personal experience, fit with historical evidence, fit with the feel of the period – and which succeed precisely because, as narrative art, they combine stories with images, poetry with prose.

However, I have jumped forward. Four paragraphs back I left myself, still 30 years ago, as a keen young historical researcher with untamed positivistic assumptions. This was why, although I had tried some interviewing with old socialists, I had been rather put off this kind of evidence by discovering how partial and in some respects inaccurate their memories could be. I was particularly shocked by an interview with Herbert Morrison, whom I knew had belonged as a young man to a Marxist socialist party, but denied this. It did not then occur to me that the problem was more with my own interviewing technique than with his memory.

By the end of the 1960s, however, I was already experimenting again with interviews, but this time from a new disciplinary perspective: for I had moved to join the Sociology Department at the University of Essex, which, to my good fortune, has been my work base ever since. Sociology at Essex has always been a broad department, encompassing social theory and policy, anthropology, and history, and it has proved an ideal context in which to develop a kind of research which, in my view, only reaches its full potential when conducted in an interdisciplinary spirit. Thus from early on I was able to think of the interview method in social scientific as well as historical perspectives. Over time I have also become increasingly interested in both the literary and the therapeutic dimensions to working with autobiographical stories. My own research, originally focused primarily on the past, has become a bridge between the two, and for this reason I now prefer to describe the field as 'life stories' rather than as 'oral history'.

Encouraged by my new colleagues, and by a handsome grant from the new Social Science Research Council, I launched a large national in-depth interview project which became a part of the basis of my book, *The Edwardians*.[3] At the time we saw the project as a novel experiment in applying social science methods to social history. Thus we took great care both to design a fully detailed interview guide which avoided the pitfalls of leading and biased questions, and to construct a representative sample. Both points remain crucial for me in designing a research project. I do not believe in rigid interviewing of the classic statistical survey type, indeed I see it as essential to the success of an interview above all to listen, and to be willing to follow what an interviewee wants to say, but nevertheless I also come with my own agenda, and I need to work out how to make sure that is addressed in the smoothest, least obtrusive way. Perhaps the primacy of this research agenda marks an important difference from the kind of listening that therapists practise. The researcher is listening for a narrative which – as a whole or in part – will 'fit' with a wider social story; the therapist is looking for a story which can heal an individual, because it 'fits' and makes sense of that suffering person's own life experience and self-identity. And sampling clearly does mark a different form of practice. Therapists cannot choose their patients as some kind of random sample from the general population, indeed the people whose stories they hear are by definition unrepresentative; but for researchers, deciding who to interview is invariably a crucial issue in designing a project, and the best stories are typically those that can be claimed to speak for a wider group.

We were well into this first project before we realized that there was already a new movement using interviews for political history in the United States, calling itself 'oral history'; and it was not until the late 1970s that I made contact with the parallel work of historians in Italy, and also the revival of the 'life stories' school of sociology led by Daniel Bertaux in France.[4] By the mid-1970s, however, oral history had become an enthusiastic movement in Britain, closely tied in its first years to the parallel genesis of History Workshop. Both shared an excitement in the rediscovery of the everyday past of ordinary men and women, and a faith that listening to their voices could not only open windows to the real experience of the past, but also help to balance the historical record by giving voice to the previously disempowered – and so contribute to the shaping of a better future. I wrote *The Voice of the Past* (1978),[5] which has become one of the classic texts of the oral history method, fully in that spirit, combining social hope with an unspoken naïve realism.

We had to put all that behind us after the late 1970s. The Thatcher government not only shattered most of our short-term social hopes, but also destroyed the funding base of the community oral history projects which had begun to be so successful all over Britain. At the same time our earlier straightforward realistic framework gave way to a much subtler appreciation of the selectivity of memory, the shaping of life stories by the context of telling in the present, the importance of narrative form, and their intrinsic interweaving of fact and fiction, of subjective and objective. While earlier we had tried to defend ourselves against accusations by sceptics that memory is too malleable to be trusted, now, while not abandoning the demonstrable position that memories include significant and reliable information, oral historians began to assert that the very gaps and distortions in memory could be equally interesting as clues to consciousness and ways of thinking: *both* aspects of memory were now recognized as being of potential value for interpretation.

From within the oral history field Luisa Passerini and Alessandro Portelli were the leading influences in first asserting the significance of 'subjectivity', shown by erasures, silences, displacements, and inventions in memories, as a crucial dimension to interpretation, often reflecting the political vicissitudes, hopes, and struggles which had given meaning to people's lives.[6] At the same time Ron Grele and Isabelle Bertaux-Wiame first highlighted the clues to understanding to be found in the literary and linguistic structures of interviews: for example, how men and women tend to speak quite differently, men telling the story in the active first person 'I' with themselves at the centre, women preferring the more collective 'we' or 'one'.[7]

Historians and social scientists using life stories have subsequently built on their insights. Two particularly important subsequent landmarks have been the 1987 international oral history conference which resulted in *The Myths We Live By*,[8] focusing on the positive importance of myths about the past, both individual and collective, as a motif force in shaping people's present and future lives; and the attention drawn to narrative forms and context by the anthropologist Elizabeth Tonkin, derived principally from her own fieldwork in West Africa but full of rich suggestions about western cultures too, in her *Narrating Our Pasts*.[9] There are striking parallels between Tonkin's argument that 'we are our memories', so that different forms of talking about our pasts structure our whole culture and our personal identities, with James Phillips' opening assertion here that narratives are with us 'throughout our lives': 'we live in and through the stories we tell and imagine about ourselves'. Roberts conversely describes solitude and silence as part of the torment of the sick, the inability to narrate memory as leaving the individual abandoned 'in a wasteland, a denarrated place'. He also suggests some of the different forms and genres of narrating which therapists regularly encounter, including children's stories, traditional tales, and family stories.[9] Significantly, the new Routledge 'Memory and Narrative' series, edited by a cross-disciplinary board which includes oral historians and life story sociologists alongside literary specialists and psychiatrists, has opened with its first volume entitled *Narrative and Genre*.[10]

The shift towards a focus on subjectivity and narrative forms was not of course peculiar to oral historians. As is clear from several of the essays in this book, the 'problem of "truth" ', as Glenn Roberts puts it in his introduction, has haunted psychotherapists for decades: indeed, as James Phillips reminds us, Freud himself was bothered by the fictional feel of the case histories that he wrote, which he thought consequently 'lack the serious stamp of science'. However – although at first without being mutually known – a parallel shift to that among oral historians had also been taking place within the psychotherapeutic world, in which the weighing of fact and fiction in patients' stories was also being changed. One of the first published recognitions from the oral history perspective of this new common ground was the inclusion in *The Myths We Live By* (1990) of an interview on family myths which I had recorded with John Byng-Hall; while from the psychiatric world a more impressive milestone was Eliot Mishler's powerful and witty argument for the narrative approach in social science research in his *Research Interviewing* (1986).[11]

I had myself become interested in the therapy dimension to oral history through my own experience, both in work and in my personal life. When I first started to interview, it did not occur to me that this could be a crucial positive experience for the person I was recording. One of the first recordings I made was with a Shetlander, and I had promised to revisit him in the following year. Sadly he died before my return. But his daughter welcomed me with special warmth, and told me that the prospect of my next visit had made all the difference to that last winter of his life. Then another oral historian told me of a woman who had been suffering from a fatal illness, but after being recorded made an astonishing recovery. And rumours of other similar incidents began to circulate. This hopeful awareness among oral historians that reminiscence might also benefit their subjects eventually crystallized in the 'Recall' project, which was led by Joanna Bornat from Help the Aged from the 1980s, and developed a form of group therapy for older people which has become widely used in health and social work, particularly in day centres or institutional contexts. This has focused on group reminiscence discussions typically initiated by the showing of tape and slide material, combining old photographs with songs and recorded memories from the past [12] It was again only once the British work was well started that connections were made with the crucial American psychiatric work of Robert Butler, who had, through his own research in the mid-1950s, stumbled on the 'quite apparent . . . therapeutic benefit in reminiscence', and launched comparable programmes as part of his own practice.[13] The essay by Errolyn Bruce here on working with older people suffering from dementia draws on this important convergence of historical and therapeutic interests.

A second professional influence came through the current of interest in psychoanalysis among social historians from the late 1970s onwards. For oral history the classic fruit of this was Ronald Fraser's remarkable autobiography, *In Search of a Past*, which interweaves three layers of memory: oral history interviews about his own isolated, upper class country childhood, which he carried out with the family's former gardener, servants, and nannies; the confused, disintegrating, fading memories of his sick father as he drove him to an old people's home; and Fraser's own diary of his conversations in therapy with his psychoanalyst. Fraser, as a historian, is bothered that his analyst is not interested in whether his memories are true, and simply demands to know how he feels about them. But in the end the analysis did bring important new insights, which helped also to make sense of the oral history interviews: he came to see how his nanny and the gardener had become a second mother and father to him. The book is perhaps in the end more artful than analytic, but it is a too rare attempt to bring the different forms of listening together.[14]

In a personal sense too, from the later 1970s I had found myself drawn towards the world of therapy, both through at times being a client, and through marrying a child psychiatrist. This has led eventually to common work on two themes. The first has been memory and trauma, and the second stepfamilies.

The issue of traumatic memories did not originally concern British oral historians, who were typically working with older people who, unless they had fought in the First World War trenches, were unlikely to have shared in a major collective traumatic experience. There was also little awareness in the early 1970s of either the extensiveness of child sexual abuse, or the severity of its impact: it was a period in which even social workers could condone incest as little more than a cultural curiosity. The past 10 years, however, have brought a much more heightened sensibility, on the one hand through the new views on sexual abuse, but also through the rapid growth of oral history work on the holocaust, and the return of genocide to shadow the contemporary world political agenda. It is symptomatic, once again, that the second volume of the 'Memory and Narrative' series is to be on *Trauma and Life Stories*,[15] bringing together research which ranges across the continents from South African townships to Guatemalan Indian civil war widows and Argentinian veterans of the Falklands war. For psychotherapists I suspect that the most interesting contribution will be the analysis by Gadi BenEzer, who has worked as a psychologist with black Ethiopian Jews fleeing to Israel, on the precise forms, including body language, which characterize their narratives of trauma.

As a whole, I am more struck by how far oral historians and therapists share a common approach to traumatic memories than by differences. Both see these as 'stories in search of a voice', and the problem of understanding silences has fascinated oral historians since the issue was raised in the late 1970s through the work of Luisa Passerini on Italian fascism.[16] One of the subjects of an Italian oral history study of survivors from the German concentration camps, Quinto Osano, a retired Fiat metalworker, sums up well the tension between needing to re-member so as to protect the future from another similar disaster, and needing to forget in order to get on with life: 'Yes, we always want it to be told, but inside us we are trying to forget: right inside, right in the deepest parts of the mind, of the heart. It's instinctive: to try to forget, even when we are getting others to recall it'.[17] But the speaker here was a man who had managed his memories well enough not to be immobilized by them, and that has been true of an over-whelming majority of those survivors interviewed by oral historians. For the British project on holocaust survivors we organized a back-up therapeutic support, but less than one in a hundred of those recorded had any need for such help. Thus while oral historians and therapists conceive of traumatic memories in very similar ways, on the whole we are listening to different people, and for different reasons. Oral historians come primarily to listen, rather than to heal, or to offer a cure for the 'curse' of a 'toxic story', as Glenn Roberts puts it; and we certainly would not wish to seek healing through 'breaking' or 'reworking' stories.[18] On the contrary, oral histor-ians typically see our own interference in the story as a problem, and seek to minimize it.

There was a somewhat similar tension, but a productive one, in the research on stepfamilies which I have carried out over 10 years with a child psychiatrist and two family therapists as col-leagues, now published as *Growing Up in Stepfamilies*.[19] We were unanimous that we wanted to write a research study on long-term outcome from stepfamily childhoods rather than a hand-book of advice, and that shaped the fundamental plan. In particular, we were determined to avoid the inherent bias of a clinic-based study, and eventually were able to carry out 50 life story interviews chosen on the basis of a representative national sample from the National Child Development Study's cohort of men and women born in 1958. We also wanted to maintain the more structural insights of social science, including awareness of class, gender, and ethnicity as crucial dimensions – the latter a point which resonates with the powerful plea for cross-cultural sensitivity here from Sushhut Judhav, Roland Littlewood, and R. Raguram – but to combine them with the therapist's understanding of the emotional structuring of families through the systems approach. The two kinds of perspectives did, in practice, prove mutually thoroughly enriching.

We also shared a common interest in narrative forms, and the relationship between early at-tachment and later coherence in narrative which Jeremy Holmes discusses here[20] emerged as a fascinating issue in interpreting our own interviews. But in the end it was easier to distinguish differences in narrative form between, for example, men and women, than to link them to early attachment, primarily because our own retrospective interviews could not contain information about the subject's earliest years. A second problem, and one which I very much hope that attachment researchers will in time address, is the need for a clearer criterion of coherence for adults in their 20s or 30s, or even later in life.

Some of our differences in approach might be seen in terms of style. Researchers still like to tease over a problem of interpretation for hours, even for days, at a stretch; therapists seem al-ways to be trying to find immediate solutions to a host of individual crises, so rarely find the luxury of a longer time space. This comes out not only in research meetings, but also in inter-viewing. Where the oral historian may take six hours to unravel a complex childhood in full de-tail, the therapist will instinctively short-cut to the heart of the issue, thus ending up with a much shorter interview which is brilliant as a diagnostic nutshell, but has too much missing for all the comparisons that are needed with other cases. It turned out, interestingly, that these differences also reflected an important distinction which we found between the evidence of therapeutic family group interviews and individual life story interviews.

We had initially been doubtful whether the systems theory of family therapists, which had been developed through the practice of the family group session, could be used effectively through the evidence of individual interviews. We therefore experimented by carrying out individual follow-up interviews with some families whose initial group sessions at the Institute of Family Therapy had been recorded, and comparing the evidence between the two. It emerged that while the group session was better at homing in on immediate problems, it did not provide the space for individuals to give coherent accounts of themselves. The life story interviews shared many similar insights on family dynamics, but traced the development of both individuals and their interaction over a much longer period and in a more sustained way, in some instances revealing sources of the present difficulties which had not been evident from the group interview. In short, the two kinds of interview were overlapping, but also complementary, in content.

The life story interview proved particularly valuable for showing, in contrast to the pessimism of much clinic-based material, the remarkable resilience of most former stepchildren and their continuing capacity for positive change into adulthood. We found that many of them, despite educational handicaps, had proved very successful at work; while others overcame earlier emotional impoverishment through a successful marriage. This connects at a humbler level with the astonishing contributions which stepchildren–such as Leonardo da Vinci or Isaac Newton– have made for centuries to European culture.

It leads me also to a more general concluding observation about the relevance of the life story and oral history approach to therapists more generally. Inevitably, because therapists spend so much of their time listening to people with recurrent or intractable difficulties, their in-depth understanding can, I believe, be broadened and strengthened by a sharing of insights with those of us who interview a more representative cross-section of the general population, and who are therefore confronted, again and again, with examples of the extraordinary capacity of ordinary men and women to overcome severe disadvantage in their lives. This resilience can be especially impressive among the old, and indeed becomes progressively essential even to staying alive. In addition to the focus on the capacity for change among younger adults in our stepfamily study, I have written myself in *I Don't Feel Old*[21] about the ways in which older people can draw creatively on the resources of their own life experience. I would suggest that this understanding of 'healthy' adaptability and resilience could also offer important insights to therapists listening to 'sick' or 'toxic' narratives, and so to the healing process.

References

[1] Paul Thompson (1991). *The work of William Morris* (3rd edn). Oxford University Press.
[2] Gloria Wood and Paul Thompson (1993). *The nineties*. BBC Books, London.
[3] Paul Thompson (1975). *The Edwardians* Weidenfeld, London, (3rd edn. Routledge, London, 1990)

[4] Daniel Bertaux (ed.) (1981). *Biography and society: the life history approach in the social sciences.* Sage; Daniel Bertaux (1997). *Récits de vie: perspective ethnosocialogique.* Nathan, Paris; Ken Plummer (1983). *Documents of life: an introduction to the problems and literature of a humanistic method.*

[5] Paul Thompson (1988). *The voice of the past: oral history.* (rev. edn). Oxford University Press.

[6] Luisa Passerini (1979). Work ideology and consensus under Italian Fascism. *History Workshop Journal,* **9**, 82–108; Alessandro Portelli (1991). *The death of Luigi Trastulli and other stories.* State University of New York Press, Albany.

[7] Ron Grele (1979). Listen to their voices. *Oral History,* **7**, 1; Isabelle Bertaux-Wiame (1982). The life history approach to the study of internal migration: how women and men came to Paris between the wars. In *Our common history: the transformation of Europe* (ed. Paul Thompson), pp. 186–200, Pluto.

[8] Raphael Samuel and Paul Thompson (eds) (1990). *The myths we live by.* Routledge,

[9] Elizabeth Tonkin (1992). *Narrating our pasts: the social construction of oral history,* Cambridge University Press, James Phillips, p. 1; Roberts (Introduction), pp. 3, 6, 12–14, 24–5.

[10] Mary Chamberlain and Paul Thompson (eds) (1997). *Narrative and genre.* Routledge, London.

[11] Eliot Mishler (1986). *Research interviewing: context and narrative.* Yale University Press, New Haven.

[12] Peter Coleman (1986). *Elderly people and the reminiscence process;* Andre W. Norris (1986). *remembering with older people;* Joanna Bornat (ed.) (1993). *Reminsicnce reviewed: perspectives, evaluations, achievements*

[13] Robert Butler (1963). The life review: an interpretation of reminiscence in the aged. *Psychiatry,* **26**, 65–76; and (1980–1). The life review: an unrecognized bonanza. *International Journal on Aging and Human Development,* **12** 35–8.

[14] Ronald Fraser (1984). *In search of a past.* Verso, London.

[15] Selma Leydesdorff and Kim Lacy Rogers (eds) (1998). *Trauma and life stories* Routledge.

[16] Passerini (1979); ref. 6.

[17] Anna Bravo and Daniele Jalla (1986). *La vita offesa,* p. 63. Milan,

[18] Roberts (Introduction), p. 21, ref. 9; Holmes, p. 22.

[19] Gill Gorell Barnes, Paul Thompson, Gwyn Daniel, and Natasha Burchardt (1997). *Growing up in stepfamilies.* Oxford University Press.

[20] Holmes, pp. 13–18.

[21] Paul Thompson, Catherine Itzin, and Michele Abendstern (1998). *I don't feel old: the experience of later life.* Oxford University Press.

Index